THE FLOWER OF PARADISE

CULTURE, ILLNESS, AND HEALING

JOHN G. KENNEDY

Depts. of Psychiatry and Anthropology,
University of California, Los Angeles, U.S.A.

THE FLOWER OF PARADISE

The Institutionalized Use of the Drug Qat in North Yemen

D. REIDEL PUBLISHING COMPANY

A MEMBER OF THE KLUWER ACADEMIC PUBLISHERS GROUP

DORDRECHT / BOSTON / LANCASTER / TOKYO

Library of Congress Cataloging-in-Publication Data

Kennedy, John G.
The flower of paradise.

(Culture, illness, and healing)
Bibliography: p.
Includes indexes.
1. Narcotic habit—Yemen. 2. Qat. 3. Yemen—Social life and customs. I. Title. II. Series.
HV5840.Y4K46 1987 362.2′932′095332 87–4676
ISBN 1–55608–011–5
ISBN 1–55608–012–3 (pbk.)

Published by D. Reidel Publishing Company.
P.O. Box 17, 3300 AA Dordrecht, Holland.

Sold and distributed in the U.S.A. and Canada
by Kluwer Academic Publishers,
101 Philip Drive, Norwell, MA 02061, U.S.A.

In all other countries, sold and distributed
by Kluwer Academic Publishers Group,
P.O. Box 322, 3300 AH Dordrecht, Holland.

Printed in the Netherlands

Dedicated to my mother
Virginia Lee Poore —
Her never failing encouragement,
enthusiasm and faith
have made this
and all my work possible —

"Qat widens the mind
It makes you remember forgotten things!
It relaxes and allows you to breathe easily.
It is a paradise of the mind.
Qat makes people strong.
They can endure hardships and climb mountains!"

Yemeni farmer on Jabel Sabr
February 1975

TABLE OF CONTENTS

ACKNOWLEDGEMENTS

Everything in this book is the result of collaboration and cooperation. The result is truly a joint effort produced by many individuals and it has only been ordered into written form by me. The people who provided the information for this study and assisted it in many ways are far too numerous to mention individually here. The many unnamed informants who participated in the study, and the many Yemeni companions who shared their good will and ideas in qat sessions in all parts of Yemen also have my special thanks. The following rendered especially important services.

During the 2 year research period in Yemen I had the good fortune of employing Mohammed al-Shamy, now of the Yemen Foreign Ministry, Abdo Ali Othman, now Professor at Sanaa University, and Fathy Salem Ali, now Deputy Director of the Central Planning Organization. Each of these competent friends agreed to serve as director of field research for a part of the study. They not only organized our research activities in Yemen, and acted as liasons between us and the Yemeni people, but each of them performed as an important teacher of Yemeni customs and history to me and to the non-Yemeni members of the research team. They each provided creative input which shaped this study in important respects, and each took initiative in solving many logistical problems.

Particular thanks go to my colleague James Teague, M.D., who designed much of the medical portion of the research and especially assisted with the analysis in Chapters 8 and 9. Together we spent many an hour puzzling over these data, and many of the ideas here are joint products of those sessions. Dr. G. J. Obermeyer introduced us to Yemen, provided initial stimulus for the research and gave consistently useful advice. My wife, Wendy Utsuki, made countless valuable contributions to the final product.

Other important members of that team at various times were Judith Obermeyer, M.A., who directed our survey activities in Taiz and helped with collection of medical data in Sanaa, Dr. Martha Mundy who assisted with data gathering in Sanaa and Wadi Dahr, Kalthum Ali, who organized medical data gathering on women in Hodeida, and Dr. Ahmad Makky M.D. who directed research in Hodeida. The other M.D.s who made physical examinations of subjects in the three cities were Dr. Jamila, Dr. Stella, Dr. Azzam, Dr. Abdul Kader Homani, Dr. Abdul Wahab Makky, Dr. Hassan, Dr. Ghorbani and Dr. Ahmad Moayad.

Mohammad Abdel Wahid, who was director of the Institute of Yemeni studies during the first half of our period of work, and Ahmad Marwani who was director during the last half, were extremely helpful in providing facilities and information for the study. Dr. Abdul Karim Iryani, who at the time of the study was Director of the Central Planning Organization and later head of Sanaa University, and Qadi Ismail al-Akwa, Director of Antiquities both provided facilities and information at important junctures of the research period. Abdullah al-Hibshi put his scholarly knowledge at our disposal and assisted us with collecting and copying older Arabic texts pertinent to qat. Other individuals who assisted in various ways with research tasks in Yemen were Hussein al-Amri, Abdul Rahman al-Moayad, Mohammad al-Wazir, Ali Agbari, Faisel Sharif, Ali Sharif and Fatma Zabarah.

Dr. Brinkley Messick, Dr. Charles Swagman and Dr. Herman Escher, each of whom wrote Ph.D. dissertations on Yemen and Ms. Shelagh Weir of the British Museum, were all kind enough to provide me with access to their comments, notes, and written works on Yemen and qat use. I owe special debt to Dr. Raman Revri, who worked closely with us on the agriculture of qat and provided much of the data on that subject which appears in this book. Dr. Haider Ghaibah was also helpful by providing access to his papers on the economy of Yemen. Others who provided specialized assistance during the field research were Professor John Neuhart, Marilyn Neuhart, Sylvia Kennedy, Fernando Varanda, Dr. Robert Burrowes, and Carla Makhlouf.

At UCLA Dr. Jolyon West, director of the Neuropsychiatric Institute encouraged the research from the beginning and recommended funds for the initial pilot visit to Yemen. Mustapha Mebarkia, Hiam Slieman and Dr. Sulayman Khalaf capably translated Arabic articles, poetry and other documents pertaining to qat. Assisting with the quantitative analysis were Elizabeth Cooney, William Rokaw and particularly Dr. Lynn Fairbanks.

I feel a profound gratitude towards the several secretaries who have laboriously typed notes, articles and drafts of this book from my poor handwriting. These were Gila Varis, Jean Samuelson, Priscilla Logue, and Vicki Stringer.

This research was made possible by DHEW Grant 5 RO1 0097403 of NIDA (National Institute of Drug Abuse) where it was supported particularly by the late Dr. Eleanor Carroll. It also received assistance from 2 small faculty grants from the N.P.I. at U.C.L.A. and from a travel grant by the Social Science Research Council. My gratitude to all the above is inexpressable, and none of them bear any responsibility for what errors may appear here.

Chapters 8 and 9 are derived from articles in *Culture, Medicine and Psychiatry* and *Social Science and Medicine*. I thank these journals for permission to reprint portions of those articles.

All photographs were taken by the author except where otherwise specified.

Note: For ease in reading, simplified Anglicized phonetic transliteration of Arabic words is used throughout, e.g., “Sanaa” instead of “San‘a’”, *Sayyids* instead of *Sada* for the plural of *Sayyid*, etc., and I have dispensed with diacritical markings. The first appearance of any non-English term is italicized: the following occurrences are not.

CHAPTER I

INTRODUCTION

This book concerns the use of the drug qat in North Yemen (Yemen Arab Republic), a country lying on the southwestern corner of the Arabian Peninsula. However, because this substance is so interwoven into the fabric of society and culture, it is also necessarily about Yemen itself. The history and culture of South Arabia are still relatively unknown to the rest of the world, and the drug qat, so widely used there, is equally unknown. Thus, the material we present here should be of interest to all of those concerned with drug use, those who wish to understand more about Yemen and the Middle East, and to the Yemenis themselves.

Another purpose is to develop some general understandings about substance uses and their effects which are less clouded by the mass hysteria and political considerations which often obscure drug issues in our own society. Examination of drug-use patterns in a country where millions of people are users on a regular basis, and where there has been familiarity with the drug for several hundred years, offers an opportunity to achieve perspectives not possible in countries with different attitudes and without such histories. I am not sanguine about the prospects of our abilities to learn from others or from the past, but I do not think we should abandon hope of doing so.

Drug use, however, is not the only interest here. The book should also shed some light on the social life of North Yemen. It is my contention that the cultures and societies of Yemen cannot be adequately comprehended without a full understanding of the role of qat in social life. Many good books and dissertations are now beginning to appear on hitherto neglected topics of the politics, economics and society of Yemen. In all of them qat is mentioned, but in *none* of them is it accorded the important place it warrants. In virtually all of these works the subject of qat-use is described in passing, and in most of them some disparaging remarks about it are made. It is my hope that, if nothing else, this book will help to instill a more adequate perspective. As will become evident, even in works focusing on history, politics or social organization, qat and the institution of using it are not a minor subject which can be adequately treated in a footnote, or in a few pages. This drug has had a profound effect on the history of Yemen; it is playing an increasingly important role in Yemeni economic and social life. There is no individual Yemeni whose life is not affected in profound ways by qat and its implications. An adequate understanding of its role should be part of all future studies of the culture and society of Yemen.

SETTING

The encounter with the ancient land of Yemen is a revelation to anyone who visits there for the first time. Approaching by air, one is first awed by its rugged and barren mountains. Crags jut up sharply like spires, and the realization dawns that the old lithographs and engravings of such "fairy tale" landscapes were really not so romanticized as one had supposed. Coming closer, it becomes apparent that the first impression of unremitting barrenness, which was reinforced by the Western stereotype of South Arabia as a total desert, is an illusion. On the very tips of peaks, tall stone castles appear. Clusters of three or four-storied houses nestle on steep mountainsides down which cascade beautiful terraces, their stone walls snaking in irregular contours along the rocky slopes. Advancing yet nearer, narrow green valleys or *wadis* can be seen between the peaks, and the recesses of canyons carved by perennial streams or seasonal floods can be discerned. It strikes the visitor that there must be enough rainfall for considerable farming here, and it is evident that every square meter of land with agriculture potential has been laboriously shaped for human use.

The Yemen Arab Republic is bounded by the Red Sea on its western side, the country of Saudi Arabia on the north, the great Arabian Desert on the northeast, and the People's Democratic Republic of Yemen (PDRY or South Yemen) on the south and southeast. Many Westerners, influenced by magazine images of Arabia, visualize Yemen as a vast and uninhabitable desert, and there certainly are some areas of it which do conform to the popular conception. However, most of the country is blessed by a healthy and agreeable climate. Up until recently it may have been on the wrong side of the peninsula in terms of oil resources, but because its mountain chains partially obstruct the paths of the monsoon winds it is the one part of Arabia which has been able to live by agriculture for at least two millenia. Two short rainy seasons enable most of its innumerable wadis to be cultivated. Sanaa, the capital city of more than 138,000 inhabitants, is situated at 2,250 meters elevation and features an average temperature of around 70 degrees. Other parts of the country are even more visually pleasing, and because of its verdant agricultural wadis, Yemen has always supported a high proportion of the population of the Arabian peninsula.

The geography exhibits great diversity, but it is generally dominated by the Serat mountains, the range running north and south through its center, and extending up into Saudi Arabia. An-Nabi Shu'ayb at 3,760 meters near Sanaa, is the highest peak in Arabia, and the average elevation in the interior Serat range is between 2,000 and 3,000 meters. The western slopes of this central spine of mountains are cut by seven major wadi systems within Yemen, through which water flows toward the coast in the rainy seasons.

Along the Red Sea Coast runs the flat coastal strip called the Tihama, a relatively barren plain between 30 and 60 km. wide and some 340 km. long. This area is the most uncomfortable part of Yemen, and though agriculture is practiced in its wadi systems by utilizing the water seasonally running off from the highlands, it is sparsely inhabited. Rainfall along the Tihama is nearly nil, temperature and humidity remain high all year, and malaria is endemic. The largest city of the coastal strip is the Port of Hodeida, which according to the first Yemen census in 1975, had 82,723 inhabitants.

On the eastern side of the Serat mountain chain the plains of the high Yemen shade off into the vast Arabian Desert and eventually into the mountains of sand in the famous "Empty Quarter" itself. Several large wadi systems lead southeastward through this region, and the run-off from the mountain floods makes seasonal agriculture possible in them. The plains along the eastern escarpment of the mountains are tillable and a considerable percentage of the Yemeni population occupy this "Central Highlands" region in such good-sized population centers as Sada, Sanaa, Dhamar, Yarim and Rida.

Some one hundred kilometers east of Sanaa, at Marib, are the ruins of the famous Kingdom of Saba which flourished between 1500 B.C. and 500 A.D. Still standing there at the edges of the Wadi Adhana are sections of the great Marib Dam which, during the time of the ancient Sabean civilization was nearly a half-a-mile in length and irrigated some 4,000 acres of desert. The desert area of that great kingdom is now inhabited by semi-sedentary sections of some bedouin tribes which still range in these eastern regions. The region will soon be the center of new activity, for it is here that oil was recently discovered, and the great dam is also being reconstructed with modern methods.

In the Yemen Arab Republic, rainfall generally increases as you move from north to south. The southern part of the country has its own distinctive geographical character, even though the same mountain range continues dividing the country before turning towards the east to continue into Hadramaut. One feature distinguishing the south from the regions to the north is the higher rainfall south of the Sumara Pass. The "Green Province" of Ibb, the most agriculturally productive region in Yemen, lies between Sanaa and the southermost province of Hujjariyya. The beautiful town of Ibb sits in the center of this rainfall belt at slightly more than 6,000 feet elevation. An hour away by road to the south of it, at an altitude of approximately 4,000 feet is Taiz, the major city of the southern region, with a population of more than 134,000. The thriving cultural capital of the Shafei Muslims, Taiz is spread at the foot of the famous mountain Jabel Sabr, one of the oldest and most productive qat-growing areas in Yemen. To the south of Taiz the mountainous southern upland country called Hujjariyya continues over the border of the People's Democratic Republic of Yemen (PDRY or South Yemen).

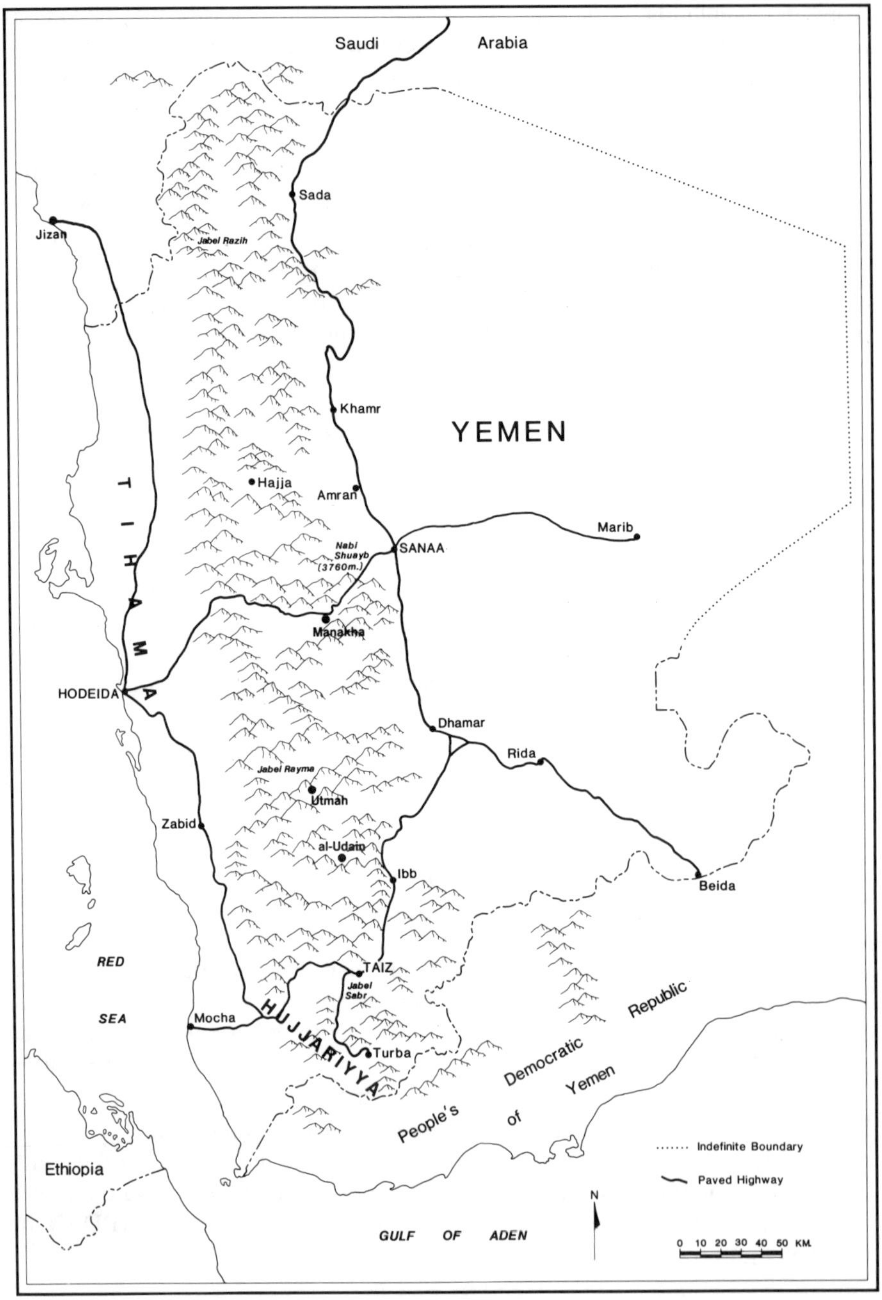
Saudi
Arabia
Sada
Jizan
Jabel Razih
Khamr
YEMEN
Hajja
Amran
Marib
Nabi Shuayb (3760m.)
SANAA
Manakha
TIHAMA
HODEIDA
Dhamar
Rida
Jabel Rayma
Utmah
Zabid
al-Udain
Ibb
Beida
RED SEA
TAIZ
Jabel Sabr
Mocha
HUJJARIYYA
Turba
People's Democratic Republic of Yemen
Ethiopia
GULF OF ADEN
Indefinite Boundary
Paved Highway
N
0 10 20 30 40 50 KM.

GOVERNMENT

From the end of the civil war until the present, the political situation in North Yemen has continued to be rather unstable. Since the revolution of 1962, the Yemenis have tried to institute a form of Republican regime in a country without a history of such a form, and to impose a centralized modern state upon a traditional polycentric group of tribal and feudal structures. There has been an effort to rapidly import social change into a situation lacking the manpower and infrastructure to deal with modern technology and institutions.

There has been a succession of presidents and prime minsters; different kinds of councils, and a number of legislative bodies have been tried. Most of them have been made up of military men along with leaders of various tribes, or representatives of various constituencies. However, none of these bodies has been elected through a plebiscite of the people. At present there is a President at the top of the Yemeni governmental structure who is selected by an elite group of power holders. He appoints the Prime Minister and a group of advisors, the most important of which have usually formed some sort of Military Command Council. There is also a Constitutional People's Assembly which assists with policy. It too, is chosen by the elite, as represented in the Military Command Council. It should be mentioned that the forum for all the meetings of the governmental bodies is a qat session. Many important group decisions are made in the context of qat chewing.

The judicial functions of the country are largely handled by two systems, one a traditional Islamic Sharia legal system, and the other a nascent state court system. The latter is trying to develop and to implement a body of civil law which can be reconciled with the traditional system. Thirty-one thousand people work in the Yemeni government bureaucracy. (For more details and references on the present government, see Cohen and Lewis, 1979:4—11, Peterson, 1982 and Burrowes, 1985).

A persisting divisive problem within the country has been the relative independence of the large northern Zaydi tribes. They are all heavily armed, and have long been in the habit of receiving subsidies, whether from the Imam, the government of Saudi Arabia, or other bidders for their support and loyalty. Individual attempts by the various local tribal Shaykhs to build their own power bases continue to reveal the weakness of the Yemeni central government. In the south and the Tihama, feudal landowners of large estates have been equally resistant to a unified government and in the late 1970s and early 1980s some of them were supported by the anti-Zaydi forces of South Yemen.

The government of Ibrahim al-Hamdi, which lasted from 1973 until his tragic assassination in 1977, was fairly successful in dealing with the multiple problems inherent in such a situation. It even succeeded in again extending the authority of the state by making agreements with some of the tribes. Al-

Hamdi was assisted in this not only through control of the army but by the economic help and modern facilities he was able to offer the various chieftains. Al-Hamdi also tried to unify the country through appointment of the Shafei Adbul Aziz Abdo al-Ghani from Hujjariyya as Prime Minister. Not only was the al-Hamdi assassinated, but his successor, was mysteriously murdered. Since then Colonel Ali Adullah Salih has been president. He has maintained the status quo by appointing a series of southern Shafes prime ministers, but little progress has been made towards his goal of a constitutional republican form of government. (See Peterson 1982, Bidwell 1983 and Burrowes 1985 for details.)

The influx of modern technology into Yemen, accompanied by foreign assistance from many countries, which have aided the forward thrust of education and health care, has created changes in traditional value systems. Even the northern Zaydi tribesmen, like the Shafei peasants of the south, have come to desire mechanical pumps, roads, schools and medical clinics in their areas. This trend has been accelerated by the exposure of several million Yemeni migrants over the past 15 years to modernizing influences in Saudi Arabia and other countries. Former president al-Hamdi's and his successors' success in procuring the cooperation of the Zaydi tribesmen has been in large part made possible by his increasing ability to offer such improvements. This carrot has been reinforced by the stick represented by an army that was better equipped than were the tribesmen or feudal chieftains.[1]

ECONOMICS

The results of the first national census in the history of the country put the number of people residing in the Yemen Arab Republic at approximately 4,705,336 persons, with some 600,000 migrants working abroad. These migrants have faithfully sent a good proportion of their earnings back home and thus have been providing enough money through remittances to more than compensate for the country's growing balance of payments deficit.

Between 85 and 90 percent of the Yemeni population is dependent upon agriculture as a primary basis of existence and between 80 and 90 percent of the farmland is planted with cereal crops. The principal grain crops are sorghum grain (*durrah*), millet, barley, wheat and maize, in that order. Modest amounts of vegetables, beans and lentils are also produced. Most of the Yemenis, whichever of the ecological zones they inhabit, live in small nucleated villages of a few hundred people. They are primarily small farmers who own their own land, or are sharecroppers or tenants who rent from larger landowners or from Islamic religious foundations (*Waqf*). Most of the agriculture is for subsistence only, and during the past 30 or 40 years at least, the Yemenis have become more and more dependent upon imported foods to supplement what they produce. Up to the time of our study, nearly all Yemeni agriculture was unmechanized, but numerous affluent countries were sponsoring aid programs, and international agencies were becoming involved in agricultural assistance. Use of pesticides and fertilizers have been increasing rapidly, and the employment of tractors and other mechanized equipment is increasing at a quickening pace, particularly in the plains areas where they can be used.

Coffee has been the most important cash crop of Yemen for several hundred years, though in recent times it has not been able to compete with major coffee-growing countries, and coffee has radically declined as a source of revenue. Another cash crop bringing in foreign currency during the latter part of the 19th and early 20th centuries was *qat*. This source of cash flow from outside has been cut off by anti-qat laws in both Saudi Arabia and the People's Democratic Republic of Yemen, but qat remains by far the major *internal* cash crop in the country (see Chapter VI).

Industrialization is yet so minimal in Yemen that the inventory of the country's factories at the time of study can easily and quickly be made: a Chinese-built textile mill in Sanaa, a Russian-built cement factory near Bajil, and another at Amran, a biscuit (cookie) factory and an aluminum plant near Taiz, an old cotton mill at Zabid, an Italian-financed cigarette factory and a soft drink bottling plant near Hodeida. This paltry list has increased since then, but it gives some indication of why Yemen has consistently been named by the World Bank as one of the six least-developed countries in the world.

The network of modern highways is still rudimentary in Yemen. Paved roads connect the three major cities of Sanaa, Hodeida, and Taiz with one another, while others now extend from Sanaa to Sada, Taiz to Turba, Dhamar to Beida, from Sanaa to the ancient archaeological site of Marib in the eastern desert, and north from Hodeida to Jedda in Saudi Arabia. There are many other good dirt and gravel roads, and many local communities have recently built barely passable tracks to isolated villages. The few roads of Yemen are traversed by the hundreds of four-wheel drive vehicles which are flooding the small country. Much of the incentive for the acceleration of road building has come from the needs to get qat to market while it is fresh.

Literacy and education generally are still rather underdeveloped. The latest census shows as literate only about 1.9 percent of Yemeni women ten years old or more, and 25.4 percent of the men. These figures should be improving because education has been stressed since the end of the civil war in 1969, and the establishment of a more modern state system. The number of primary schools was almost doubled through the financial assistance of other Arab countries (from 821 in 1970 to 1,528 in 1977), but at the time of the census, girls still made up only 13.6% of the primary school population of 221,482.

Meager as all these numbers seem, they are major improvements over the situation during the Imamic regime prior to the revolution of the 1960s. At that time only about four percent of the children between five and fourteen were in school. All but a very few of these received only verbal religious instruction for at most six years, i.e., some reading of the Quran, and some arithmetic. A select few boys from rich families went on to higher religious schools, and some even were sent abroad to study, primarily in Egypt (Steffen *et al.*, 109—110).

Despite some steps forward, the outlook for economic development in North Yemen must still be considered fairly bleak. It is true that there are unprecedented amounts of foreign currency coming from labor migrants and from the many development projects. This has created a flurry in building and high demands for consumer products such as cars, trucks, and electronic products, and allowed many people to open small shops, etc. It has also created increased demands for qat and assisted the spread of qat plantations, as we shall see. However, these economic changes must be viewed as shallow and temporary. They create an illusion of economic prosperity which is not underpinned by the fundamental changes necessary for sustained economic development. Because of this the rosy picture of "economic revolution" painted by Weir (1985:19—22) must be placed in perspective. The country is still predominantly rural and remains one of the poorest countries in the world. Up until 1984 there were really no exploitable minerals, with the exception of some inferior salt deposits near Salif on the Red Sea coast. Recent discoveries of oil in the eastern desert have raised hopes, but so far these have not been developed. The relatively low price of oil at this time does not bode well for those hopes in the near future, but eventually this new source of revenue should provide significant benefits.

There is little potential for industry in Yemen, due to a lack of infrastructures and of trained personnel in all fields. Until the 1970s the gross national income was less than $100 per capita per year. With the opening up of the country and the migration abroad of almost half the labor force per capita income has recently increased sixfold, but the generally gloomy economic prospect is well summarized in the following quotation:

> The time required for manpower training and institution building will limit the speed of change in agricultural production techniques. Self-sufficiency in food production appeared years away to many observers but some industrial processing of cotton, oilseeds, tobacco and hides could be developed. Expansion of the fishing industry (including processing), tourism, construction and trade had fewest constraints and therefore the best prospects, but these sectors were starting from a small base. Even with rapid growth it would take several years for them appreciably to affect the economy and employment (Nyrop *et al.*, 1977:207).

Apart from the new oil discoveries, the only areas where there seems to be come hope on the economic side are in the improvement of agricultural potential and in tourism. Yemen's impressively beautiful landscape, its picturesque architecture and the monuments of its almost unknown civilizations are drawing larger numbers of visitors as better hotels and other facilities are becoming available.

THE CONTEXT OF THE STUDY – SANAA, HODEIDA AND TAIZ

Unlike the situation in most countries of the Third World, many of the poor farmers of Yemen live in beautiful multi-storied structures. The spectacular architecture of Yemen has captivated most of its foreign visitors, including many architects who have had the privilege of visiting this land of castles. South Arabia was probably the first area of the world to develop multi-story buildings for the people's use as common dwellings, as well as for public buildings, and the walled city of Sanaa is one of the most unique and distinctive of the several South Arabian cities still preserving the ancient skyscraper styles. Yemen has been a "land of builders"[1] from time immemorial, and the houses of old Sanaa, tall, brown, and fancifully decorated with white, testify to the truth of this with an unforgettable impression. The multitude of graceful and distinctive minarets of its many mosques, the old Turkish baths, and the winding narrow streets, all contribute to the medieval quality, and complete the effect of transporting the visitor back through the centuries.

While the old section of Sanaa retains the qualities of a medieval Arab medina, the city has not been left untouched by change. During the recent civil war, Egyptian army engineers imported concrete building techniques and quickly created a replica of some of the more nondescript parts of modern Cairo. Fortunately, this "modernization" was applied outside the walls of the old city, but the influx of returning migrants from abroad following the civil war created new and pressing needs for living and working space, and drab suburbs sprung up all around Sanaa. Fortunately, some of the Yemenis returned to their crafts after the Egyptians withdrew from the war in 1968, and some of the new buildings were quite well constructed with the older stone techniques. Others are of inferior quality. The old city is now enclosed within a vast new one, and the unity of style which traditionally characterized the city of Sanaa is being destroyed.[1]

Sanaa is unique, but other parts of Yemen have their own beautiful and distinctive architectural styles as well. Sada, on the border of Saudi Arabia, and the other towns in the extreme north are distinguished by majestic, slightly tapering, multi-storied buildings with tan mud-plaster facades graced with small irregularly spaced windows. These, too, are decorated by lacy white designs differing from those of Sanaa. The Tihama plain along the coast also has a characteristic style of mud-brick buildings decorated with intricate friezes of ancient Islamic design. Zabid, the old capital and university town of the Tihama, is notable for its hundreds of beautiful mosques, many of which are now in ruins. Most of the wall which used to surround the city is also gone, but from an architectural standpoint Zabid is perhaps the most interesting city of the coastal plain.

Hodeida, the only port of modern Yemen, due to its commercial activities is much more bustling and active than any other coastal town, but many of its fine large Turkish-style houses have fallen into disrepair. Within other sections of Hodeida one finds straw African-type huts of the poor, like those of typical Tihama villages. New buildings continue to be hastily erected as well to handle the increasing business of this steaming port city. Mostly they are of the concrete style which the Egyptian Army left as its dubious legacy.

In the busy Hodeida market, men in the tall, finely-woven tarbush-shaped hats of the northern Tihama villages mingle with those wearing the orange or purple turbans of Hujjariyya, and with men in the red and white or black and white Palestinian scarves so popular in Sanaa and the highlands. Besides their dress, the curved knives (*janbiyyas*) symbolizing male status among the mountain tribesmen also set them apart from the dark people of the coast, who are mostly unarmed. Here in the crowded Suq, where the smells of the odorous fish market belnd with those of fragrant spices, Indians in long robes rub elbows with Yemeni doctors in business suits, and beautiful dark Yemeni women pass slowly in their long, loose dresses. Some balance baskets on their heads, others are covered with black robes and completely veiled, like their sisters of Sanaa, whom they are emulating. Many wear tall straw hats or head scarves.

Taiz, the major city in the southern part of the country, is distinguished by the magnificent mountain, Jabel Sabr, which hovers over it. As one ascends this living mountain, villages and houses appear everywhere along its hundreds of ridges and terraces. It is one of the oldest qat-growing areas of Yemen, and virtually all its lower slopes, up to the level of nearly 8,000 feet, are primarily devoted to growing the drug which gives the "sabris" their livelihood. Above the 8,000 foot level on Jabel Sabr, where qat cannot grow, large terraces of durrah and wheat are found.

The old City of Taiz is distinguished by its two beautiful Turkish-style mosques, and its colorful market stretched between two ancient gates of the city. Farther up the hill are several "Sanaa-style" palaces built for Ahmad, the last Imam. The people of Taiz resemble those of Aden, and indeed many of them have spent long parts of their lives there. A good number of them are merchants, and the "taizis" commonly wear a more richly colored *futa* (wrapped skirt) from Indonesia which distinguishes them from the Northern Zaydi tribesmen. In Taiz, one sees many women from Zanzibar, Mombasa and Aden, clothed in stylish European dresses, and even slacks. In the bazaar between the two old city gates they unconcernedly mix with the unveiled countrywomen from Hujjariyya or Jabel Sabr, who in their brightly colored dresses, walk proudly with clusters of shining bangles clicking on their bare upper arms.

Hallmarks of Yemen are its local diversity and its individualism, and many smaller towns are equally unique in flavor and qualities to the larger ones I have mentioned. For example, Ibb and Jibla stand like two jewels in the green province (*liwa akhdar*) just to the north of Taiz. Bayda and Marib in the eastern desert, Yarim and Dhamar in the highland plain, Wadi Mawr of the Northern Tihama, Manakha and Mahwit, Thula and Shibam, Shahara and Suda of the central mountains; each sub-region has a distinctive character of its own.

WHY STUDY QAT?

Carsten Niebuhr, the great traveler sent to Arabia by the King of Denmark in the mid-18th century, recorded the widespread use of qat in Yemen, and nearly every visitor since that time has commented on the ubiquity of this Yemeni "national drug." When we visited Yemen in 1972 we were impressed that the reports of the travelers were not exaggerated. Walking through the busy qat markets, which are found in every town of any size, we were assailed from all sides by merchants waving green leafy bundles in our faces. "Yemeni whisky" was the gleeful call, "Chew this and see your home in America!" or "This is our oil." We later discovered that this last phrase referred to the fact that though Yemen still has not been able to produce oil, the drug qat brings considerable revenues to the merchants who sell it, and to the farmers who grow it. As later chapters of this book will show, it is entirely reasonable that they regard qat as a basic resource.

We were invited into many houses by the hospitable Yemenis and in the early stages of our research we would be given generous amounts of the qat leaves to chew. Our hosts were proud of their qat, and they wanted us to appreciate it too. We soon learned that the majority of the Yemenis chew the tender leaves and generally claim to derive great satisfaction and enjoyment from the practice.

The common people extoll the virtues of qat, which is said to relieve colds, fevers and headaches. It can brighten the sad one and give confidence to the unsure. One chews a little qat to climb mountains. "You can go right up, like that!" exclaims the Yemeni, snapping his fingers twice and pointing to the crags above. It enables endurance and perseverance in difficult physical toil, concentration when mental effort is called for, and maintains alertness when fatigue threatens. It relaxes the body and stimulates the mental faculties. Qat "widens the mind," is a common saying. The scholar uses it to concentrate, and the pious to remain awake. The businessman chews to comprehend, quickly and alertly, all nuances of the transaction at hand. Qat "gathers people," as the phrase goes providing the forms of social intercourse and the matrix for the communication of gossip and of general information. "Without qat what would we do for entertainment?" ask many of the young Yemeni men. "We have no cinema, theater, bars or clubs, as are found in other countries."

On a Friday afternoon, more than eighty percent of the nearly five million people in the Yemen Arab Republic are to be found sitting in small groups, chewing the tender leaves of the qat plant. On any other day of the week, the percentage of the population chewing these leaves may range between fifty percent and sixty percent. This high proportion is even more impressive when it is realized that in most areas of the country children below the ages of ten or twelve do not chew, that in some regions, particularly the eastern desert and parts of the Tihama, it is fairly difficult to get qat, and that in some places women still do not chew at all.

During the hours of early afternoon, many businesses are closed and the streets of towns and cities of Yemen are empty. However, in the interiors of thousands of dwellings activity is in progress. The president of the country and his council chew qat as they conduct their afternoon deliberations. Religious leaders and scholars use the forum provided by the qat session to advance their views and discuss their latest writings. Business leaders deliberate on market changes and conclude financial arrangements. Students of high school and university chew during their examinations. Women chew in afternoon neighborhood gatherings. Merchants chew as they sit for hours in their tiny shops. Laborers, drivers and stonecutters all say they cannot do a good day's work without qat.

What is this qat which is so loved and so much a part of Yemeni life? The answer to this is not simple, but we may begin by saying that it is a perennial plant which may take the form of a small shrub or of a thin tree. In some areas of Yemen groves are found as tall as 25 or 30 feet in height. In present-day Yemen, in parts of Ethiopia, and in several areas of Kenya and Somalia, the tender leaves of qat are chewed primarily for their stimulant, euphoric and social properties.

There are many names of the qat plant, and a variety of transliterations of these names. The reader should be warned that several variations will be encountered in the many citations I will make in this book. These are not inconsistencies on my part, but are largely ad-hoc transliterations, some of which have crept into the literature to be repeated again and again.

Here, we use the "qat" spelling. This is based on the logic that the original Arabic word utilized the inital letter *qaf* (ق), which is probably best transliterated with a "q". This spelling is usually used by authors familiar with Arabic, but not invariably so. The most common spelling found in the English literature is *khat*, and even some scholars of stature, such as Tigani El-Mahi, who will be cited extensively later, used the *kh* initial letter. This is, I think, an error since in Arabic the qaf is never transliterated by *kh*, whereas the *Kha* (خ), which is not used in the Arabic spelling of qat, nearly always is. In English such variations as *kat, cat, kaht,* or even *quat*, are frequently seen.

Another confusion in the literature comes from the fact that in many dialects of Yemen, the Arabic *qaf* is pronounced as a hard English "g." For example, in most of Yemen north of Taiz, you hear gat, even though it is known that the spelling is *qat*. In Hujjariyya south of Taiz, the classical Arabic pronunciation of the *qaf* is preserved.

Many of the other words for the plant are found in other languages. It is known as *chat* in the extensively qat using Harrar province of Ethiopia and in Somalia, though sometimes one encounters the transliterations of *tschat* or *ciat*. In Kenya the plant is known most commonly as *miraa*, or *marongi*, and many other tribal names for it are found there and throughout southeastern Africa.[1]

Almost without exception, the benefits of qat are extolled by Yemenis, but the majority of foreigners who have visited Yemen and written about life there have viewed it as a pernicious influence — an evil habit which should be rooted out. The following are representative examples of outsiders' opinions:

To the Southern Arabian, Kat is as important as the Koran. It is a poisonous drug, but he calls it an essential stimulant. Kat-chewing is practiced by everyone. Men, women and children are kat-addicts without exception. It is a habit possessed by king or sultan down to the poorest beggar who can afford a few coins to buy this priceless stuff. It is said that the Yemenites can, in case of need, do without food for several days, but that it is impossible for him to exist a single day without Kat (Helfritz 1936: 184—185).

There can be no doubt, though, in the long run it is an injurious habit. It gradually impairs physical efficiency, and the man who has long been addicted to the drug is easily to be recognized by the inanity of his expression and by his protruding eyes. The body, too, loses its power to resist the attacks of tropical diseases, such as typhus and dysentery . . .

. . . If the people of Yemen appear degenerated and weakly, it may be attributed to this widespread evil. Therefore, it is no matter of surprise that the Yemen soldiers, all of whom are Kat addicts, were no match for the powerful warriors of the great King Ibn Saud (*Ibid.*:187)

By and by the habitue finds himself incapable of clear and consecutive thought without the herb, and its deprivation engenders much mental discomfort and nervous irritability. Further addiction induces marked symptoms such as constipation, insomnia and finally impotency. The teeth are much affected becoming permanently discolored and loose, for the gums become flaccid. By this time the victim of the habit is incapacitated for real thought or efficient work by any accidental deprivation, which is bound to occur at intervals, for the supply of Kat is by no means regular, and it will not keep (Bury, 1915:152).

Dorothy Ingrams, wife of a British adminstrator in Aden, after a short trip to Yemen felt herself qualified to make the following declaration:

They might have been a far more prosperous community than the Hadhramis as they lived in a fertile country, but there was at that time no apparent desire to leave the Middle Ages for the twentieth century and benefit from the know-how of other countries. One reason for this apathy of the average Yemeni was, I am sure, due to their addiction to *qat* (catha edulis), the most debilitating, time-wasting scourge of Yemen. The leaves of the shrub are chewed to give the addict a feeling of being on top of the world, of being able to solve all problems, but the after-effects are lassitude, apathy, and depression. Every Yemeni who can afford it, and most of them got ahold of *qat* somehow, spent the afternoons with his friends chewing, spitting, drinking water and chewing again. These sessions inspired a great deal of talk but no action and I saw no possibility of Yemen developing into a prosperous country so long as qat was allowed to exhaust the people's talents and sap their vitality" (1970:113)

Even the well-known Carleton Coon, the first anthropologist to visit Yemen, made the remarkable judgment that:

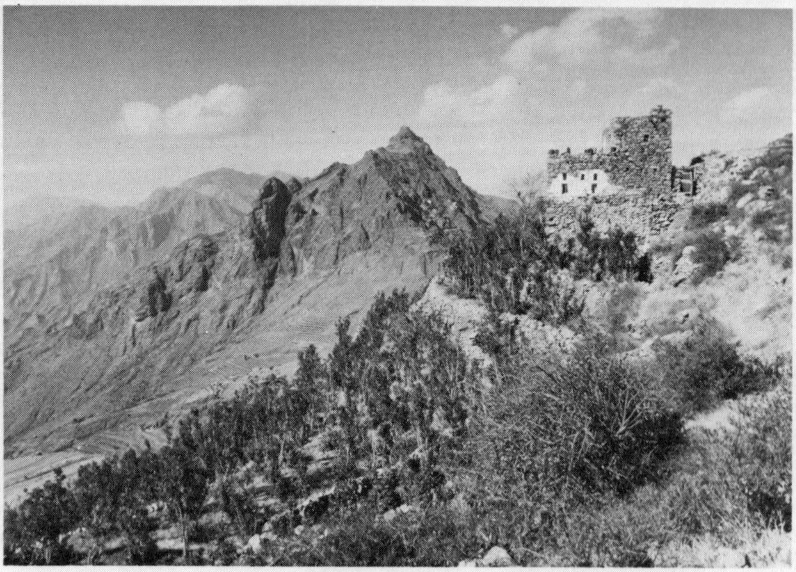

Qat Orchard on the Sanaa-Hodeida Road

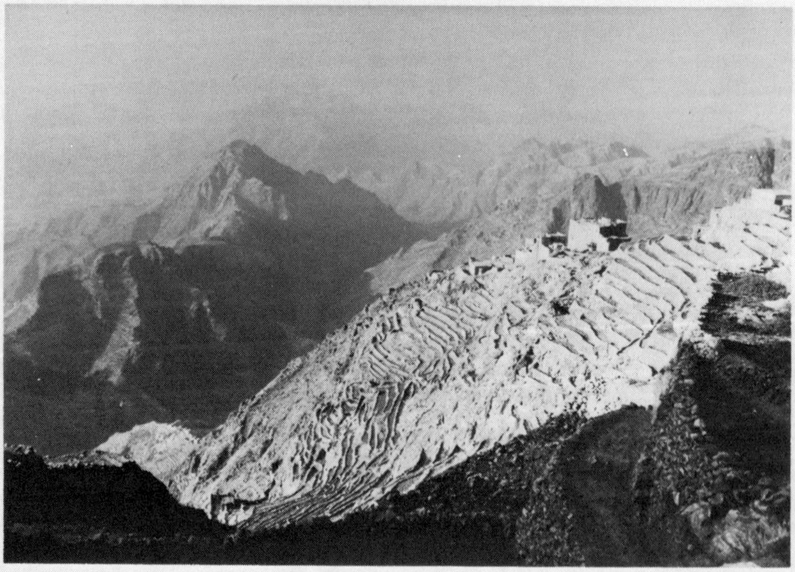

Terraces at Shahara

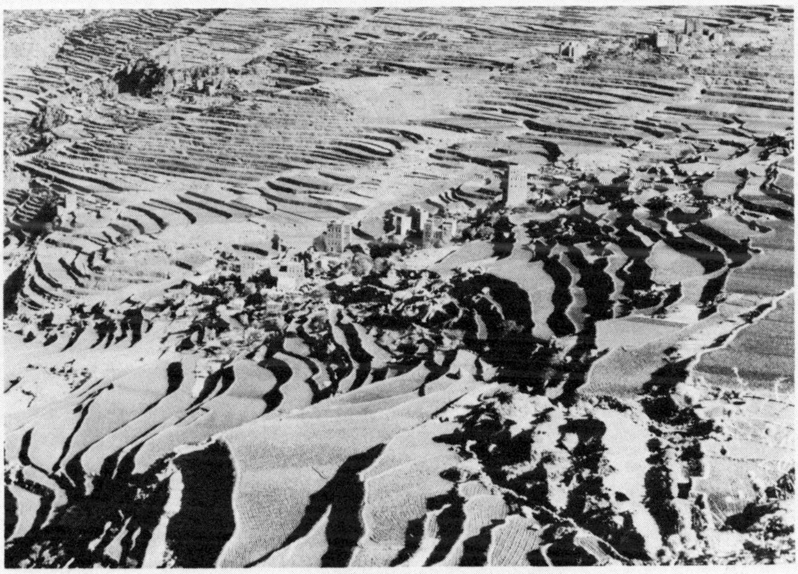

Terraces at Hayma

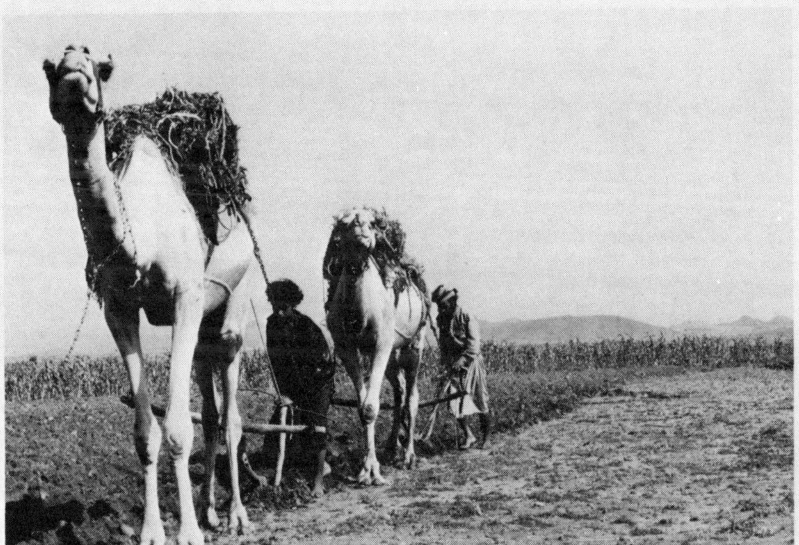

Cultivating Durra on the high plains near Dhamar

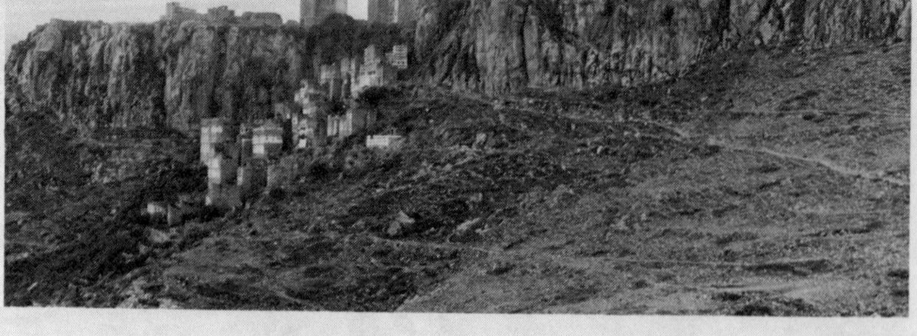

Al Hajar — a village near Manakha

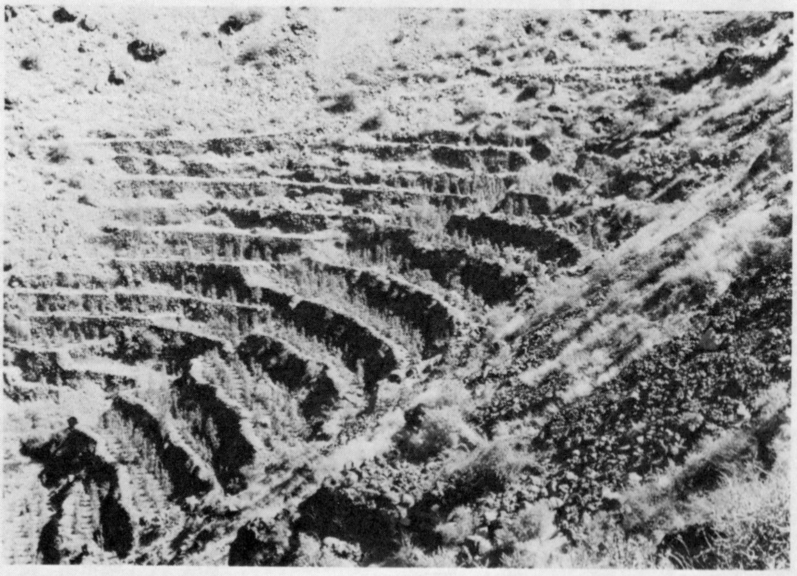

Qat on abandoned grain terraces

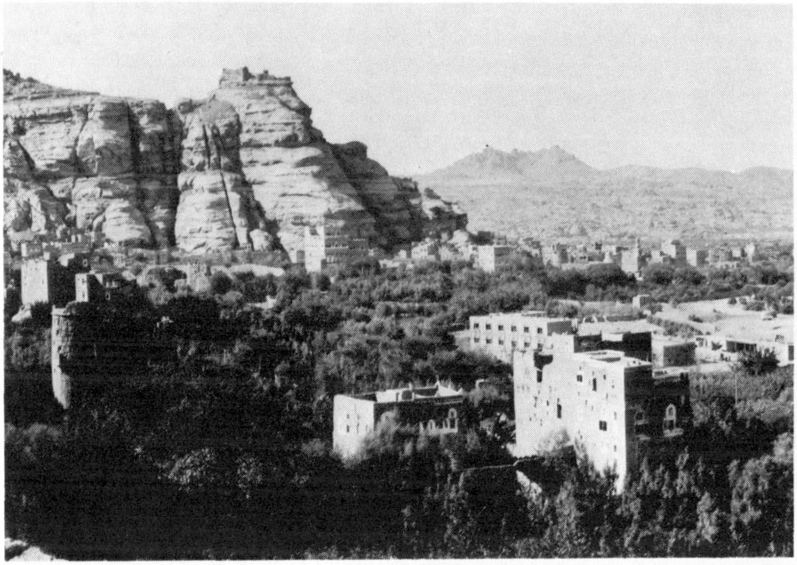

Qat orchards at Wadi Dahr

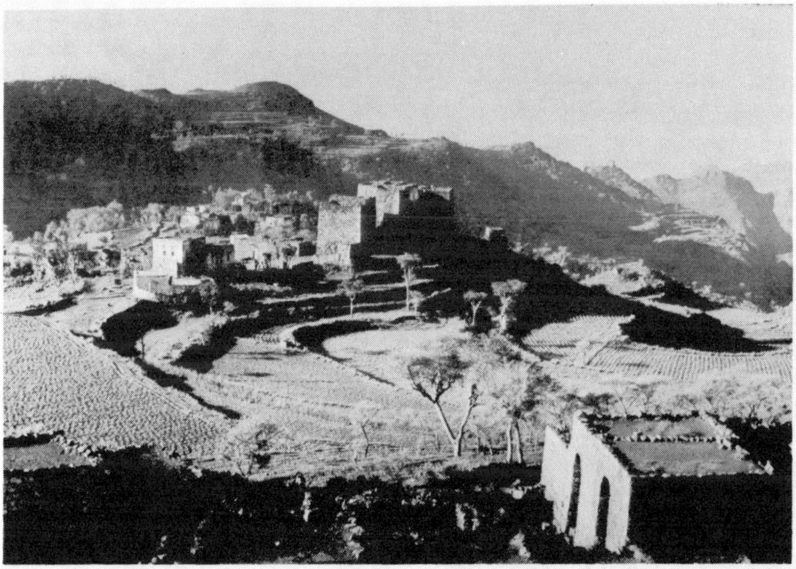

Village in Utmah

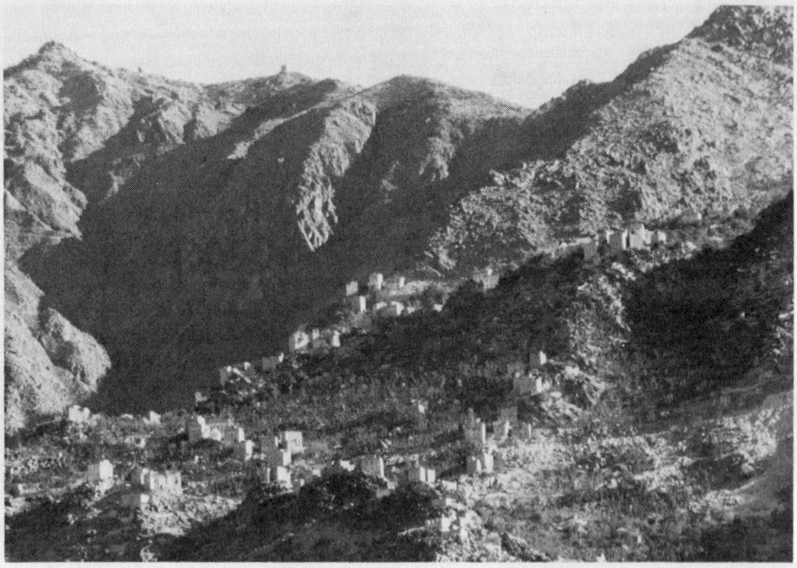

Jabel Sabr — mountain behind Taiz

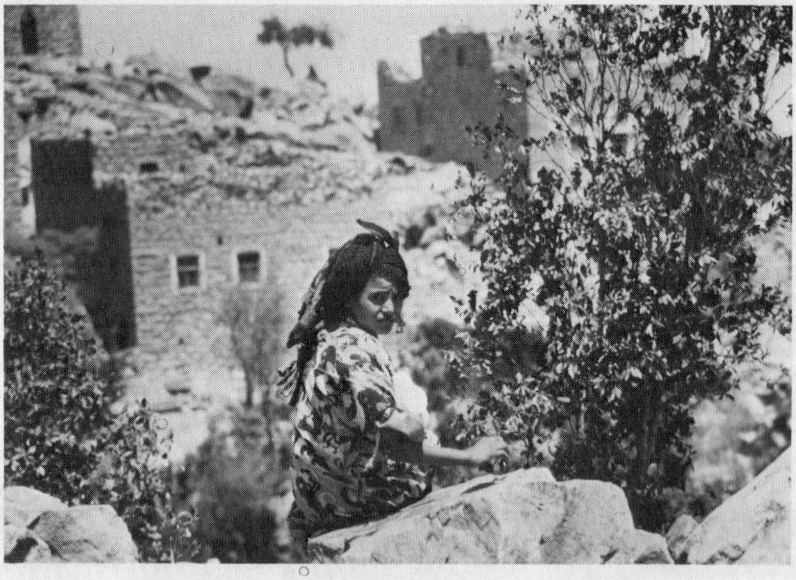

Qat seller on Jabel Sabr

> Like nicotine, it does not seem to be a drug. It is much worse than nicotine, however, in its ultimate effects, for it definitely reduces strength and vigor, and addicts who are deprived of it lose their ability to think clearly without it; they tremble and sweat and are very difficult to cure (1943:202).

Such "expert" opinions could be cited endlessly, but it would be a tediously repetitious exercise. My companions and I visited Yemen prepared for the worst. However, after participating in a number of qat sessions, we found it difficult to reconcile the uniformly negative foreigners' opinions with our own experiences, and with the conditions we observed. On one side there is an entire nation of people who appear as active and healthy as any other nation of the same economic level, who nearly all use the drug on a very open and regular basis, and who swear by its beneficial effects. On the other side, you have the nearly unanimous opinions of many intelligent travelers that the use of this drug is "addictive" and a great bane, totally harmful to health, debilitating to family budgets and inhibiting of economic development. Can such wide divergencies of perception and opinion be reconciled?

This contradiction seemed to us to offer the conditions for meaningful research. Was it possible that the Yemenis could be so drug-addicted that, as a nation, they could delude themselves into believing that what was really extremely dangerous and debilitating to them was actually beneficial? Could they have persisted in this delusion for centuries without recognizing that they were being damaged so severely? In fact, how could they have continued as a nation at all under such conditions? The logic of the experts would lead to the conclusion that such a society of stumbling "drug addicts" would have perished long ago and disappeared from the earth. Yet we heard many accounts of how during the recent civil war the Yemeni tribesmen were extremely brave, and resourceful. With our own eyes we observed a busy, ongoing society.

The general question arose in our minds: what might be the effects of institutionalized drug use on a country as well as upon individuals in it? It occurred to us that the mass use of amphetamines in the United States and elsewhere is increasing, and that since Yemen presents a natural experiment of a similar drug over a period of generations, here could be a unique opportunity to learn something of broad practical value.

We also became aware that the World Health Organization was making inquiries about qat with the stated intention of demonstrating its harmful characteristics, and with the specific intent of initiating action to forbid its growth and use. Yet in Yemen, as in the other countries where it is found, thousands of merchants and farmers depend on it for their livelihoods and the qat session is a focal institution of social life.

Dr. Teague and I saw the potentialities for doing some research on these questions during a visit to Yemen in February 1972 in the company of Dr. G. J. Obermeyer of the American University in Beirut. Our first trip for six weeks in that year was made by possible by the Neuropsychiatric Institute of U.C.L.A. Dr. Teague and I traveled to many parts of Yemen, meeting farmers, laborers and officials, as well as foreigners working there. We concluded, after this trip, and after considerable library research on the country and consultations with colleagues, that a study of qat-use could be important to the people of Yemen, and that it would have some potentiality for throwing light on general questions of drug use and abuse as well.

Initially we used the knowledge and enthusiasm about Yemen we had developed during our six weeks survey visit to the country to work up a proposal for a more extensive project, and our work was rewarded by a grant from the National Institute of Drug Abuse. We worked under the direction and encouragement of the late Dr. Eleanor Carroll of that agency, a person of powerful mind and personality who understood the value of cross-cultural work in the drug field.

When I finally reached Sanaa in October 1974, I found that the research situation was in reality more complicated than had been anticipated — that will become evident to those who continue through this book. There were many difficulties in doing research in a country formerly isolated from the outer world, in which such work had never before been tried. Furthermore, the qat issue is a politically sensitive one in Yemen.

Among Yemeni people everywhere in the country we found an extremely high interest in our research. The common people have never experienced European colonial domination and they are uniformly proud of their customs, including those of qat-use, even though some doubts about it are developing among educated sectors of the population. After the opening up of the country following the long civil war of the 1960s, many Yemenis who had lived in exile in East Africa, Aden and elsewhere during the days of oppressive monarchy, returned with ideas and values absorbed from the changing world outside. Students who had gone out to study during and after that time were also returning to practice medicine and other professions, and to participate in the exciting tasks of introducing and mediating change to the formerly closed and traditional country.

Many of the ideas and opinions concerning the negative effects of qat being brought back by the migrants from abroad were acquired in Aden during the last three decades, particularly by Yemeni and Adeni intellectuals who were influenced by European opinion. In the British colony these North Yemenis were exposed to Western notions of drug abuse and to values of economic development. Articles in the Adeni newspapers regularly argued that qat is bad for health, and that its economic effects are disastrous. These articles appeared from the late 1930s onward in many Adeni periodicals, but particularly in *Fata'al-Jezira*.

An important influence upon intellectuals in Yemen has been Said al-Attar, a Yemeni who in 1956 wrote the book *Le Sous-Développement Économique et Social du Yémen: Perspectives de la Révolution Yémenite.*

Many of al-Attar's opinions are repeated today in an almost formulaic way by officials in Yemen. Most common among these is his calculation that two million hours per day wasted on the drug, and the inference drawn from this that the economic backwardness of the country is importantly attributable to it.

In 1972, the Prime Minister of Yemen, British educated Mohsin al-Aini, instituted a campaign against qat. Though he stopped short of attempting to pass laws or decrees against it which would have had to be enforced, al-Aini banned its use among all government employees during business hours, forbade its use in all governmental buildings, and prohibited its planting and growth on *waqf* (government religious trust) land. He also began a strong propaganda campaign about its deleterious consequences. This included radio programs, newspaper articles, poems and skits put on at public holiday celebrations.

According to some young educated Yemenis, this campaign was ill-conceived and ill-timed. One informant, a member of the government at the time, told me that al-Aini had been losing influence, and while casting around desperately for an issue to divert attention from his detractors, struck on the qat issue almost by accident. Opportunistically, he seized upon it as a crusade.

Qat is certainly of great interest to all Yemenis and their attention was galvanized by this campaign. However, they were not ready for al-Aini's propaganda blitz, and they refused to go along with it. In fact, he was turned out of office within three months after beginning his anti-qat efforts.

Certainly it is not correct to take a simplistic view of this. Obviously there were major political reasons which contributed to his resignation at that particular time. Among these was a brief war which had just occurred with the People's Democratic Republic of Yemen. Nonetheless, many prominent Yemenis insist that al-Aini's campaign against qat was not negligible among the reasons for his political demise. For example, it is said that part of his campaign was an attempt to withdraw some agricultural subsidies from some qat-growing areas, and that powerful Shaykhs and other rich qat farmers united their efforts against him. Knowing what we do about the prevalence of use, the economic importance of the drug and the emotional values related to it in Yemen, it is a reasonable conclusion that al-Aini's anti-qat campaign contributed to his fall in 1972.

Slightly after this in 1973, a journal founded by intellectuals in Yemen called *The New Yemen* (*Al-Yemen al-Jadid*) devoted a whole issue to qat. Although a few of the articles dealt with basically neutral topics such as the history and poetry of qat, most of them expressed opinions against chewing, and many supported al-Aini's aborted anti-qat campaign. One of the strongest of these was an article by Abdel Salam al-Muqbel in which an argument was made that qat is antithetical to economic development. His reasoning was that it makes people less ambitious, makes them concentrate on single ideas or activities, makes them stupid, hinders scientific thinking, wastes a great deal of time which could be spent productively, hinders savings because people spend their extra money on it (and, thus, money is not used for investment), occupies land that could be used for productive crops, and produces no foreign exchange. This article repeated many of al-Attar's ideas, but it added some new ones as well.

Another article by the late Dr. Omar al-Abass, M.D., reviewed historical and chemical data on qat and then listed a long catalogue of bad physical effects. Most of the authors in this edition of *Al-Yemen al-Jadid* proposed solutions to the qat "problem", and there was much similarity among these. Recognizing the importance of the drug to many segments of the economy, these Yemeni writers did not, as do most foreigners, push for delegalization or for harsh restrictions. Instead, they recommended such measures as government subsidies to farmers who are heavily dependent on qat income, substitutions of equally remunerative crops, mass education about the harmful effects of the drug, and provision of alternative forms of rewarding work and entertainment to occupy the time now devoted to chewing.

All during our two years of research in Yemen, articles and poems repeating the same laments, arguments and proposals continued to appear in the newspapers from time to time. Meanwhile, the use of the drug continued to spread to parts of the country where it had been relatively unknown before, even though prices rose continuously. The building of each new paved road allowed the qat merchants faster access to more and more areas, stimulating more farmers to grow the drug. The influx of money from the many new development projects sponsored by oil-wealthy Arab neighbors, Western and Eastern bloc countries and international agencies, as well as from remittances sent back by Yemeni immigrants abroad, made it increasingly possible for many more people to purchase greater amounts of qat. This, in turn, stimulated more farmers to plant it, making it potentially remunerative for more people to buy trucks and go into the delivery business, and so on. This typical capitalistic cycle still continues.

When we reached Yemen in 1974 to begin the study reported in this book Mohsin al-Aini was again back in the Prime Minister's post. After a two-year absence he had recovered from the political debacle I mentioned above. In order to get more effective official sanction for the study, I wished to secure his approval and the Prime Minister granted me an interview. He began by asking a rhetorical question about what my study was going to be about, but before I could do more than barely state our intentions he began praising the campaign he had initiated against qat during his prior tenure as Prime Minister. He spent much of the interview admonishing me about how to carry out the research and listing the kinds of results which the study should produce.

> You must come to the conclusion that qat is harmful to the health and economy of Yemen because it *is* harmful. Be sure that this is your result.

Impatiently he listened to my reply that we were trying to carry out an impartial scientific study, and that we could not predict at the outset whether we could conclude that the use of qat was entirely detrimental.

"I know that you will find, and it is your duty to help us stamp out this evil,"

he insisted.

I replied that we were hoping the study would yield more reliable knowledge about qat, and that our project would be of some benefit to the people of Yemen. Though he did not change his position, Prime Minister al-Aini gave our project his blessing.

RESEARCH METHODS

From the very beginning of our stay in Yemen, until the end, we tried to participate in qat-sessions on a regular basis. Thus, I attended more than 100 chewing sessions during the 2 year field period. Dr. Teague also participated in more than a dozen sessions in the nearly 3 months he spent in Yemen. This first hand experience was extremely valuable for a number of reasons. First, the qat session is a primary institution of Yemeni society. In the near absence of public entertainment and also the other institutional means for people to gather and interact, the chewing session has developed into the most important social form serving the ends of both sociability and the transmission of information. Participation in sessions was thus necessary in order to obtain a first-hand understanding of the role and the uses of the drug in Yemeni society. Through actual experience we were better able to interpret the impersonal answers found on our interview schedules, but additionally, attendance in a number of sessions during our first six months provided a background which made it possible to design the interview schedules for the quantitative parts of the research to be used later.

It had become immediately apparent during our preliminary visit to the country in 1972, that it would be impossible to use drug studies done in the United States as the basis for designing the study of qat. Though, of course, we would use available knowledge of the drug field, we were immediately made aware that there is a vast cultural gap and that much groundwork had to be done without prior assumptions about drugs. The first six months of participant observation enabled us to learn the norms of qat chewing in various social classes, the beliefs of the people concerning its effects, good and bad. This experience helped us develop a more realistic idea of the role of the drug within the culture as well as learning many specific features of the qat chewing institution. With this information in hand, the interview schedules could then be designed to fit the parameters of the question, rather than being attempts to impose assumptions and ideas derived from drug studies in the West upon the Yemeni situation. We got an idea of the real variation in ages of beginning to chew, so that we could pre-code the range. We got an idea of the relationship of eating and smoking to qat-use and concluded that it was necessary to ask about these relationships. The relationship of qat to work was found to be important in a situation where the drug is completely legal. We learned the range of ailments for which qat is considered to be a remedy by segments of the population, and this list was then included in the interview schedule, etc.

One unexpected fact we learned was the great and growing importance of alcohol in this totally prohibitionist Muslim state. We gradually became aware of the fact that, in addition to locally made distilled beverages, a vast amount of Scotch whisky is smuggled into the country and that its use is related to qat use. The latter drug produces insomnia and, in many subjects, a loss of sexual desire. Alcohol is used to negate or reduce these effects. Thus, if an individual has access to alcohol he can experience the rewarding features of qat use without suffering many of the short-term negative effects. However, because of the circumstance that, in contrast to our own norms, alcohol is the illegal drug in Muslim Yemen, it was impossible to approach its use in a straightforward way. We included questions in the schedules which attempted to get at it indirectly, but answers tended to be evasive. Most of our knowledge of this phenomenon thus comes from informal interviewing and participant observation with groups following qat sessions. Because it is expensive and since alcohol is still used by only a minority of men; members of the educated elite and some returned migrants seem to be the primary users.

THE SOCIOMEDICAL SURVEY

The sociomedical survey was the "centerpiece" of our study of qat use in North Yemen and it consisted of two main parts. The first was what we termed "the sociological interview" which took about an hour to administer. It probed many characteristics of the respondents, e.g., age, sex, class affiliation (*Sayyid, Qabili*, etc.), religion (*Zaydi, Shafei, Ismaili*, etc.), occupation, father's occupation, ownership of land and other items, income education, literacy, marital status, household composition, etc. The next section was an extended inquiry into habits of chewing qat, attitudes about it, its relation to eating habits, and opinions as to its effects on life and health. The final part of this schedule probed habits of eating and costs of food.

The second part of the sociomedical survey involved the more difficult task of getting already interviewed respondents through a two step medical screening process to be described later. There was some attrition of the sample with each succeeding step.

We designed the medical component to yield a health profile which could then be compared with chewing habits, with economic level, with attitudes about qat, with dietary habits, etc. While it was not easy to get a large sample of sociological interviews, the problems of getting each respondent through a full physical examination, and a further set of laboratory tests, created extremely heavy logistical problems for the study under the conditions in North Yemen.

Demographic data on Yemen are sparse, and we were not funded or equipped to carry out the large epidemiological survey which would have been desirable. Instead, we elected to study a sample chosen primarily on the basis of people's qat-chewing habits (heavy users, moderate users and non-users), in order to directly assess health effects. The general population from which the sample was drawn constituted an extremely broad spectrum of the Yemeni population in and around geographically separated cities of Sanaa, Taiz, and Hodeida, the three major population centers in the country.

In each of these cities many of the people are recent arrivals from a large hinterland, and thus each city is "representative" of its region. Our sample thus includes individuals from all parts of Yemen. Problems of poverty, illiteracy, limited medical personnel and laboratory resources, and the lack of census or population registry data, made random sampling impossible. No modern census had ever been made until February 1975. A convenience sample was therefore required, and a quota sampling scheme was utilized.

The recruitment of participants was accomplished by a group of native interviewers trained for the purpose, according to a specified group of quota factors. The interviewers numbered four males and four females in each of the three study areas. The quota factors were level of qat use, gender, age, and socioeconomic status. Preliminary participant observation revealed several distinctive patterns of frequency of chewing, along with some variance by season, and these factors were taken into account in our interview schedules.

Age was dichotomized into over 30 and under 30 groups. Rural participant selection was originally planned, but proved unfeasible because of the unavailability of doctors and laboratories in rural areas. Children under 14 were excluded because regular chewing generally begins around that age, and only one interviewee was selected from any given family.

Interviewers were required to select participants from multiple neighborhoods. Subjects were compensated for their cooperation with a payment of 10 Yemeni rials (a sum equivalent about one quarter to one half day's income for unskilled laborers), enough qat for a day's chewing (for users), and for those submitting to physical examinations, the results of their diagnosis were supplied to them gratis. Since many of them proved to be in need of some sort of treatment, this was of some value to them.

Some potentially biasing problems were encountered in several areas of selection. Recruitment of females was difficult in socially conservative areas, particularly Sanaa, where we were only able to secure a sample of 81 women. We were able to partially flesh out the total female sample by getting slightly enlarged samples of women from Hodeida and Taiz.

With respect to our attempt to achieve equal numbers of rural and urban respondents, we were also not successful. This resulted from the fact that our operation was largely confined to the three cities where there was access to laboratories and doctors. Because we could not carry out medical examinations or laboratory tests in rural areas, only 19% of the sample is "rural" by our standards. However, contrary to our initial assumptions, our experience leads us to believe that the rural-urban contrast, which is so meaningful in other areas of the world, is not yet significant in the Yemeni context. This is because life differences between people in "urban" and rural areas are minimal in a country where the largest "city" (Sanaa) only contained some 138,000 people, and the other two "cities" possessed about 80,000 and 134,000, respectively. When we scrutinized this "rural" 19% closely for differences, we concluded that much of the style of life, in what are really large towns, is not significantly different from that in the smaller towns and villages of Yemen. Even though there are elite groups, large markets, etc., true urbanization has still not occurred. The rural-urban distinction does not have the sociological significance it does elsewhere.

The drug user categories were eventually constructed from answers to a series of questions pertaining to chewing in the interview schedule. They probed: (1) the number of chewing days per week, (2) the number of times chewed per day, (3) the number of hours per chewing session, (4) the number of bundles (*robtas*) chewed per session, and (5) the amounts paid for qat per session and per day. Another set of questions attempted to get at the length of time the respondent had used qat. All of these questions were asked for every season during the past year, as well as for the prior month. Chewers, therefore, had no idea how they were finally categorized.

TABLE I

Sample distribution in user categories

User	Males		Females	
categories	Number	%	Number	%
Non-chewers	96	21.9	93	25.5
Light chewers	141	32.1	143	39.3
Heavy chewers	202	46.0	128	35.2
TOTALS	439	100.0	364	100.0

Another important set of categories are those derived from dividing the study population into socioeconomic levels. These were constructed from answers to a series of questions in the sociological portion of the interview schedule. Being based on on self report data the economic categorizations cannot be taken as absolutely accurate, but we believe they are consistent relative to one another, and that they are a fairly accurate approximation of reality.

The natural reticence of people to divulge information on their personal finances was exacerbated by the not unreasonable suspicions that our interviewers might be from that perennial drain on income, the government. Fortunately, we asked a whole series of questions which allowed us to estimate various aspects of household economics. The answers to these were used in combination for constructing reasonable estimates. For example, data on property owned, houses, vehicles, occupations, income from remittences, amounts spent on qat, food, meat, etc., were used for this purpose.

After the income estimates had been made using all available data, and an initial computer run made, cut-off points were drawn according to breaks in the distribution and our knowledge of Yemeni society. The income categories that emerged are presented in Table II.

TABLE II

Yemeni rials per month[a]

Level 1:	0—800
Level 2:	801—1500
Level 3:	1501 and above

[a] The Yemeni rial remained at 4.5 to the U.S. dollar throughout the period of the study.

The distribution of those in the total sample who completed sociological interviews is presented in Table III.

TABLE III

Economic categories

Level	Males	%	Females	%	Combined	%
1	153	34.9	147	40.4	300	37.3
2	188	42.8	156	42.9	344	42.8
3	98	22.3	61	16.7	159	19.8
TOTALS	439	100.0	364	100.0	803	100.0

The heaviest representation in the sample is clearly in the poorer categories, i.e., of individuals whose incomes are less than 1500 rials per month. Our distributions thus are probably fairly indicative of the population of all of Yemen in this regard. We were attempting to get nearly equal proportions of rich and poor distributed among non-chewers, light, medium, and heavy chewers, but were unable to achieve this. It was extremely difficult to persuade wealthy people to be interviewed and to submit to health examinations.

A survey of this sort had never been carried out in Yemen and we had great problems in interviewer recruitment and turnover. In Taiz, we had to throw out one whole series of some thirty forms which we finally discovered were filled out falsely by one interviewer. We had trouble with several doctors also. One did his examinations in a perfunctory and unacceptable fashion, while another after a period of two months, had done none at all. We replaced these, but they wasted valuable time and then demanded payment.

The interview work in the southern city of Taiz was directed by Ms. Judith Obermeyer, who also assisted with the design of psychological tests. The survey in Hodeida was under the direction of Ahmad Makky, M.D. The overall research supervisor, Mr. Fathy Salem Ali and I supervised the interviewers in Sanaa. Without the unceasing efforts of these individuals it would not have been possible to achieve our goals. Every two weeks, Mr. Ali and I made visits of several days duration each to Taiz and Hodeida to check on the interviewing, make payment, etc.

MEDICAL ASSESSMENT

Though we secured data on chewing habits, attitudes and experiences with qat, and household economics, etc., from 803 people (439 males, 364 females) as described, we were only able to get 711 individuals (374 males and 337 females) through the entire medical screening steps of the study.

The medical forms were developed by Dr. James Teague after consulting with several European-trained M.D.'s in Yemen. The examination included recordings of height and weight, reflexes, presenting symptons (if any), a medical history designed to cover the major physiological symptoms, a present examination of all major physiological systems, (cardiovascular, respiratory, skeletal, etc.), and a global assessment of overall health.

After each respondent had been interviewed, he or she was personally escorted to the office of one of the doctors participating in the study. This was found to be necessary early on in our experience, when we noticed that a number of those interviewed failed to appear for medical examinations as they had promised. Additional delays often ensued because the doctors sometimes found it difficult to work our respondents into their own schedules. Naturally, they had to give first priorities to severely ill patients, particularly as there is a critical shortage of physicians. A number of our potential respondents grew tired of waiting to be examined and left. They did not regard themselves as ill and decided that they had no further time to lose.

The third part of the total process was seeing that the respondent, after being medically examined, was taken to one of our cooperating laboratories for some tests, mainly urine and hemoglobin. The laboratory in Taiz also made faecal examinations.

The three broad health categories (well, moderately ill, severely ill) were finally constructed from the medical protocols which had been filled out by the 11 physicians who did the physical examinations. The examining physicians remained blind to the chewing habits and other characteristics of the respondents they were examining.

ECONOMIC ASPECTS OF THE STUDY

The economic data which we gathered is of four different types. It pertains to qat agriculture, qat selling, governmental figures (e.g., taxes, etc. and family budget data). Most of the family budget information was collected on the sociological interview schedules of the user survey which is described above.

QAT AGRICULTURE

After being in the field a short while I realized that agricultural data was more important than I had originally anticipated. During the first months of the study, I interviewed a number of farmers in various parts of the country, and as I did this I began to understand how more detailed data would be of great value. Fortunately, early in the second year I was called upon by a young agronomist named Raman Revri who was working at the German Agricultural Assistance station in Sanaa. He informed me that he intended to do a doctoral dissertation on qat agriculutre for Hohenheim University in Germany, and asked my advice and assistance. I agreed to cooperate and gave him what financial assistance I could. He was able to pay a part time Yemeni assistant, and I provided him with access to aerial photographs of different qat growing regions in Yemen which I had obtained. He in turn, promised to provide us agricultural data that we needed.

These data came in several forms. Using the aerial photos as guides, Revri made overlay maps of the several important qat-producing regions of North Yemen. These were based upon his observations and sampling on the ground, in which he was able to estimate the distributions of various crops, percentages of which kinds of land are devoted to qat in proportion to other crops, etc.

He also did interviews with samples of farmers in the same areas. These schedules were drawn up with my collaboration and included questions on marketing and chewing, in addition to those specifically on agricultural practices. Revri collected a third set of systematic data on the selling prices of qat in the qat markets of Sanaa. On a weekly basis for more than a year prices were checked in four locations in the city. From this he was able to chart the seasonal fluctuations in the market.

Revri's dissertation (1983) has now provided access to his studies on soil, water, etc. and much of this valuable data is included in Chapter VI of this book.

QAT SELLING

In addition to the weekly sampling of prices mentioned above, we designed an interview schedule for the two major categories of qat merchants: street sellers and stall sellers. We managed to fill nearly 300 of these schedules, mainly in Sanaa and Taiz.

GOVERNMENTAL FIGURES

We collected as much data as we could from the government offices concerning taxes, revenues for qat, etc. Because of the abysmal record-keeping practices which characterized the Yemeni government during the Royalist period, this data is very uneven. Much of it is probably unreliable, but still there is some useful imformation, especially when used in conjunction with data from other sources.

THE YOUTH SURVEY AND THE SECRET POLICE

During our final year in the field we discovered that there is a group of young modernizing people in Yemen, who in the future will be making decisions about the directions of the country. These people are mostly males who work in government offices and private businesses, or attend the University of Sanaa. Since these young people are literate, we decided to sample their attitudes by questionnaires.

In the spring of 1976, I developed forms which covered basic data about background, place of origin, etc. and attitudes and practices relating to qat. Fathy Salem Ali, our field surpervisor, then began distributing the forms in banks, government offices, and the new Sanaa University. To our dismay, after about two weeks Fathy was called in by the secret police to be questioned intensively about our activities and our purposes in distributing such a document. All of the forms of the Youth Survey were confiscated. We were informed to cease that activity and were ordered to appear before the head of the secret police at a certain time. The situation appeared ominous. It looked as if the project as a whole was going to be halted and that all our data would be confiscated.

It was at this critical juncture that the careful groundwork with officials which was carried out at the beginning of the project paid off. When this crisis arose, I called on various officials whom I had kept apprised of the progress of the project and let them know of our dilemma. A number of phone calls were then made, and within three days all our confiscated material was returned and we were told that our scheduled interrogation by the police was cancelled. However, we were advised not to continue the Youth Survey. We were careful to heed this advice, and thus emerged with only a few completed forms for this particular survey. We had wanted to obtain at least 500.

THE DOCTOR SURVEY

The Doctor Survey was an attempt to get a sample of the beliefs and opinions of Yemeni doctors on the questions of qat and qat use. There were some difficulties due to reluctance of some doctors to talk, and to problems with fitting us into busy schedules. Twenty brief interviews were carried out with a spectrum of doctors whose training countries included Czechoslovakia, Egypt, Germany, Iraq, Italy and Russia.

PSYCHOPHYSIOLOGICAL TESTING

Late in the research process we did some psychophysiological tests on 60 subjects before, during and after controlled qat sessions staged in the field station in Sanaa. The tests consisted of monitoring EKG, EEG, temperature, blood pressure, pulse, pupil size, and a series of simple psychological tests. Though some of these data are presented here, equipment problems posed by the physical activity of chewing (movement artifacts) have prevented a complete analysis of this aspect of the study up to this time.

HISTORICAL DATA, INFORMATION FROM LITERARY SOURCES AND FOLKLORE

This material was gathered largely from old books written in Arabic, and from literary magazines and newspapers from Aden and Yemen dating back about 40—50 years. In Sanaa, we were directed to Mr. Abdullah al-Hibshi, who worked at the Dar al-Kuttub library, and who has a local reputation as a scholar. He agreed to scan the older historical works, as well as modern periodicals for references to qat use, legislation, etc. Mr. al-Hibshi collected quite a body of materials which he copied by hand in Arabic from the many sources. Most of this material was translated at UCLA by Mustapha Mebarkia and Hiam Slieman. Much of it is repetitive but it does provide us with some historical context regarding attitudes and laws pertaining to qat-use in the past. It adds a dimension to the written sources available.

This book does not make use of the entire corpus of material gathered in the study. It does, however utilize much of it. No claims are made that this is "the definitive work" on the subject of qat in Yemen. However, it is hoped that it will stimulate further more extensive and intensive work on this socially important drug.

It should be mentioned that, despite the lag of several years between the research reported here and the appearance of this book, the substance of it remains accurate. I have kept track of conditions in Yemen through many Yemeni friends and several researchers. During the interim the prices of qat have continued to rise parallel with inflation, and plantation of the drug has increased. These trends are confirmation of the essential correctness of the account presented here.

Chapter II sets the stage for the later ones by briefly outlining the historical and social context within which the institution of qat use arose. An understanding of the role of qat in Yemen society must be founded upon a broad historical and cultural base.

VIEWS OF SANAA, TAIZ AND HODEIDA

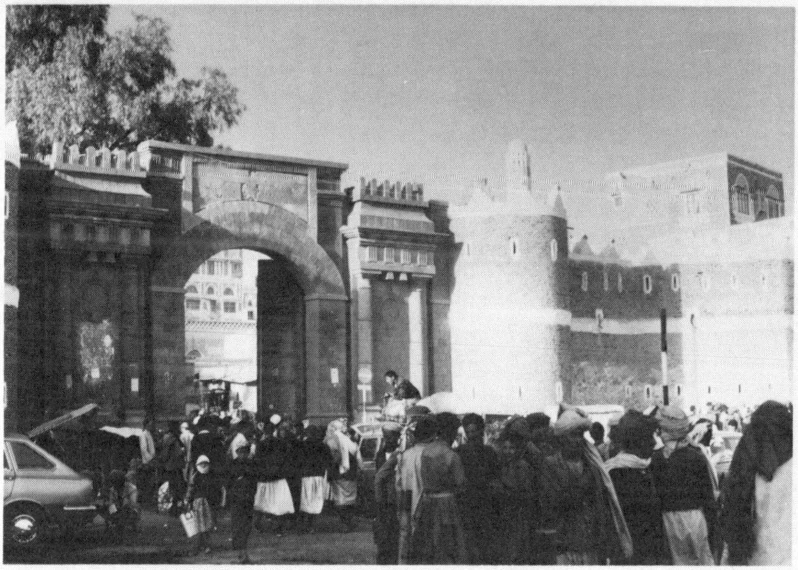

Bab al-Yemen — (Gate to old city) at Sanaa

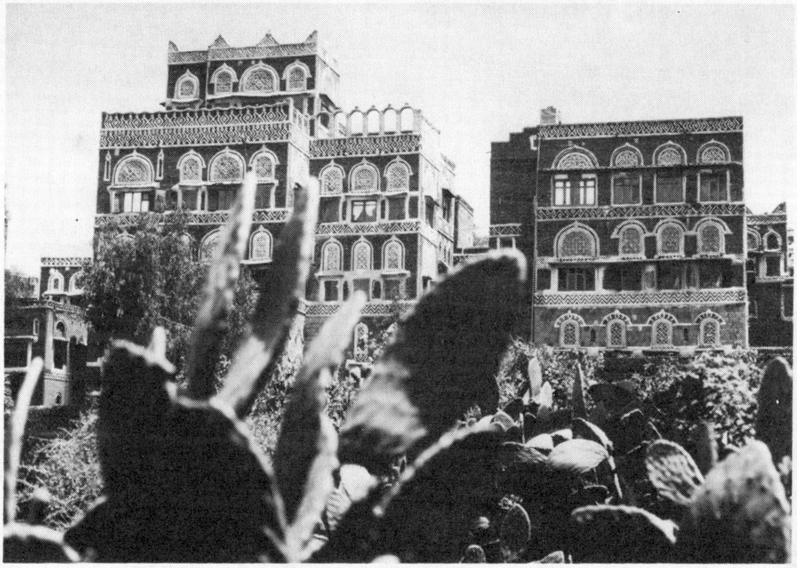

Houses — old city of Sanaa

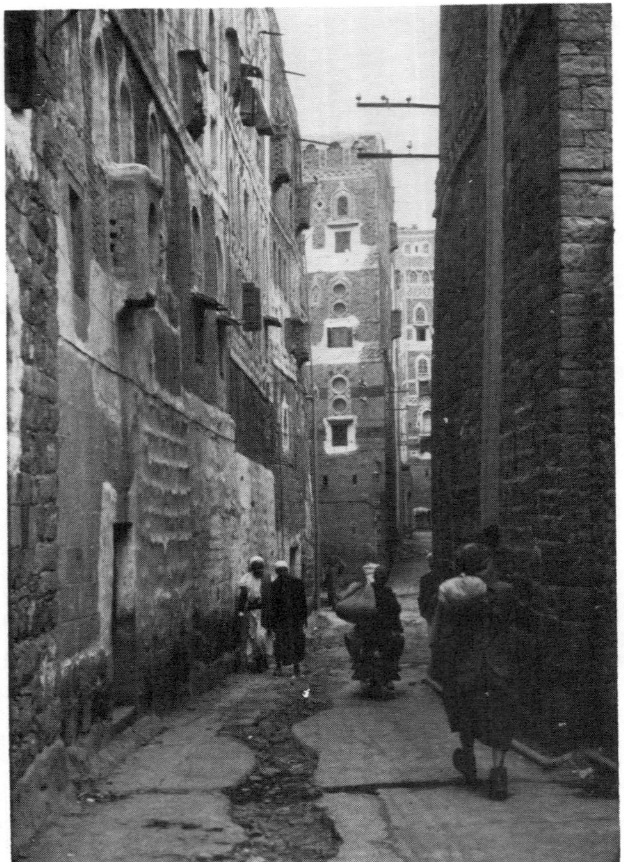

Street scene old city of Sanaa

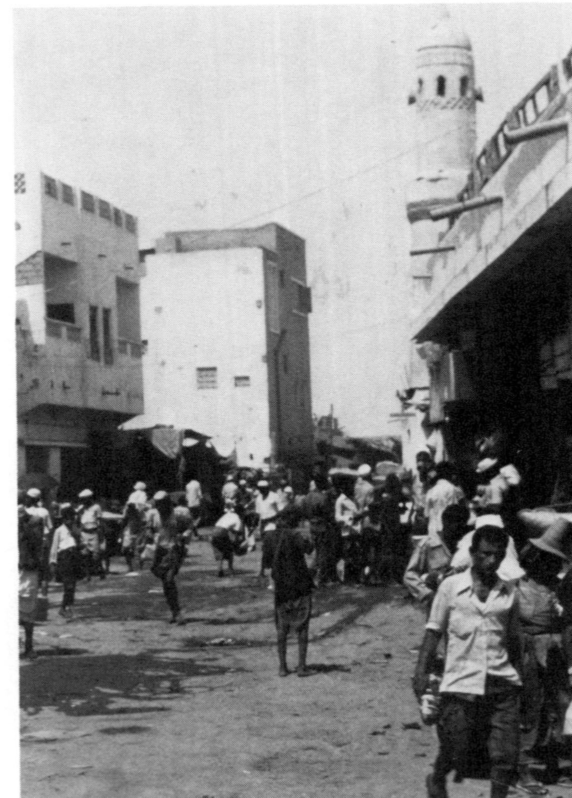

Photo credit Sylvia Kennedy

Street scene new market of Hodeida

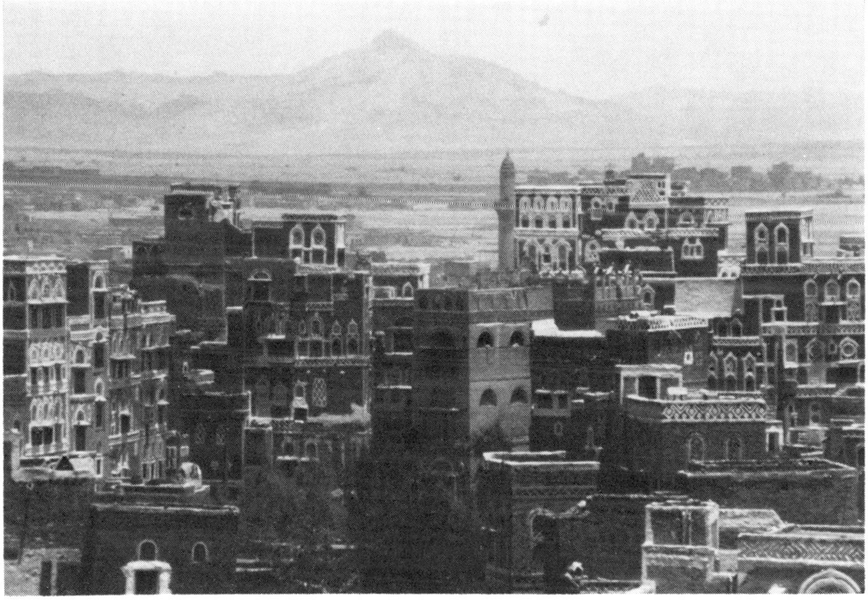

Photo credit Marilyn Neuhart

View of old city of Sanaa

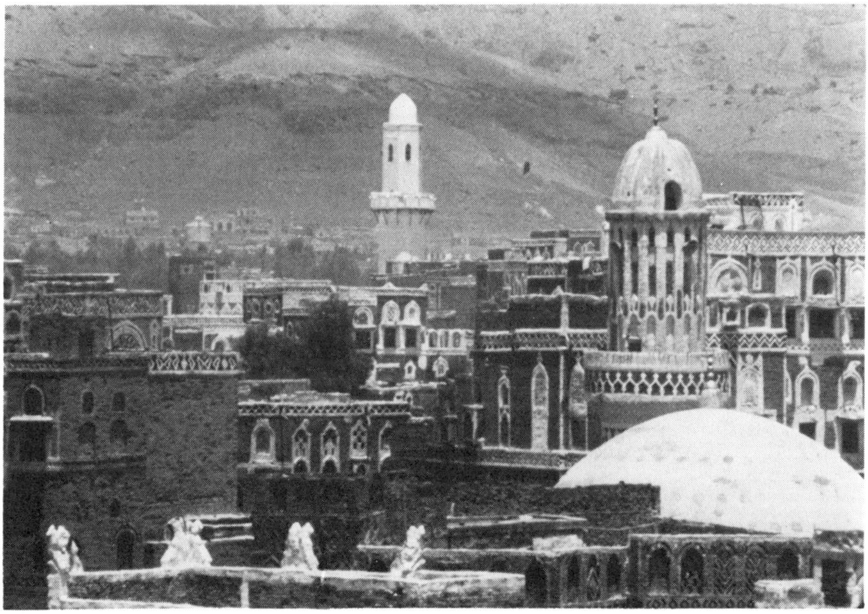

Photo credit John Neuhart

Old city of Sanaa (with mosques)

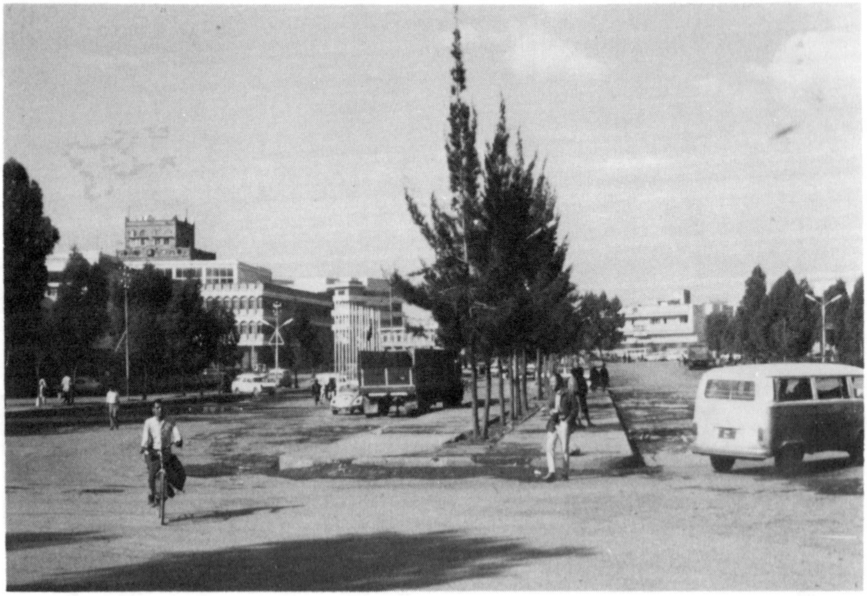

Photo credit John Neuhart

New city of Sanaa

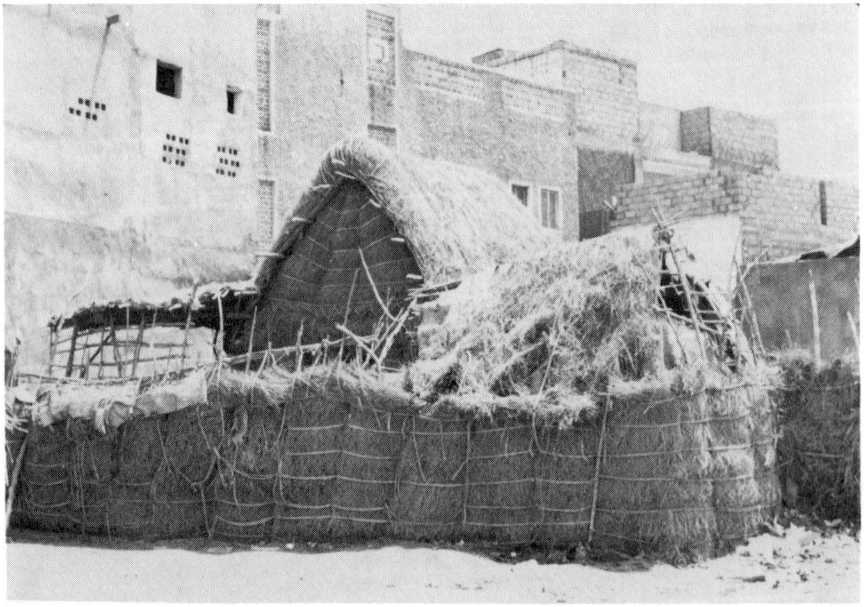

Thatched houses with buildings in Hodeida

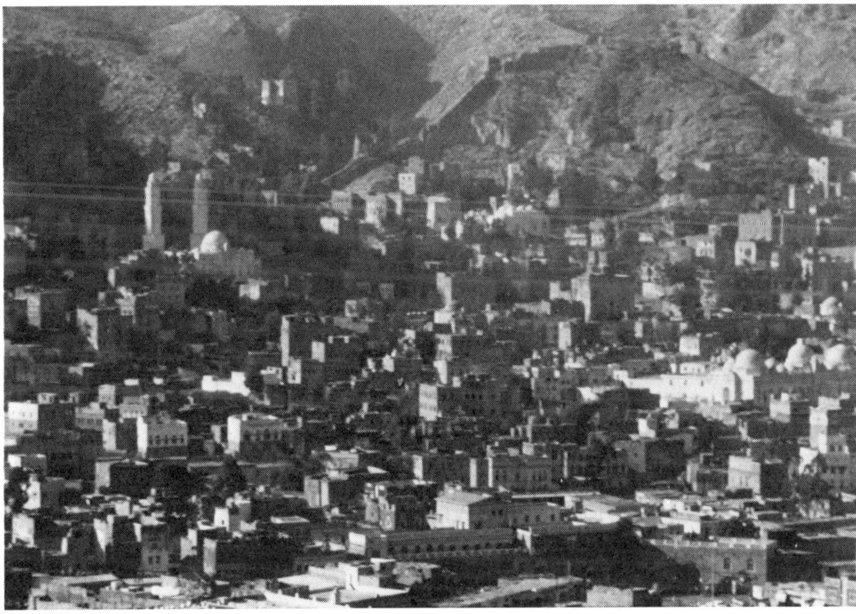

View of city of Taiz

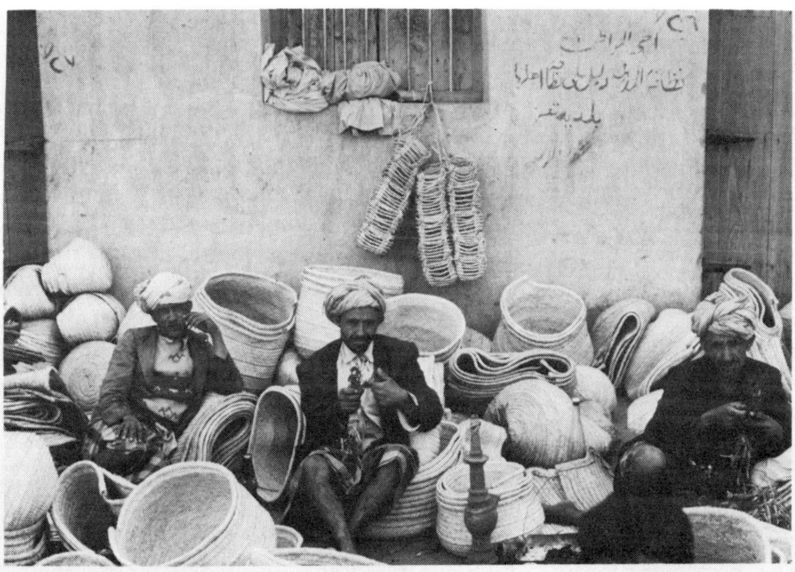

Photo credit James Teague

Merchants chewing qat in the Taiz market

CHAPTER II

HISTORY AND SOCIAL STRUCTURE OF NORTH YEMEN

HISTORICAL SKETCH

Ancient civilizations flourished on the southwestern part of the Arabian Peninsula, but they remain almost unknown. We have learned something about them from surface inscriptions, coins, a few partial excavations, and some fragmentary reports in Greek and Roman historical literature, but no full-scale archeological work has yet been completed in the heartland of these complex cultures.[1] The area now covered by the Yemen Arab Republic (North Yemen), and the People's Democratic Republic Yemen (South Yemen) was known in the pre-Islamic times as Arabia Felix, or Happy Arabia. This name referred to its reputation as the source of some of the materials most highly-prized in the flourishing civilizations of Egypt, Greece, and Rome, but just as justifiably the name could have arisen from the happy circumstances of its beautiful green wadis and the salubrious climate of its magnificent mountains.

The civilizations of South Arabia were based largely upon trade, supplemented by an agricultural system made possible by impressive irrigation works. They appear in the record at nearly the fullest complexity of development ever reached by them i.e., about 1400 B.C., and they continued for nearly 2000 years. Well into the early Christian era they were in decline, and after a weak struggle against the forces of the new and dynamic Islamic religion they were eclipsed in the early eighth century A.D.

The economic source making possible the emergence of complex kingdoms in this region was the hospitality of the climate to the frankincense tree, which may have originated in Dhofar, a province of present-day Oman, or in Somaliland, the other of the two areas where it flourishes. South Arabia is also an area where myrrh, another highly valued commodity of the ancient world, is found in abundance. The domestication of the camel in this region sometime before 1000 B.C., coupled with the rising demand for frankincense and myrrh for rituals and embalming in Ancient Egypt and Sumer, and later in Greece and Rome, created the conditions that attracted relatively large numbers of people from Mesopotamia into South Arabia in the middle of the second millenium B.C. These migrants apparently subdued some of the native Bedouins and intermarried with them while establishing caravan routes northward through the peninsula. Beginning at Dhofar, the main road led through Marib, Najran, Mecca and Medina, and thence either west to Alexandria or northeast to Petra, Damascus and Babylon.

A number of kingdoms grew up along these routes whose economics were based primarily on taxes from these incense caravans, which also carried silks, spices and other rare commodities from India and the Far East. Since each kingdom extracted its toll, by the time they reached their destinations the values of all these substances were elevated to a level nearly comparable with gold.

Each kingdom on this "Incense Route" experienced periods of autonomy and fluorescence, but Saba (Sheba), whose capital city of Marib was located in the eastern desert of Yemen, dominated the area longer and had hegemony over a broader region than any of its sister states of Hadramaut, Qataban, Ma'in, and others of lesser importance. Though built upon trade, all of these states were theocracies ruled by priest kings, and their spiritual lives centered around cults to the Moon and Sun gods.

The South Arabian cultures were at first entirely derivative from those in Mesopotamia, but as time went on they showed strong influences from the civilizations of the Mediterranean, from whom they imported sculptural styles and technology. Their trade positions made these states extremely wealthy. When the Queen of Sheba (Saba) made for famous pilgrimage to visit King Solomon of Israel, the legendary riches of her caravan became part of the mythology of the world.

The Kingdom of Axum which arose in Ethiopia during the first millenium B.C. seems to have been directly stimulated by the Sabean conquerers and artisians there, and the ancient script of Ethiopia derives from South Arabia. In 24 B.C. the Emperor of Rome sent an expedition under the direction of Aelius Gallus, prefect of Egypt, to conquer Saba and bring it under the control of the Roman Empire. His expedition, though it reached to a point south of Najran before turning back, became a fiasco for Rome.

Probably the most noteworthy technological achievement during the period of great kingdoms in South Arabia was the construction of the great Marib dam. The massive stone and masonry ruins of this ancient architectural masterpiece still tower impressively at the edges of the wide wadi Dhana near Marib in the eastern desert of Yemen. The mute splendor of these ruins gives immediately understandable testimony to why the Marib dam was one of the wonders of the ancient world. The richness of the civilization making such an engineering feat possible is clearly revealed.

This dam did not create a reservoir, as do modern dams, but diverted the waters from the yearly floods in the wadis to irrigate more than 4,000 acres nearby. Scattered throughout the northern and eastern part of Yemen are ruins of several hundred smaller dams which utilized the same methods, providing more evidence of the large number of people who once lived on this now barren part of the land.

By the fourth century A.D., the wealthy south Arabian states had begun a steep decline. Apparently, this was due primarily to the fact the caravan routes for incense, myrrh, and spices were being superseded by sea routes. Greek sailors by accident had discovered how to reach India and return via the monsoon winds, and thus had learned that many of the spices, silks, rare woods and other goods brought via the camel routes of South Arabia actually came from India and the Eastern Orient.

When Christianity officially became the religion of the Roman Empire in 325 A.D., frankincense was banned in ritual, and demand for the only truly native resource of the region ceased entirely. The entire economic base which had enabled these states to develop beyond the potentialities which their agriculture could provide finally was cut off. The last 300 years before the advent of Islam were marked by political instability, declining adherence to religious values and relative anarchy. The great Marib dam had broken and been repaired several times in its 1500 year history, and the last time it was reconstructed was in 543 A.D. by the Abyssinian Christian governor Abraha. However, by that time, due to general cultural decline, many of the Sabeans had already migrated in all directions. Some of these early-migrating groups were ancestral to some present-day tribes in Syria, and others settled in Yathrib, which after Muhammad took refuge there was renamed Medina.

In the latter stages of the pre-Islamic era, the Himyarite tribe built a capital at Zafar near present day Yarim, and for a short period their kingdom incorporated the Sabeans. The main center of power in Yemen remained primarily with the Himyarites from 300 A.D. until 570. Then cultural decline became even more pronounced and, at one point, the area was even ruled by a Jewish king, Dhu Nawas, who became famous for massacering the Christians from across the Red Sea. Yemen finally became a Persian satrapy shortly before the Prophet Muhammad loosed the Islamic religious and military forces which swept the peninsula and beyond.

Due to its proximity to Mecca and Medina, and to the circumstance that Yemeni tribes were already established in the latter city, Arabia Felix felt the impact of the Prophet Muhammad's message very early in his career. The first mass conversion of Yemenis took place in 628 A.D. among the Ash'ira, a Tihama tribe. The following year, the great Hamdan tribe of the north capitulated, and then others quickly came over (Stookey 1978:20).

The conversion, however, of the southern part of the peninsula was not a smooth and uniform process. The first two centuries of Islam in Yemen were turbulent and uncertain as false prophets contended with the followers of Muhammad, and as leaders of various sectarian offshoots built up followings in all parts of Arabia. The major doctrinal and institutional cleavage which eventually divided Islam as a whole — that between the Sunni and the Shi'a sects — also came to be represented in Yemen at this time. This religious division still demarcates the major sociopolitical regions of the country.

In the early phases of the Islamic empire, i.e., during the Ummayyad and Abassid periods, the country was ruled from Damascus and Baghdad through the governors of the Islamic Caliphs. However, there was always opposition to centralized control. At times this was led by independent Yemeni tribes of the mountains, while at others resistance was manifested by a rebellious Ziyadi state in the Tihama Plain, by the Himyarite tribes of the southern mountains, and by various sects of Qarmatians, etc. None of the great ancient states of Saba, Ma'in, Qataba and Hadramaut ever really unified the mountains and plains of Yemen in earlier times, so it is not surprising that tribes and groups with histories of relative autonomy frequently broke away from the yoke of Islamic governmental authority.

Aside from the Ziyadi state which had independent control of the Tihama for the short period between 822 and 889 A.D., the most important though short-lived dynasties of this early Islamic period were the Yufrids and the Qarmatians. Both of these appear to have been forms of Ismailism, a branch of the Shi'a which is still important in other parts of the Islamic world. The Yufrids gained partial and uneasy control over an area of the highlands stretching from Kawkaban and Shibam in the north, as far as Janad in the south, and kept it for more than 150 years (861 to around 1014 A.D.). The Qarmatians had a brief period of power when, near the beginning of the 10th century, a leader named Ali bin al-Fadl conquered parts of the Tihama as well as the region around Udain and Ibb, and even Sanaa for a short time. In Yemeni history, the Qarmatians are generally castigated because they are alleged to have approved of fornication, incestuous marriages, wine drinking and abandonment of the pilgrimage — all terrible crimes against Islam. The ascendancy of the Qarmatians was brief indeed.

The Fatimid conspiracy to take over the Islamic Caliphate was strongly representing itself in North Africa in the year 910 A.D., and a Fatimid Dynasty called the Sulayhids was established there around 1056. The Sulayhids lasted from 1056 until 1152, that is, until just before the Fatimid Caliphate in Cairo fell to the Abuyyids led by Saladin. The Sulayid regime in Yemen is perhaps most noteworthy for the period of it which was marked by the reign of Queen Arwa, who moved her capital from Sanaa to Jibla where her mosque with her tomb inside it still stands. Queen Arwa's long incumbency was relatively peaceful and productive, especially when judged by the standards of those warring times. Today, even uneducated Yemenis know that she or her engineers performed the feat of laying out the course of the road between Sanaa and Taiz, essentiallly the same route which was only recently paved for vehicular traffic.

Zaydism, a branch of the Shi'a sect, was founded by Zayd ibn Ali Zain al-Abdin who was killed in Kufa, Iraq in 870 A.D. It was introduced into Yemen by Yahya bin Hussain bin Qassim al-Rassi, one of Zayd's followers, who in 893 was asked to come to Yemen to settle persistent disputes between the tribes around Sada. He is known as "The Guide to Truth" (*al-Hadi ilal Haqq*), and through his influence the tribes of the northern area were rather quickly converted to Zaydism over the next decade.

The Zaydi sect had been established in Yemen in 893 A.D., i.e., even before the Fatimid period there, but in the early phases the Zaydi state was confined largely to the northern region around Sada. Except for a brief conquest of Sanaa in 900, during the Sulayid's time, the Zaydis were never able to gain ascendency over most of the country until 1152. From then until 1962, when the final Imam was overthrown, the Zaydis have been predominant in North Yemen, even if rarely in full control.

The leader of the Zaydi sect is known as the Imam, and he has always been chosen by and from the descendants of the Prophet Muhammad, who are called Sayyids. Zaydism has been called "pragmatic shiism," and actually it differs from orthodox Sunni Islam only in minor ritual prescriptions, some minor legal points, and its concept of the Imamate. The Zaydis reject the orthodox Iranian Shi'a notion of a "hidden" Imam who is supposed to reappear with the prophets on Judgment Day, and they do not accept the associated Shi'a doctrines of an esoteric or occult exegesis of the Qur'an. Unlike other Shi'a legal schools, the Zaydis have never embraced sufism. Rather they have many times moved to stamp out sufi sects when they appeared.

The Zaydis often have been in command of major portions of Yemen, but at least half of the country, and frequently a much higher proportion has always followed an orthodox Sunni form of Islam called Shafeism.[2] The Tihama has been Shafei since earliest times, as is part of North Yemen south of Sumara Pass. This landmark is the traditional boundary between the two sects. The division of the country along Zaydi-Shafei lines has constituted a major fault line along which political and economic oppositions have historically developed.

Many times the warlike Zaydi tribes have conquered parts of the Tihama and the Shafei areas south of Sumara Pass. From one perspective, the political history of Islamic Yemen has been a continuous attempt by the Zaydi Imams to unify the whole area under their control. Occasionally they have accomplished such unity, as with one of the most successful Zaydi states, the Rassulid Dynasty (1232—1454). For a time it controlled not only the most traditional Zaydi area north of Sanaa, but also the Tihama, the southern mountains and plains all the way to Aden, and even the regions east through part of Hadramaut as far as Dhofar. It was probably during the earlier part of this dynasty that the custom of qat use became rooted in Yemen (see next chapter).

The fall of the Rassulid Dynasty was followed by a considerable contraction of the Zaydi state, a situation which lasted more than a hundred years. During this time the country was not only torn by internal dissension, but had, by the beginning of the 16th century, suffered invasions from Egyptian Mamelukes. Later, it was invaded by the Turks, who captured Taiz in 1545, and then seized Sanaa and the Tihama.

The Ottoman Turks unified the administration of the country and kept relative order in the cities and towns, but they were never able to subdue the northern and eastern tribes. The famous Zaydi Imam, Sharaf al-Din led the tribal resistance against the Ottomans all of his life, as did his successor

Qassim bin Muhammed, the founder of the Qassimi Dynasty (1598—1892). Sharaf al-Din issued a ban against chewing qat, indicating that it was in widespread use by this time. It was the third Imam of this dynasty, al-Mu'ayyad Muhammad, who finally drove the Ottomans out in 1635, and again unified Yemen under Zaydi control.

The details of the history of the Qassimi Dynasty until its rule was interrupted by another Turkish invasion in 1872, are somewhat unclear. However, it was during this period that Carsten Niebuhr and his group of scientists and scholars made their famous trip to Yemen. King Frederick V of Denmark sponsored the expedition of scientific exploration in which all the senior members but Niebuhr died of disease. Niebuhr's account of the group's ill-fated sojourn in Yemen in 1762—63 is an invaluable and incredibly vivid record of some aspects of Yemeni society and culture during the Qassim Dynasty.[3] There is evidence (cited in the following chapter) that qat was now widely used in large areas of the country.

The early part of the 19th century was a period in which Britain, France, Egypt and the Ottoman Empire were contending for colonial interests in the Red Sea area and the Indian Ocean. At the same time, the Qassimi Imams of the highland Yemen were following the Zaydi pattern of extending their hegemony over the Tihama and the Shafei parts of Yemen, only to lose control over some of them again as local leaders rebelled and as internal weaknesses allowed competition among heirs to the Imamate to develop.

Muhammad Ali of Egypt, who had imperialistic designs on Arabia, sent armies which occupied Tihama from 1835—1840. This provoked retaliation from the British who staked their claim in the area by occupying the Port of Aden and the adjacent shaykhdom of Lahej in 1839. Aden first became a British port and later was made a Crown Colony, a status which lasted until the recent independence movement ended British control in 1963.

Returning to the 19th century, the Asir Sharifs, based in the province of Asir, now a part of Saudi Arabia, were allowed governance of the Tihama when the European colonial powers forced Muhammad Ali to retire from the region. From then until the Turks again occupied Yemen in 1872, the Zaydi Imam, using tribal warriors from the Hashid and Bakil confederations of the nothern mountains, fought sporadically with the Asiri Sharifs for control of the Tihama. He also had to deal with uprisings among Ismailis and various insubordinate tribes. Eventually, he was unable to maintain any semblance of control. Chaos became so extensive that the Ottomans were actually invited back in by Sanaa notables to restore order in the country (Stookey, 1978:159).

In 1872 began the final Turkish occupation, which lasted until World War I. As in the previous Ottoman occupation three centuries before, the Turks were never able to completely rule the country. They were again incapable of conquering the unruly Zaydi tribes of the north, but were able to govern the Tihama and to control the large cities and the roads. This time the Ottomans did introduce some modern administrative forms of government, establish a few schools, and they kept a temporary peace, but their rule was extremely oppressive. Thus they were soon opposed by both the Shafeis and the Zaydi tribes, and this opposition assumed the proportions of a liberation movement.

The resistance crystallized around the Hamid ad-Din family, from which Mohammad bin Yahya was elected Zaydi Imam in 1891. He led the tribes in successful guerilla warfare against the Turkish occupying forces until his death in 1904, and through his efforts, many concessions were gained from the Ottoman government. However, it was his son, Yahya, who continued the battle and finally completed the task of again expelling the Turks from Yemen in 1918. Yahya was greatly aided in this by the defeat of Turkey during World War I, a circumstance which led to the diversion of much of Turkish military power to other areas.

Imam Yahya, a veritable model of an anachronistic medieval king, ruled North Yemen from 1904 until his assassination in 1948. Again, a large part of his long reign was occupied with the Zaydi dreams of extending the power of the Imamate and reunifying the country. Like all Yemeni rulers, Yahya had severe problems with the Northern Zaydi tribes from time to time, but he had considerable success in keeping their rebelliousness under control by shrewdly balancing alliances, and by keeping the sons of leading Shaykhs hostage in Sanaa. Many Yemeni people believe that he encouraged the use of qat by the people to help keep them pacified and acquiescent to his restrictive policies.

The Yemeni social system since the pre-Islamic kingdoms has been based upon a near subsistence agricultural economy. The kingdom produced most of what it consumed, and minor exports of coffee, hides, salt, and qat (for a few years) brought sufficient revenues to satisfy the wants of the nobles for a few luxury goods. The very slow pace of change, which outsiders tended to view as stagnation, was maintained by the Imam's policies of rigidly restricting foreign influences and exiliing or killing opponents of the system. As Robert Burrowes has pointed out, the theocratic Imamic state, ruled by a small elite was thus a good example of a “”patrimonial” political system, in Max Weber's terms (1978:7—8).

As was stated, a central motivation of Imam Yahya and later of Ahmad his son, was the centralization of state power, and the extension of governmental control over wider and wider areas. The extent of this ambition was not unlimited, however; it was guided by a historical ideology relating back to the periods of Sabean and Himyaritic hegemony over most of the southern end of the Arabian Peninsula. By the time of the revolution of 1962, the combined successive efforts of Yahya and Ahmad were successful in gaining uneasy control over the entire area now comprising North Yemem.

A cardinal feature of Imam Yahya's policy, as it was also of his son Ahmad, was the isolation of Yemen from the rest of the world, and most particularly from Europe. The idea which they overtly articulated to rationalize this policy was that foreign ideas would contaminate the Islamic purity of the people, bringing immoral decadence and stimulating religious apostasy. However, in retrospect, it is evident that this rigidly imposed policy of isolation helped the Imams to control their people, and thus to maintain and consolidate their power.

One effect of social and cultural isolation was that North Yemen did not participate in the economic development so rapidly accelerating in the rest of the world. The country remained preserved as a preindustrial backwater, a condition from which it is still trying to emerge. As Fred Halliday so correctly states: "The poverty, misery, ignorance and disease of his [Imam Ahmad's] people as well as the emigration of possibly one million, i.e., 11 percent of the whole population, were eloquent evidence of the policies pursued by the Hamid ad-Din family" (1974:86)

During the early part of this century many Yemenis fled to escape the oppressive monarchy. They had long wanted their country to participate in the social and economic changes they witnessed going on in other countries and as the century wore on, some of them founded groups to oppose the Imamic regime. The most important of these was the Free Yemeni Party founded in Aden in the 1940s which from its base in the Aden Colony, tried to influence the people of North Yemen through newspapers, pamphlets and books.

The Free Yemenis were closely associated with the underground opposition to the monarchy in Yemen, led by Abd Allah ibn Ahmad al-Wazir. This Sayyid leader led a rebellion against Imam Yahya in 1948, in which the old Imam was killed in an ambush. In spite of a short-lived initial success, the uprising led by Wazir was crushed by Crown Prince Ahmad with the help of certain tribes, and the Hamid ad-Din regime continued under his autocratic rule. However, Imam Ahmad no longer trusted the people of Sanaa because of the rebellion formed there aginst his father, so he established his capital in Taiz.

For 14 years Ahmad unsuccessfully attempted to preserve order, maintain control and keep the status quo. Until 1962 he managed to fend off rivals (mainly by assassinating his brothers), and to keep most innovation and change from his people. In his later years, he reputedly became a morphine addict and there is evidence that he may have suffered from mental disorder as well. He perpetuated a multitude of harsh injustices and promulgated myths of his supernatural powers among the ignorant populace.

Imam Ahmad was shot by an assassin in 1961 in Hodeida, but he did not die until a year later, his death partially a result of the complications of the wound. In that year Yemeni revolutionary forces assisted by the Egyptians finally ousted the Imamate and eventually set up the Yemen Arab Republic (YAR).

After the fall of the Muttawakkilite monarchy of the Hamid ad-Din family the country of Yemen was wracked by seven years of civil war between 1962 and 1968. Because of the difficult terrain, the conflict consisted primarily of guerilla operations, which raged in various parts of the country at different times. The split among the Yemenis between the "Royalists" (mostly made up of norther Zaydi tribesmen), and the "Republicans" (composed of most of the Shafeis of Taiz and Tihama areas, along with tribes of Harraz and of the eastern desert), was exacerbated by the intervention of Egypt on the Republican side, and Saudi Arabia on the side of the Royalists. King Saud, viewing his own kingdom to be threatened by the forces of socialism, armed and paid the northern tribesmen.

Egypt supported the largely Shafei Republicans. Motivated by Nasser's imperialistic plans in the area, Egypt had participated in the planning and accomplishment of the Republican uprising and, though resistance continued in the northern part of the country for some years, Nasser's puppet Sallal in 1962 became the brief first president of the new regime in Sanaa.

It took more years of sporadic bloody battle for the Yemenis of both sides to grasp the nature of the outside interventions in their country, but eventually many of them formed a "Third Force" which was successful in expelling both the Egyptians and Saudi elements. They were materially assisted in this by the defeat which Egypt suffered in the 1967 war with Israel. Although the major brunt of hostility was directed against the Egyptians, the Saudis, too, lost out because they had solidly backed their sister Royalist regime, which was permanently overthrown. Though the Saudis have since regained an important degree of influence on Yemeni affairs through grants of assistance and subsidies to the new government, the Yemenis still fiercely maintain political independence.

Since the end of the civil war and the establishment of a different form of government, the history of politics in Yemen may at one level be described as a continuation of the perennial attempts by the central government to extend state control over the many semi-autonomous groups which have so long characterized the Yemeni scene. The big difference is that with the influx of modern technology, modern arms, and ideas from outside, the political struggle for unification has taken on new dimensions and assumed a complexity of character which is partly determined by forces in the larger world.

THE TRADITIONAL SOCIAL STRUCTURE AND CHANGE

Though change from the outside world is now striking Yemen with particular force, much of the traditional social structure remains, along with the accompanying traditional attitudes and values. In order to talk meaningfully about social behavior in the country or about social change now occurring, it is necessary to outline the main characteristics of this structure as it was in the immediate past. Most features of this system extend back several centuries and many of them still persist.

There has been some confusion in the descriptions of the traditional social system of Yemen. This is partially a reflection of regional variation, since each author tends to present the structure which *he* found as "the" Yemeni system (See al-Attar 1964:103, Chelhod 1970:63, Glaser 1885:202, and Gerholm 1977:103—158, Stevenson, 1985). In all accounts, however, there is agreement about the upper and lower levels of the stratification systems. This indicates that, although we may be dealing with regional differences, the upper and lower groups probably were generally similar throughtout Yemen.

At the highest level were the *Sayyids* (also called *Sharifs*). Throughout the Middle East Sayyids are people regarded as the descendants of the Prophet Muhammad. In Yemen, the Sayyids claiming descent through the Prophet's daughter Fatima and his second cousin Ali, constituted a hereditary elite. Though many were poor and had no power, a number of them particularly those in the Alid line, managed to accumulate large land holdings and a group of these aristocratic families dominated many aspects of political life in Yemen for centuries.

Originally, in many parts of the Arabian Peninsula, the Sayyids were invited mediators between warring Southern tribes. They were given sanctuary in certain towns under a rule called "*hijra*," and were accorded special respect as the Prophet's descendants. Over generations their preferential status enabled their major families to attain a level of power and its perquisites which was considerably above that of the average Yemeni tribesman.

Their hijra (sanctuary) towns often grew into trading centers and larger towns in an area intermediate between two or more tribal regions. The Prophet Muhammad himself utilized the role of "holy man", and the town of Medina (originally Yathrib), to which he was sent as a mediator, was the prototype of a Islamic religious sanctuary and market center.

As noted earlier, in general Islamic history the question of succession of Imams was the matter which gave rise to the schism between Sunnis and Shi'a sects. The Zaydis always insisted that the Imam be selected on the basis of a specified set of twelve specific qualities, rather than on the criterion of heredity. Still a major criterion was that he must come from the line of Sayyids, decending from Ali and Hussayn through Zayd.

The "*Qadis*" constituted another nearly parallel segment of the ruling class, but since they were not descendants of the Prophet, they could never achieve equality with the Sayyids. The word qadi in most of the Arab world simply means "judge," but in Yemen it came to be associated with a class of people.

Historically, the people of the Arabian Peninsula trace their ancestry through either of two lines — those of North Arabia claim descent through Adnan and are known as *Adnanis*, while those of the southern part of the peninsula trace through Qahtan and are known as *Qahtanis*. The Qahtanis, however, also produced holy men who, like the Adnani Sayyids, also became established in sanctuary-market towns, and the clans and lineages composed of their descendants came to form what is known as the Qadi class in Yemen. This group is smaller and not nearly so widespread as are the Sayyids, and they have always ranked slightly below them, but Sayyid and Qadi families frequently became allies and developed similar privileges and wealth. However, since they are not descendants of the Prophet, the Qadis were always excluded from the highest offices of the society. They had no part in selecting the Imam, and he could not come from their ranks.

Ironically, the tables were temporarily turned when the regime was overthrown in the later 1962 "revolution." While Sayyids were unceremoniously rejected and demeaned, the Qadis were untouched, and in fact many of them found prominent places in the succession of post-revolutionary governments. For a while, the appellation "Qahtani" was resusitated as a sloganary symbol which referred to a kind of indigenous, and more legitimate South Arabian identity, as opposed to the Northern Adnani "intruders." However, this identity never took on much importance outside of the intellectual circles which, for a short while, tried to promote it.

One reason why there is such confusion in the literature regarding the Qadi class in Yemen is that many times Qadis have actually performed as judges. In Yemen, however, the term *hakim* is the more general term in use for judge, and Qadis, like Sayyids, may or may not be hakims.

Though the Sayyids and some Qadi families were recognized as being at the top of the social pyramid in pre-revolutiolnary Yemen, in actual practice the great Shaykhs of the larger tribes in the north often equalled these hereditary elites in prestige, and frequently surpassed them in political power. A major difference was that since the power, prestige and authority of a Shaykh had largely to be achieved through military deeds and charismatic political leadership, it was inevitably more ephemeral. Such status, which under tribal mores may be earned by any tribesman, could not transfer to the offspring, as did the hereditary rights and status of the Sayyids.

The next lower level in the hierarchy contained the mass of the people. Here were the tribesmen (*Qabilis*) of the north, and the peasants (*Fellahin*) of the south. The Zaydi tribesmen, most of whom derive their livelihood from the land, actually have viewed themselves and have been viewed, more as warriors than as farmers, and therefore their prestige is higher than that of the peasant farmers of the Tihama and those south of the Sumara Pass. The tribesmen of the Yemeni north see themselves as blood descendants of Qahtani, the putative ancestor of all southern Qahtan peoples and as members of particular tribal confederation. In other words, they maintain a kinship idiom and can still be rallied for war by leaders appealing within that idiom. The tribesmen subscribe to a tribal ethos, and a tribal law code, embracing such values as protection of fugitives, feeding guests, defending territory to the death, responding to insults on one's honor, bearing arms for brother tribesman, etc. (See Adra 1982 and Stevenson 1985 for full descriptions of Zaydi tribalism). Tribesmen honor the Adnani-descended Sayyids, but also protect them and in many ways consider themselves superior to them. However, the positions of both the tribal cultivators of the north and of the peasant cultivators of the south are superior to those of a group of occupations and ethnic groups which from demeaned, if not despised, stratum below them.

These are "people of the *suq*" (market,) i.e., townspeople who engage in a number of disvalued occupations which have different names in different parts of Yemen. Regardless of name, their low positions in the local hierarchies remain fairly constant. The important thing in Yemeni eyes is that they have no honorable descent. Some of the names given them in various areas are the *Bani al khums, Bayya', Anadil,* and the *Nuqqas*. Occupations included in this category are the butchers (*Jazzara*); the barbers (*Muzayyen*) who peform such roles as circumcision, the potters, weavers; bath attendants (*Hammami*), *Gisham*, (vegetable growers and peddlers), *Khadem*, (servants), and the semi-nomadic public criers (*Dawshan*). The inferior groups generally can marry among themselves, but not outside this low-status group of occupations. They lack the pedigree and values of tribesman and historically their functions have been to provide services for the Sayyids, Qadis and Qabilis. Thus, they have always been under tribal protection.

The Jews (*Yahud*), have occupied a social niche parallel to these disvalued groups, but though the occupations they performed were not especially respected, the criterion for their low status was not occupation, but ethnic origin. Jews were the principal artisans of Yemeni society; they crafted the intricate jewelry which is still highly prized, made the elaborate stained-glass windows which grace the best of the old Sanani houses, and were merchants of certain products. They also made the wine which many wealthy Yemenis drank in secret. Only a few thousand Jews still remain in Yemen, the majority having left in 1948 on the "magic carpet" for Israel.

Below the Suq people and Jews are the true pariah groups, the *Abid* (formers laves), and *Akhdam*. The Abid are an extremely tiny group, since there were never many slaves in Yemen, where accumulation of wealth by the elite has never equalled the levels of the rich in other Arab countries. The Akhdam, on the other hand, are fairly numerous. They are black, like the Abid, and apparently came from Ethiopia at some undetermined early date.

The Akhdam have been almost as despised as the untouchables of India. They have always performed the most defiling and unwanted tasks, such as cleaning the latrines of the mosques, and sweeping the streets, and they are strictly compelled to marry within their own group. Gerholm and others do not believe the hierarchical status system in Yemen should be called a caste system. I agree that it fits uneasily in such a classification, but the Akhdam are an exception; they are indeed a caste in the strictest sense.

The hierarchy I have sketched should not be taken entirely literally. It represents an idealization which was always partially realized but never met with in full detail in any region of Yemen. For example, in many areas, such as parts of the highlands, there have never been Abid or Akhdam. In others, such as parts of Hujjariyya or of the Tihama, the "suq people" are not found, etc. Butchers and craftsmen in these areas sometimes have as high a status as the peasant farmers.

Another feature of the status system which has led outsiders to conflicting conclusions is that, according to situation, at least two sets of criteria often are operating. Tribal Shaykhs have great status and power in certain situations, and their degrees of authority are directly dependent upon their charisma and ability to rally the tribesmen. On the other hand, in situations of intertribal mediation, or in matters of religious law of learning, etc., the Sayyids clearly have taken precedence. Their high prestige has been legitimized by their holy descent, though in some cases it has come to be reinforced by wealth and special prerogatives.

The differential operation of status criteria may be illustrated by the fact that people may verbalize in ideal fashion that the Sayyids are the highest prestige group, while their actions of adulation and loyalty in a particular choice situation actually may go to a tribal chieftain. At the lowest level of the system, however, there is no ambiguity. The Akhdam are a clearly-marked caste. They have not been able to rise, or marry outside their status group, and their complete lack of prestige values and power is still evident today.

For traditonal Yemen, then, to describe a single hierarchy is misleading. Clearly the society was hierarchically ordered, but not only were there considerable regional variations in status systems, but prestige wealth, power, and influence, and the prerogatives of these, did not necessarily coincide. The mid-level positions of the system are particularly unclear, perhaps because the members of these and the customs regarding them were more variable from place to place and from situation to situation than they were at the other levels. In the part of the country just south of Sumara Pass, the northern tribesmen are paralleled by peasant farmers who, like their Zaydi counterparts may be called Qabilis. More often they are called fellahin (peasant farmers) in areas where tribalism is weak. In this region when the word "tribe" is used it usually refers only to an extended family. In the north, on the other hand, it is a widespread socio-political unit whose members claim strong tribal identity.

The tribesmen of the northern mountains have always been warriors as well as farmers, and they have traditionally provided the Zaydi Imams with the military force to subjugate both the southern peasant regions and the peoples of the coastal plain. At the call of one of their tribal chieftains, these mountain farmer warriors have always been ready to drop their plows and hoes to unite for battle. The aristocratic and scholarly Sayyids as well as the non-military tradesmen, craftsmen, suq people and other town dwellers, historically have been under the protection of these Qabilis during centuries of endemic warfare, and this military role has given the tribesmen their position above the town dwellers in the status hierarchy. However, in spite of their arrogance and command over force, both Qabilis and other peasants have been generally thought of as country bumpkins by the Sayyids and Qadis of the city and town, as well as by the sophisticated merchants and professional people.

Within the general class of other groups in the middle ranges of the status system, relative rankings were not always clearly defined. For example, the Jews were marked by mandatory special clothing, long side curls, and were prohibited from riding horses or building their houses more than two stories in height. However, in some ways they enjoyed advantages over the butchers, barbers and other low-status occupational groups. Because of the services they could provide, the Yahud were sometimes accorded special privileges, and some attained wealth and even prestige far beyond that of average townsmen or tribesmen.

As in any truly hierarchical society, symbols marked various classes and groups and their prerogatives. For example, the *janbiyyas* (ceremonial daggers) of the noble Sayyids were of elaborate decoration and worn toward the right side of the front of their bodies. Those of the tribesmen, called *asib*, were encased in wrapped leather and worn upright at the very center of the body. Butchers and other lower-status groups were distinguished by a lack of janbiyyas, as were the Jews and the Akhdam. The elaborate embroidered caps under the head-dresses of the Sayyids and Qadis were quite distinct from the loose cloth turbans of the Qabilis or the dark indigo ones of the Suq People.

An abundance of honorific titles in speech and writing were common in traditional Yemeni society, and customs of deference were particularly elaborate towards the Sayyid and Qadi classes. Even in the middle of the 1970s it was not uncommon to see a country Qabili, or a woman kneeling to kiss the feet or knees of a Sayyid or Qadi, and then to proceed through a ritual of kissing his robes and hands. When individuals were allowed access to the Imam these self-degradation rituals were carried to extreme lengths. Another prerogative of the elite classes was that they had greater access to qat and that its use by them was an emulated status marker. As well will see, however, this should not be overemphasized since use of the drug was also fairly widespread among tribesmen and peasants for at least two centuries.

Perhaps enough of the traditional Yemeni status system has been described to show that there were many local variations, but essentially it was a hierarchy on the medieval pattern. With the passing of the monarchy much of this is breaking down, and no doubt it will fast disappear. However, so much of the system still remains intact that it is necessary to have some understanding of it. Much current Yemeni behavior and the nature of presently ongoing social change in the country cannot be grasped without at least a rudimentary knowledge of the partially intact structure of beliefs and customs which still govern much Yemeni behavior.

One of the main motivations of the revolution of the 1960s was the overthrow of the Sayyid class. Therefore, while some individual Sayyids and their families have re-emerged since that time, they have generally been kept out of governmental posts and away from the seats of power. Pure wealth as the main criterion of status is rapidly assuming the importance it has in the West, while the older criteria of religious descent and charismatic tribal leadership have declined.

The rules which traditionally defined the relationships between the various Yemeni groups have become attenuated, though they certainly have not disappeared. For example, the Qahtani Qadis, in a sense, became status beneficiaries of the Adnani Sayyids when the latter were stripped of wealth and power. During the 1970s, many Qadis in full traditional dress could still be seen in Sanaa and other cities, and they were still being accorded considerable deference by tribesmen and Suq people. With regard to status symbolism, an interesting sign of change is the fact that many young men of Sayyid or Qadi classes are now wearing vertical tribal asib-type janbiyyas. This is a popular democratic fashion. Many members of the suq classes, who previously were forbidden to carry weapons, also now may be seen with large vertically-worn daggers in plain view.

There are now in Yemen considerable numbers of young men of all groups who have gone abroad. They have returned with new ideas, and government and business offices, business and Western clothing are replacing both the ordinary male skirt (*futa*) and the elaborate robes and head-dresses of the Qadis and Sayyids. However, on returning home after their daily activities, or for chewing qat, the more comfortable traditional dress is still preferred.

In addition to the political changes emanating from the civil war and otherthrow of the Imamate, many other important changes are taking place in the traditional stratification system. As modernization penetrates the country, and the inflow of ideas from abroad becomes a flood, the resulting social transformations and dislocations are reflected in changes in deference behavior and in dress.

One change in the power structure has been the development of the army as a kind of elite. Additionally, it has become an avenue of status achievement in itself. For example, a number of butchers and others of disprivileged backgrounds have risen to fairly important military posts. Abdullah al-Salal, a member of the Muzzayen, became Prime Minister in the early stages of the revolutions, and I even learned of one Akhdam who became our equivalent of a captain. In keeping with these changes, the army uniform has become another status symbol.

Education abroad has become another criterion of status in Yemen, and the college graduates are now on their way to becoming a new elite group.

As it faces its new role in the international community, Yemen needs technocrats who speak the language of world politics, and as yet it has few of them. An interesting struggle and potential shift is going on in this sector, since up to now most of the educated Yemenis have been Shafeis from Hujjariyya. These men have taken on important roles in the Ministry of Economics and the Central Planning Organization, which handles foreign assistance, foreign loans, development projects, etc. Their skills in dealing with matters of finance and administration have given them new opportunities to wield influence.

The Shafeis are reinforced in the economic arena by the fact that the majority of merchants handling the importation and merchandising of goods from abroad are from this Sunni sect. These men learned their business skills in Aden and East Africa. Thus, the Zaydis, though still politically powerful, are feeling the pressures deriving from new economic criteria of status, and new avenues available for the attainment of influence and power.

At this point it is not possible to predict how the social pyramid will be reconstituted in Yemen. However, the histories of other countries provide the basis for broad predictions, and it is clear that due to the outlined combination of political shifts and economic development, the higher levels of the socio-economic system are definitely being restructured. The central section of the pyramid is also going through profound reordering.

Contibuting to a reshuffling here are (1) the farmer-warrriors (Qabilis) are gradually losing their status. Their claims to superiority founded on a tribal ethos and upon their fighting function is now losing its vitality. Their fighting role is gradually being absorbed by the army; (2) many Qabilis as well as the southern peasant farmers are now migrating to the cities, as much greater proportion of them will be exposed to some education. Thus, some of them will be added to the proletariat poor, some will become clerks or merchants, etc., but in any case many will leave the land.

These trends toward development of new views and skills are being hastened by the opportunities for labor migration, which is exposing vast number of Yemenis to another kind of educational process, the long-term effects of which are not likely to be reversed. Additionally, there are now many more opportunities for members of the disprivileged groups (the Bani al khums, Akhdam, etc.) to become absorbed into the general urban population. As the old status symbols break down, and as some of these people utilize their new wealth to gain access to new roles, to marry outside their groups, etc., such trends gain momentum.

This is all a familiar pattern in the Third World, and I need not detail it further here. The important point is that, in comparison to almost any other country, Yemen is still nearly at the beginning of these change processes.

It has been briefly indicated that qat plays a role in all this, and this will be discussed in more detail later on. Due to new roads and the influx of automobiles and trucks, more qat can be transported greater distances to markets much more rapidly. More varieties are available to more people, and due to migrant remittances and the influx of foreign aid capital, more money is available to buy it. It is thus ever more profitable for farmers to grow more qat, and ever more profitable for those who market it. In turn, such conditions make some wealthy people more wealthy, and allow mobility opportunities for many others who previously never had any chance to get parts of the economic pie. These new economic conditions also assist the other forces already tending in that direction in creating possibilities for graft and corruption as well as accumulation of legitimate wealth. Thus, qat has its part within the total pattern of interrelated socio-economic forces.

I have so far spoken only of the more obvious male spheres of social organization, since the overt social structure of Yemen is one determined by male concerns. However, women are certainly affected by the conditions and processes I have described, and though we still know less about them it is necessary to indicate some features of the structure where women's interests are predominant.

WOMEN AND SOCIAL STRUCTURE

As in most Middle Eastern societies, Yemeni women are, for the most part, excluded from the arena of public events. Their places within the larger stratification system of the society and within local institutions are ascriptively determined by the statuses of their fathers. Later, they are influenced also by the social position and attainment of their husbands. They play no overt part in politics, and are not found in any major economical roles. However, women have charge of the domestic sphere and most of their lives are played out within the confines of the household, family and neighborhood. It has not been generally considered seemly for women of good reputation to go to market, so men traditionally do most of the shopping. As would be expected in such a situation, with the exception of some matriarchs, women often have little control over the family budget except through personal influence on their husbands.

The separation of male and female areas of activity is extreme in comparison with any country in the West, and most women form their closest attachments with members of their own sex. This is demonstrated by the fact that in many areas, distinctively female verbal accents and special vocabularies exist which men of the same communities often do not understand (Makhlouf 1979:28)

Women's sphere within the household has a certain privacy which must be respected by males. Particularly in Sanaa, males, even of the immediate family, must signal their entry by loudly repeating "Allah! Allah!" as they ascend the stairs. This warning enables the women to either cover their faces or to quickly retreat to another part of the house. Surprise encounters between men and unveiled women may be quite embarrassing.

Such restrictions are less evident at the lower rungs of the social ladder; lower-class women go out more, are less likely to veil, more likely to work, etc. For example, the textile mill in Sanaa employs several hundred women, all from the lower classes, and many of them widowed or divorced. Also, one sees many women assisting with cleaning the streets, but of course these are dark women from the Akhdam, the despised caste of Yemen.

Many women in Yemen today still veil, and in the capital city of Sanaa it is still unusual to see the face of a mature woman. Sanaa is one of the most conservative places in Yemen in this regard, and the wearing of two veils is a common practice there. One is the *lithma* or light underveil which covers nose and mouth, and the other is an overveil of gauzy material which is dropped down from the top of the head to cover the whole face. The outer veil may even be doubled if this material is particularly thin.

When women venture out of the sanctuary of their houses into the streets of Sanaa they are covered from head to foot with long flowing robes of either shiny black taffeta (*sharshaf*), or of a typical combination pattern of red and blue. With the black outfit goes the sheer black overveil (*khunna*), while with the red-and-blue combination a black veil with large triangular design of white and red (*sitara*) is worn.

Veiling allows the women moving through the streets of Sanaa to be anonymous, though within their own neighborhoods they may be recognized by small individual differences in veil style or by familiar shoes or socks. At home the outer veils may be shed, though the lithma is retained in readiness to be raised over the nose if there is a possibility that males outside the nearest degrees of kinship may appear. It is extremely important that good Sanani women conceal their faces in a large number of contexts, and they are raised to feel vulnerable and embarrassed if caught with face uncovered. Such occasions provoke nervous laughter or shameful panic. Girls begin to be socialized in this about the age of six or seven, and anonymous female bundles of miniature size are commonly seen in the streets.

In the villages and towns of Yemen many variations on the theme of veiling are found, and we could discern few patterns common to the whole country. For example, in many villages of the north and east we encountered women wearing a lithma covering the lower face, but with no overveil. In many areas of the Tihama and of Hujjariyya most women do not cover their faces at all, though a layer of yellow face powder almost achieves the same effect. These more relaxed village practices appear to be related to the fact that rural women are responsible for a high proportion of agricultural work. Besides being inconvenient for farm labor, elaborate veils and head coverings are not as necessary to protect the village women from the gazes of males. Also important is that many men in the local area are relatives, and due to labor migration there are often few men around at all.

Down on the coast in Tihama towns such as Zabid and Bayt al-Faqih, where veiling has been rare until recently, quite a few women may be now seen covered from head to foot in the Sanani fashion. Only the black skin of their feet allows the observer to know that they are local dark women of the coast, and not visiting Sananis. However, in the remotest villages of the Tihama, not only do the faces of the women remain uncovered, but their breasts are sometimes revealed as well.

One might be tempted to try to correlate the degree of veiling with the degree to which women are disprivileged in Yemeni society, but this would only lead to confusion. There is undoubtedly considerable variation in the relative status of women in the various parts of Yemen, but this appears to have only a very rough correlation with veiling practices. In the Tihama and in Taiz, women enjoy more freedom of movement than those of Sanaa, but this does not mean that they therefore enjoy much higher positions in society.

In all areas, females are generally not directly concerned with public decision-making processes, but overt social subordination does not necessarily translate into docility or a sense of personal inferiority. There is certainly a pride and strength of character in many Yemeni women from all regions. Perhaps most outstanding in this respect are the women from the mountain, Jabel Sabr. Sabri women, who are famous for their independence of action and strength of personality, bring qat down from the mountain terraces to peddle in Taiz. They wear no veils and are forthright, bold, and sometimes a bit flirtatious in their dealings with men.

Neither are the heavily veiled women of Sanaa in any way a depressed class. On the contrary, an argument could be made that the institution of veiling has fostered a feminine freedom not found in unveiled parts of the Middle East. These women go out almost daily to visit or to their own social gatherings called *tafrita*, where they chew qat, smoke the water pipe, dance and converse. On several afternoons a week they are out of the house at these events for several hours at a time. The street anonymity provided by the veil enables those who desire to go to alternative destinations a latitude to do so, and there are many reports that frequently these opportunities are not wasted.

There are, of course, many regional variations in the details of the patterns of women's activities, but something of the general quality of women's life in Yemen can be gathered from the following description by Anika Bornstein:

> The women meet in each others' homes, spending the time after lunch until late afternoon sitting together, drinking tea of qisher (the national beverage, prepared from a decoction of coffee husks), some smoking the hubble-bubble pipe like the men, and chewing qat. The town women in particular have a very intensive social life; there is hardly an afternoon that they do not spend in each other's company. The occasion may be a marriage, a childbirth or just a coming together. A marriage includes several days' celebration before and after the wedding, when female friends and relatives of the bride gather in her home, entertaining themselves with songs and dance. A childbirth is an even bigger feast: 40 days after delivery, the mother receives her female relatives and friends every afternoon in her home to celebrate the birth. It is not without reason that the Sana' anis say: 'Two marriages rather than a childbirth,' thinking of the cost of entertaining all the women during the 40-day period (1973:21).

The social changes now affecting Yemeni society must have their impact upon the lives of women, and as the figures quoted earlier show, many more of them are getting some schooling than ever in the past and a few are moving into the job market. Foreigners are now often startled to see veiled girls operating switchboards, working in hospitals, and attending classes at public schools. The number of foreign women now present in the country for various reasons, and the considerable numbers of Yemeni girls raised in East Africa or Aden who have returned to Yemen also must eventually have some impact on female status. Many of these refuse to veil, and some boldly move about the city streets. Television, which was established in Yemen in 1975 during our stay, will also certainly be influential, since foreign fashions now flit across the screens in the houses of the most wealthy and fashion-setting families. There is also now a nascent women's organization which is still focused on minor advances but which as yet touches the lives of very few women. The goup will surely be an eventual vehicle for more radical change.

Some of the initial female responses to changing conditions have not been in a direction that most Westerners would predict. It is often supposed that one of the first traditional elements which women would discard would be the veil, but at least initially, the reverse is true. With increases in income provided to country women through remittances from abroad, more widespread sales of qat, etc., and with greater mobility to cities provided through the development of transportational facilities, there are now more opportunities to imitate social superiors. Thus, there has been an actual *increase* in the proportion of women who use the veil. Following apparently universal laws of prestige emulation, veiling is being adopted by women who can afford it. It provides the protective rewards of anonymity and defense against unwanted male aggressiveness in public places, and it is approved by men. Males have their fears of promiscuity assuaged and at the same time see themselves as supporting Islamic tradition.

FAMILY

Yemeni families generally conform to the pattern which is found throughout the Middle East. Ideally, they are extended families organized on partilineal and patrilocal principles. Where sizeable wealth and property make it feasible the extended group tends to remain together as a social unit, but in many cases, economic necessity forces (or allows), the young married couple to establish its own household as soon as it can afford to do so.

The average family size in a survey of Sanaa was 5.2 persons, and even in the countryside nuclear families appear to outnumber extended ones at a proportion of about two to one. Marriage to relatives is fairly common, though perhaps the custom of cousin marriage is not as strong in Yemen as in other areas of the Middle East. Bornstein, in a survey of 11 villages scattered thoughout the country, found that in 30 percent of the families husband and wife were relatives (1973:5).

Yemeni women have much more ability to influence the choice of their marriage partners than is commonly supposed by Westerners, particularly through the communication of preferences to the men, and also through influences upon the decision by the older females of the family. There is some evidence that most of the initial arrangements of Yemeni marriages are actually carried out by women (Fayein 1957:96, Dorsky 1986:99).

Marriage involves a *mahr*, or marriage settlement, which the husband must provide to the father of the bride. Part of this generally pays for the wedding, part of it goes for the "wife's insurance" in the form of gold jewelry and clothing, and the remainder is kept by the bride's father. These marriage payments have become more and more extravagant as inflation has escalated and many young men are finding it increasingly difficult to marrry. Presidential decrees attempting to limit these payments have been largely unsuccessful. It seems that the amount of the payment is judged to reflect the beauty of the bride and the worth of the groom's family. Also, the amount of money now floating around in the economy stimulates greedy fathers-in-law to extract the maximum. A cultural pattern with this degree of power cannot be so easily legislated out of existence.

As elsewhere in the Third World, the changes consequent upon exposure to the forces emanating from the industrialized world are affecting the structure of the Yemeni family and the definitions of its roles. This is not the place to dwell on this, but it can be simply stated that from the female side, the roles of mother, wife and daughter are undergoing redefinition and strain (Makhlouf 1979:65—95). As we would expect, these changes also reflect and affect the transformations of male definitions, male roles, and male insititutions.[4]

NOTES

1. Brian Doe's work was in Aden, which was out of the mainstream of the history of civilizations in the area (*Southern Arabia*, 1971), and the work of Wendell Phillips' expedition at Marib (*Qataban and Sheba*, 1955) was interrupted midway. Most of the recent work has been surface collecting and epigraphy.
2. Orthodox Islam is divided into four main divisions based upon schools of jurisprudence named after their founders. There are Shafei, Malki, Hanifi, and Hanbali.
3. This important expedition will be discussed more fully later in the chapter.
4. The reader interested in delving more deeply into historical political, or social structural matters should look at Robert Stookey's *Yemen*, Manfred Wenner's *Modern Yemen 1918—1966*, Eric Macro's *Yemen and the Western World*, and *Handbook for the Yemens* by Nyrop, *et al.* The recent civil war is well covered in *Yemen, the Unknown War*, by Dana Schmidt, and *The War in Yemen*, by Edgar O'Balance. Recent political events and changes are well discussed in *Yemen, The Search for a Modern State* by J. E. Peterson, *The Two Yemens*, by Robin Bidwell, *Yemen: Tradition and Modernity*, by Mohammed Ahmed Zabara, and The Yemen Arab Republic and the Ali Abdallah Salih Regime: 1978—1984, by Robert Burrowes. Recent works which are very useful in clarifying aspects of the social structure are: *Transactions in Ibb: Economy and Society in a*

Yemeni Highland Town, by Brinkely Messick, *Women of Amran, A Middle Eastern Ethnographic Study* by Susan Dorsky, *Social Change in a Yemeni Highlands Town*, by Thomas Stevenson, and *Qabayla, The Tribal Concept in the Central Highlands of the Yemen Arab Republic*, by Najwa Adra. The best discussion of recent socio-economic changes in rural areas is Charles Swagman's *Social Organization and Local Development in the Western Central Highlands of the Yemen Arab Republic.* In 1985 *Qat in Yemen*, by Shelagh Weir appeared. It is a fine description largely concerned with aspects of qat consumption, treating a few of the issues dealth with here, but from a different perspective.

CHAPTER III

A SHORT HISTORY OF QAT AND ITS USE[1]

The origins of the qat plant are obscure, and much of what has been surmised about the early history of its use is speculative. As presently known, the most ancient mention of a drug which may have been qat comes from Egypt. R. Cotterville-Girandet theorized, on the basis of linguistic evidence, that qat was the drug which was forbidden to the priests of Isis at the ancient Temple of Philae at Aswan. He attempted to identify the letters kd, which designated the forbidden plant, with the Arabic letter q (qaf), and t. This linguistic hypothesis is strengthened by the fact that the rites of Isis emphasized sleep as therapy required for seeing divine revelations in dreams. Since qat use inhibits sleep, its interference with sleep therapy would naturally arouse opposition. However, Rodinson feels that the linguistic evidence for this is too slender (1977:76). It must also be noted that the environment around the Philae Temple at Aswan does not seem the proper one for the plant's growth. Despite such doubts, however, it would seem that the idea does warrant further investigation.

Even more speculative is the Yemeni legend that qat was brought to Ethiopia by Alexander the Great (Dhu l'Qarnayn the Two-Horned), to whom God had given it as a gift for Yemen (Schopen 1977:52). The French scholar Merab proposed this theory and attempted to identify qat in Ethiopia with the sacred laurel of Delphi on the basis of legends recounting how Alexander the Great had sent the leaves to Harrar, Ethiopia to cure an epidemic of melancholy (neurasthenia). Commenting on the unlikelihood of this, Rodinson however points out that the similarity of names Du l'Qarnayn (Alexander) and the shepherd, Awzulkernayen, are historically intertwined. In legends in both Ethiopia and Yemen Awzulkernayen is said to have discovered both coffee and qat (1977:80).[2]

The earliest materials with more factual basis are Arabic sources which indicate that perhaps qat was known as early as the beginning of the 11th century in Turkestan and Afghanistan. Schopen reports that in a book on materia medica called the *Kitab-as-Saidana fi Tibb*, written by Abu Raihan Muhammad ibn Ahmad al-Biruni 362—443 A.H. (973—1051 A.D.), it is stated that:

> Al qat is something that is being imported from Turkestan. It tastes sour and is artifically refined in the same way as the known batu-alu. It is red, it discharges heat. It calms the gall bladder, refreshes the stomach and bowels.

However, since qat is not mentioned in the slightly earlier pharmacopeia of Ibn Baitar (died 1248 A.D.), Schopen reasons that it probably had local importance in only a few areas of the Persia-Afghanistan area (1977:45).

Another mention of the plant from the same regions, and at about the same period, appears in the famous book of compound drugs Kitab al Qarabadin written by Nagib Ad-Din as Samarqandi (died A.H./1222 A.D.). Tigani El-Mahi, the Sudanese psychiatrist who wrote an interesting paper on qat and coffee stated that he had examined an early manuscript of this book:

> In this work, the author Nageeb Ad-Din of Samarkand gives what is so far the earliest notice on Khat in a prescription for euphorizing purposes, useful, as he contended, for the relief of melancholia and depressive symptoms. A marginal note, apparently in a different hand, juxtaposed to the text reads as follows: 'Khat is a shrub of Kilwa of Yemen, popularly known as kafta' (1962:3).

El-Mahi goes on to note that a later copy of this work, the Kairouan Edition, does not mention qat at all.

Rodinson, who has more recently examined the evidence on this point, notes that the editions of Samarqandi's work which he and other scholars could locate do not mention qat. Apparently, unaware of the Biruni reference mentioned above, Rodinson thinks it strange that a mention of qat should appear in Eastern Iran at the time of Samarqandi. Noting that El-Mahi, who is now deceased, provided no information on the manuscript cited, Rodinson implies that it may not exist, and concludes that it is better to consider this mention of qat as a posthumous addendum to the text by an unknown person at a much later date (1977:76).

This conclusion seems unwarranted, since El-Mahi clearly stated that the reference to qat was within the text of the manuscript he examined. On the other hand, the addition, which he noted on the margin referring to Yemen, may well be of later date.

Even if qat was used medicinally in northeastern Iran or Afghanistan in that early period, there is still no evidence that it was used there for pleasure, recreation, or general stimulation. However, that is remotely possible since a chemist reported that in 1910 it was used east of Kabul as a tea to combat fatigue (Owen 1910).

The first known mention of this drug being used for recreational purposes is in the chronicle of the "wonders and deeds" of the Christian Ethiopian King, Amda Seyon I (1314—1344 A.D.), who fought several wars against the Muslims. The author of the chronicle quotes his enemy, King Sabr al-Din, as boastfully proclaiming:

> I will make the churches into mosques; I will lead the King of the Christians and all his people over to my religion, I will make him one of the governors. But if he refuses to accept my religion, I will turn him over the shepherds of cattle who are called the Wargey, so that they will make him a camel driver. Likewise, I will put his queen, Jan Mangasa, into the grinding mill. And as for Mar'adi its capital, I will make it mine and I will plant qat there, for the Muslims love this plant (from A. Schopen who quoted A. Dillman's translation 1889).

Rodinson and El-Mahi cite another 14th century source, the *Masalik al Absar* by Ibn Fadlallah al Umari (1301—1348 A.D.) which recites some of the same events and speaks of the passions of the people of Ifat (called Aufat in the chronicle) for qat (Rodinson 1977:77, El-Mahi 1972:2—3). The famous historian Maqrizi (1364—1442 A.D.) also apparently relying on Umari as well as other sources, clearly describes qat in the same Ethiopian area. Maqrizi's description, which is the first to depict some of the behavioral and experiential effects of qat, implies a fairly extensive use of the drug in Ethiopia at least as far back as the 14th century. Schopen not unreasonably concludes from this evidence that we can assume that it may have been introduced there by the 11th century.

When did knowledge of this plant and its effects then reach Yemen, and how? Or did it originate there? Most historical and folk sources in both countries agree that the drug was discovered in Ethiopia and imported eastward into Yemen, though this is disputed by some local legends in Ethiopia which reverse the direction. Most authors accept an Ethiopian origin, but the matter is not as clear cut as modern writers assume. Here I take the opposing view.

Getahun and Krikorian recount the following legend which they collected in Ethiopia:

> Its use was discovered by a Yemeni herder named Awzulkernayen, who noticed the effect of the leaves of this plant on his goats and tried them himself. He experienced wakefulness and added strength, and took some home and consumed a small amount before retiring for the night. He had no sleep that night and was able to stay up and pray and meditate for long hours (1973:354).

As mentioned earlier, variations of this legend are frequently heard in Yemen also, but sometimes it is set in Ethiopia or Somaliland. However, Getahun and Krikorian report another, even more interesting account, in which qat travels westward to Ethiopia from across the Red Sea:

> The legend of the introduction of chat into Harrar tells of a group of religious and civic leaders who met one day to determine a suitable site to establish a new city. They chose four sites. After long argument, a choice was made and Harrar was built on the site of the present old walled city. The choice was made because of the suitable elevation, the splendid landscape and the many rivers and streams in the area, but it was also discovered that the air of the new town had a depressing effect on the people and made them tired and very lazy.
>
> The council met to discuss the problem. They agreed that the holy tree of Awzulkernayen was the cure. A mission of merchants was dispatched to Yemen to fetch the chat, and thus the first chat is said to have come to Harrar and indeed to Ethiopia (1973:354—5).

As I stated, most authors believe that its origin was Ethiopia. Some even surmise that qat came to Yemen from there as early as the last conquering invasion of the country by the Coptic Christian Ethiopians in the sixth century A.D. Mancioli and Parrinello mention this possibility, citing the unconvincing evidence that Jabel Habashi (Ethiopian mountain) near Taiz has long been a center of qat production.

Mancioli and Parrinello cite what they call "a little-known tradition," but one supported by the undisputed authority of some unnamed "Taiz experts" that it was first introduced from Ethiopia into Yemen by the famous Sufi, al-Arasi, around 1222 A.D. His burial place is supposed to be preserved in a mosque at the foot of Jabel Sabr. There is no written evidence or this, but if it were true, it would be earlier than any established date we have.

Both Schopen and Rodinson are among those who think that Ethiopia is the source of Yemen's qat , but they do not accept such an early date. Each cites the lack of mention of the drug in the works of Arab authors in the period between the sixth and 13th centuries A.D. as evidence that it was unknown there prior to the latter period.

This "negative evidence" argument was also made previously by Abdullah al-Hibshi (1972), who makes the telling observation that qat was not mentioned in the famous dictionary of plants in Yemen written by (or for) the King Umar II bin Yusuf al-Malik al-Ashraf, who died in 1296 A.D. Al-Hibshi mentions a number of other observant historians of that early period who also failed to mention the drug. Most important of these is al-Hamdani, who in his great 10th century geographic work on the Arabic Peninsula makes no mention of qat, even though he describes a great number of plants in his native Yemen (al-Hibshi 1972; Schopen 1977:48— 49).

Rodinson noting some of these same facts, adds that Ibn Batuta who traveled through Yemen around 1330 does not speak of qat, though he should certainly have noticed it if it was there, especially since he carefully described piper betel in Somaliland. The absence of references to qat in these early sources, in addition to supporting the theory that it was not used in the latter part of the first millenium A.D., also casts further doubt on the opinion sometimes heard that qat might have come to Yemen in the sixth century during the Ethiopian invasion just prior to Islam.

Rodinson believes that the evidence points to an introduction of the drug into Yemen around 1300 A.D., but Schopen places the entrance early in the 13th century (1977:47—49). Schopen also points out that early traditions regarding the saint Ibn Alwan, who is now known to have lived in the 13th century, considered qat as one way to turn away from wine, which is forbidden by the Prophet. There are similar traditions about the 13th century scholar Said al-Miswari, who is buried in Taiz. One poem attributed to him praises the indispensability of a qat potion (*qahwat al qat*) for scholarly research, for the student in his studies, and for the pious in his devotions (Schopen 1977:49).

Further indication of an introduction to Yemen earlier than 1300 has emerged with the discovery that the Saint Ibrahim Abu Zarbita (called variously Zaharbui, Zerbin, Zarbei, etc.), who has been thought to have been one of the 44 saints sent from Hadramaut to missionize Ethiopia in the 15th century, actually lived in the 13th century. This may be important because many traditions have Abu Zerbin becoming a heavy user of qat in Harrar, then bringing it into Yemen. Richard Burton heard this tale in Harrar in

1855, and said it was in the common folklore (1856:75). If there is any substance to the earlier date for Abu Zarbita, it adds evidence for the hypothesis of a 13th century date of introduction to Yemen.

Much available data thus seems to support Schopen's opinion that knowledge of the stimulant existed in Yemen early in the 13th century, and that its initial use was as a "tea" among Sufis and religious men to intensify their mystic experiences (Schopen 1977:52). This cannot be considered established by any means, but the data certainly point to presence of qat in Yemen at a much earlier period than the often cited 1543 date in the reign of Imam Sharaf Al-Din.[3]

The theory of an Ethiopian origin for Yemeni qat is also given some support by the fact that Catha edulis grows profusely wild in the Ethiopian mountains and in several places in East Africa, while in Yemen the wild plant is rare. However, the possibility must be considered that even if it was growing wild its use could have been unknown in Ethiopia, and that the knowledge of what to do with it could have diffused from central Asia to either Yemen and Ethiopia, or to both during the same period. Thus, it should be emphasized that, in spite of the preponderance of folklore and of scholarly opinion, there is as yet no hard evidence that the use of qat in Ethiopia actually preceded that in Yemen. It is true that most oral traditions speak of passage from Ethiopia to Yemen, but we have cited some which claim the opposite, and there is other evidence. Some recent botanical (cytogenetic) data adduced by Raman Revri supports the case for a Yemeni origin. Because of its recency and importance, I cite his conclusion on the matter *in extenso*:

> Contrary to the general opinion, that qat is indigenous to Ethiopia, is our study on cytogenetics (Chapter 5.2) of the two species *catha* described by Forsskal, 1775. The species of *Catha spinosa* Forssk., to date found wild in the Serat Mountain range of Yemen is probably a diploid ($2n = 26$). Whereas, *Catha edulis* Forssk. is triploid ($2n = 3q$). According to Darwin's theory on descendants, *Catha edulis* Forssk. appears to have evolved from the ancestral *spinosa* which is more adapted to the lower elevations with pronounced warm arid conditions. It is quite possible that *Catha edulis* Forssk., known to the Arabs as a medicinal plant (Margetts 1967) was taken by the Ethiopian conquerors (525—575 A.D.) to Ethiopia and it later returned as a social stimulant from Ethiopia in the 14th century. According to this hypothesis the primary origin of qat is probably Yemen while the secondary origin is Ethiopia (1983:4).

Without further confirmatory research this conclusion cannot be taken as certain, of course. In addition to replication of Revri's findings, it would be convincing if it were shown that *Catha Spinosa* is not found in Ethiopia. The issue is still in doubt, but my interpretation of existing data inclines me to accept a Yemeni origin for Catha edulis and particularly for its use as a stimulant. At any rate, there is enough evidence to throw into question the generaly accepted dogma of the Ethiopian origin of the drug.[4]

Whatever may be its origin it seems that perhaps even before the 12th century the use of qat was known to small groups of individuals on both sides of the Red Sea. Certainly, the lack of mention in historical sources alone is not a very convincing argument. The absence of such citations probably means that knowledge about qat was not prevalent among the privileged classes from which the authors came, but its use among the obscure subgroups or in areas personally unknown to the writers in those times of difficult transportation and minimal communication is not precluded by any means.

While qat may have been in limited use in the Red Sea areas as early as the 13th or even the 12th century, it is clear that it became much more widespread during the 13th and 14th centuries, the period in which it came to the attention of many contemporary historians and scholars. In this period, however, its use was probably still confined to small numbers of sufis, some wealthy individuals, and perhaps some of the farmers who grew it.

It seems probable that the idea that qat was introduced to Yemen in the 15th century comes more from its historical and cultural relations with coffee than from the legends of Abu Zerbin. Some traditions, for example, attribute the introduction of both qat and coffee into Yemen to the Shaykh Ali Ibn Omar al-Shadhili, a famous Yemeni mystic who reportedly died in Harrar in 1442 A.D. The ruins of the beautiful mosque built in honor of al-Shadhili still stand in Mocha. The most frequently recounted legends state that al-Shadhili advocated the substitution of the coffee drink for that of qat, which would indicate that the latter had been in use for some time before coffee. Given the fact that qat is now always chewed as the only method of ingesting the alkaloids, it is interesting that in the earliest accounts it was generally referred to as a tea.

Early travelers also reported that Yemenis made a hot drink (*qisher*) from the husks of coffee, rather than the coffee beans themselves, which they still do today. A drink made from the coffee beans was used early in Arabia and Ethiopia. Saints and holy men around Mecca drank it, both for medicinal purposes and to keep awake during their devotions. The same word *qahwa*, which has always been applied to the beverage of coffee, was also used for qat.

Despite this, however, the original stories of the shepherd and his goats refer to the mastication of the leaves, as is the current method. The legend of the discovery of coffee is precisely the same shepherd story as for qat, and it seems that coffee beans were also at first chewed before it was discovered that a brew could be made from them. Other legends recount that Shaykh al-Shadhili, the reputed founder of Mocha and patron saint of coffee, first brought coffee and qat to that town at the same time, and one of his nicknames is Abu Zahrain, or Father of Two Flowers. However, most of the legends about al-Shadhili connect him with coffee only.

It is also said that the Yemeni town of Udain (which means the two branches), was named in honor of the two cuttings, one of qat and one of coffee, which were planted there when they were first brought to Yemen. At the present time, neither qat nor cofee is grown in the immediate vicinity of Udain, though coffee is still found farther towards the east up the Wadi Dour towards Ibb, while Bilad Sharr on the same road is an important source of the supply of qat in Ibb province.

In may be historically significant that the names for both qat and coffee might have a similar origin. El-Mahi states that these names derive from a place in Ethiopa called *kafa*, and he also suggests that the Arabic word *kahwa* derives from the Ethiopian Galla word *qofa*, which is apparently a word for qat. Rodinson, however, adduces evidence from several sources to buttress an opinion that the Arabic word *qat* designating *catha edulis* may well be older than the Ethiopian *chat*, and by extension older than the Galla word qofa as well. This discrepancy may be construed as further evidence of a Yemeni origin of the drug.

Rodinson points out that a shift from the *q* to the *ch* is difficult if not impossible to accept in terms of linguistic laws of change; yet to support his belief in an Ethiopian origin he is led to a rather tortuous attempt to reconcile the contradictions. He reasons that perhaps the word qat was an ancient Ethiopian term which at first existed along with other forms such as chat. Later, according to this reasoning, it was somehow dropped in Ethiopia, but this was some time after the word (and its referent plant) had been diffused to Arabia where it has been retained until the present (1977:75—76). Why the Arabs would not have taken over the word "chat" is not explained, nor is it very plausible that "qat" should have dropped suddenly from Amharic. Such a history seems unlikely unless new linguistic evidence is adduced. It seems more economical to assume that perhaps the word qat was originally used in Arabia, while chat was the term in Ethiopia. If the origin of the word is Arabic, an earlier date for the drug in Yemen than in Ethiopia would be likely. We await new data and more penetrating philological analyses.

In any case, in the Arabic historical literature the term kafta is frequently used for both the dried leaves of qat, which were used to brew a drink, and for the drink itself (El-Mahi 1962:2). As the above discussion has demonstrated, the written historical materials on qat and coffee are clearly interwoven. Both drugs are alleged to have come from the highlands of Ethiopia; they are similar in their stimulating effects; they were both used first by Sufis and religious scholars for purposes of prayer and concentration; and they both became extremely important in the societies of Yemen and Ethiopia.

It is not appropriate to recount a detailed history of coffee here, but it has such a significant place in the history of Yemen that a few words on it are in order. During the 15th century, coffee drinking spread from Yemen to other parts of the Middle East. It became popular in Istanbul during the reign of Sulayman I (1520—1566 A.D.), and it was also known in Cairo during this period (Schopen 1978:55).

During the seventeenth century, coffee became common in Damascus and Mecca as well, and its use became a focus of controversy throughout the Muslim world. El-Mahi describes how the coffee houses became social clubs where political and social discourse took place which frightened authorities. At the same time, theologians debated whether its psychic and physical effects put it in the class of the "forbidden" (*haram*) or the "permitted" (*halal*). Well up into the 19th century harsh measures were taken against coffee users at various times by governments in all these countries.

Europe discovered the virtues of the coffee beverage from traders who had been initiated when passing through the port of Mocha in Yemen, and it was being sold in European shops around the end of the sixteenth century. Sir Henry Middleton of the East India Company was sent to Mocha in 1600 to make commercial arrangements, but it is commonly accepted that the European coffee trade was really opened up by the Dutch merchant Pieter Van de Broecke who traveled to Mocha in 1616. By the middle of the seventeenth century a regular trade had been established with several ports in Europe, and the numbers of coffee trees in Yemen had increased tremendously to meet demands. The coffee trade became the most important source of foreign exchange in Yemen, and the source of most of its contacts with the world outside the Arabian peninsula.

The greatest early setback to the coffee trade of Yemen came when Dutch traders took the plant first to Holland, then to Ceylon in 1696 where coffee plantations were established which soon began to outproduce Yemen. The French also planted trees from Yemeni stock in the Antilles in 1715, and from there coffee spread throughout Latin America in response to the continuously rising demands of Europe and America (Wellman 1961:18–21). Yemen's coffee trade has never really recovered from these competitive blows.

In spite of the competition, Yemen's famous mocha coffee remained its primary export up until the U.S. Civil War. There were many fluctuations of price and production due to market vagaries and to internal political problems, but it generally brought significant tax revenue both to the Imam and to local authorities in such areas as Beit al-Faqih, as well as steady profits to the growers and merchants of Haraz, Rayma and other coffee growing areas.

Exploitation by the Ottomans during their periods of control of Yemen, corruption at various times by local authorities, and unpredictable shifts in prices on the world coffee market all produced temporary economic problems at various periods, but more significantly, these historical conditions have resulted in a persistent three-century decline in the importance of Yemen as a coffee producer.

The history of qat paralleled that of coffee in many respects up until the 16th century, but then it diverged from that of its brother stimulant. Dry coffee beans could be easily transported and stored, and this facilitated the diffusion of the practice of coffee drinking. In contrast to qat, coffee developed into a commodity of world-wide economic importance.

The tea made from the dry leaves of qat was weak by comparison to the coffee drink. The green qat leaves only remain fresh for 48 hours at most, and the drying process results in a loss of some volatile alkaloids. Knowledge of its satisfying qualities therefore remained confined within the areas where it was produced, the countries bordering on the Red Sea, and to this day these qualities are unknown to most of the world.

After its discovery or introduction in the immediately succeeding centuries, the spread of qat use in the country of Yemen was apparently very slow. However, by the middle of the 16th century it was common enough among the upper classes and the pious to have stimulated legal and religious commentaries. The best-known example of these is a book called *Tahdir al Thiqat al Kafta wa al Qat*, (The Authoritative Warning Against the Use of Kafta and Qat), by Ibn Hagar al-Haythemi (died 1567 A.D.). Contrary to the implications of the title, this is not a polemic against qat. Instead, it is a wonderfully objective assessment based upon empirical inquiry.

Haythemi began by noting that the previous literature attempting to ascertain whether qat should be forbidden or permitted was unclear and contradictory. In conducting his own investigation, he collected accounts of experiences with qat from many people. What he found was that the confusion in the literature reflected an actual diversity of experiences among users. Haythemi's informants reported all of the various negative symptoms which are reported today: loss of appetite, digestive disorders, loss of sexual drive, semenorreah, lightheadness and "cheerless countenance," but these were not reported as occurring uniformly, nor necessarily simultaneously. On the other side, he collected data from long-term users who not only claimed to experience no negative effects, but reported that their piety was enhanced, their happiness increased, and their energy sustained.

He compares the reported effects with those of alcohol, hashish, and opium and concludes that qat is different from these and milder. Observing that differences in experience may be due to factors of individual makeup, etc., rather than to drug effects themselves, Haythemi finally leans toward the opinion that qat should be avoided, but concludes that it cannot logically be equated with hashish. It cannot be forbidden on the same grounds, and no firm judgments can be made at all without further conclusive evidence.[5]

This document seems to indicate conclusively the extensive spread of qat use in the mid-sixteenth century, and it is remarkable in its objectivity and reliance upon empirical evidence. The discussion in it presages much of the later legal debate which attempted to fit qat into the existing legal categories of things forbidden or permitted by Islamic law. The arguments Haythemi recorded sound nearly identical to those which may be heard at the present time in Yemen, and in the countries bordering on the Red Sea.[6]

There are other indications that the use of qat had become widespread in

Yemen by the time of al-Haythemis' report. Both Barraduni and Rodinson cite documents reporting the sales of fields of qat from this time, and Rodinson also points out that the oldest poems about the drug come from the same time period (1977:78). Qat use was the source of so much controversy that Imam Sharaf al-Din is said by several later historians to have issued a decree during his reign (1543—1544) to destroy the qat fields. The order was said to have been precipitated when he observed a person who had become mentally disordered after chewing the drug. He rescinded the order a short time later, after observing a number of cases of use where no such effects occurred (al-Hibshi 1972:20).

At least one of the historians recording Imam Sharaf al-Din's reign claimed that qat was only introduced to Yemen about 15 years prior to that ruler's order of prohibition (*Ibid.*: 20), but, given the spread of use in the country which seems indicated by the cited decrees, and in light of the evidence we reviewed earlier, this seems highly unlikely. The common opinion, still frequently heard in Yemen, that qat is only 400 years old in the country, seems to derive from this source. Most authors on this subject agree that, while qat may have been in common use among the upper classes, it was relatively unknown to the common people until the recent civil war.[7]

For example, Barraduni holds to this view, citing a sixteenth century document which claims that qat was too expensive for the peasants and was thus only available to the elite. As further evidence he quotes poems of praise of the drug to argue that its scarcity and the difficulties of acquiring it led to a poetry of longing (1972:4).

Certainly, there are not many data relating to qat use in Yemen during the sixteenth and seventeenth centuries, though poems praising it were written by two sixteenth century sufis of Taiz and Mocha. However, the conclusion that it was confined almost entirely to esoteric religious groups, and to the upper classes until the present century seems to be based exclusively upon negative evidence. This is not at all convincing because, at least in the agricultural areas were it was grown, many people certainly would have had opportunities to imitate practices of the elite. People generally avail themselves of such opportunities unless there are strong restraints, none of which are apparent in any of the evidence so far put forward.

Krikorian has noted that probably the first information about the drug to reach Europe may have been the report of Barthelemy d'Herbelot de Malainville in 1697 in a work called *Bibliothèque Orientale*. Barthelemy had never been to Yemen or East Africa and his account is somewhat confused, but he does seem to distinguish what may be a qat drink *Cahuat al Catiat* (maybe a corruption of *ad-Qahwa al Qatia* or qat coffee) from both coffee (*bunn*) as such (*cahwa al bunnait*) and *Cahwa al Caschriat* (qisher, a Yemeni drink made from coffee husks) (Krikorian 1983:9).

A later French traveler, Jean de la Roque, visited Yemen on two extensive trips between 1708 and 1713, which he reported in the book *Voyage del'Arabic Heureuse*. He described Yemeni coffee in some detail and mentioned a drink "made from the beans of a certain plant called *cat*, which we cannot suppose to be tea . . ." (quoted in Krikorian 1983:9).

These brief mentions of the drug apparently made little impact in Europe and the first more informed knowledge concerning qat that came to the notice of Europeans apparently was through the writing of Carsten Niebhur, along with the botanical descriptions which Forsskal, his naturalist companion, made during their famous expedition in 1761—1763. Pieter Forsskal died in Yarim, Yemen during the expedition, but Niebhur, the only survivor among the major members of the group, preserved the botanical notes of his friend and published them posthumously. Qat was among the many plants first described in Forsskal's famous *Flora Aegypto-Arabica*, and Linnaeus, the father of modern botanical classification, who was also Forsskal's teacher, named the plant after his student: *Catha edulis Forsskal.*

In Niebuhr's account of the great expedition *Travels Through Arabia* there are only a few references to qat, but these are enough to reveal something about the extensiveness of use in Yemen in the middle of the eighteenth century. For example, about midway through the description of that part of the trip which was in Yemen, Niebuhr and Forsskal with their entourage arrived at Taiz:

> Immediately after our arrival, we sent out a letter from the Dola [*Dawla*] at Mokka, to the Dola of Taoes [*Taiz*], who straightway required us to wait upon him at his house. He seemed to be in a very good humor, and made us an offer of Kisher [*qisher*], pipes and Kaad [*qat*], the buds of a certain tree which the Arabs chew, as the Indians do Betel; but we did not relish this drug (Niebuhr 1792:V.I:334).

Niebuhr's group remained in Taiz for some time, attempting to get permission to travel north to Sanaa, and they were still there for the Small Feast at the end of Ramadan. Within the report of these festivities is this comment: "The Dola striving to show his address, was thrown from his horse. However, all returned home, made good cheer, chewed *Kaad* and burned spices in their houses" (*Ibid*.:334). These statements have been taken by some writers to mean that only the upper classes used qat, but while it is a reasonable conclusion that they did use it, I do not believe that it follows that the poorer people of Taiz did *not* chew it. In the second volume of his work, Niebuhr makes two more comments on the drug which seem to refer to widespread use:

> Catha is one of those new genera peculiar to Arabia. The tree which is improvable by culture, is commonly planted among the coffee shrubs in the hills where these grow. The Arabians are accustomed constantly to chew the buds of this tree, which they call Kaad; they are as much addicted to this practice, as the Indians are to that of chewing betel. To their kaad, they ascribe the virtues of assisting digestion, and of fortifying the constitution against injurious distempers. Yet its insipid taste gives no indication of extraordinary virtues. The only effects we felt from those buds were the hindrance of, and interruption of our sleep (*Ibid*.:351-352).

I never say the Arabians use opium, like the Turks and Persians. Instead of taking this gratification, they continually chew *Kaad*. This is the buds of a certain tree which are brought in small boxes from the hills of Yemen. Persons who have good teeth chew these buds just as they come from the tree. For the use of old men it is first brayed [ground] in a mortar. It seems to be from fashion merely that these buds are chewed; for they have a disagreeable taste; nor could we accustom ourselves to them. I fould likewise that Kaad has a parching effect on the constitution, and is unfavorable to sleep (*Ibid*.:224—225).

In both of these statements, Niebuhr makes the generalization that "the Arabians" chew qat. Nowhere does he refer to differences by class. His inability to understand why the Yemenis were so fond of this drug is echoed in many later European travelers' accounts, but what I want to emphasize is that he appears to be saying that use of qat was general.

The historical sources we have quoted earlier point to the regions near Udain and Taiz as being among the first areas of Yemen to grow quantities of qat. Niebuhr's comment that the plant was found among the coffee trees appears to give some corroboration to this, since it indicates extensive growth on Jabel Rayma or near Udain. He could not have found it on Jabel Sabr, the other likely candidate, because the Dawla of Taiz prohibited him from climbing the now-famous qat mountain behind the town, as he wished to do (1792:55).

Barraduni does not adduce written evidence for his statement that the first areas in Yemen where qat was plentiful were Utmah, Jabel Rayma, Udain and Jabel Sabr, but in light of the above he is probably substantially correct (1972:4). With the exception of Jabel Sabr, these areas apparently were the first in the growth of coffee as well. Given the interlocked history of these two plants, and the circumstance that a generally similar ecology favors them both, it is probably safe to infer that by Niebuhr's time qat was in common use at least throughout the southern part of what is now North Yemen.

The dates of qat's entry into the Zaydi highlands of Yemen are still very problematical. There is as yet a singular lack of evidence on the subject, but most authors seem to agree that it did not diffuse into this region until much later than in the south. Barraduni even claims that qat only appeared in Sanaa around the latter part of the 19th century A.D. (1972:5). However, he gives no evidence for this, and there are data indicating that it was regularly used in the highland regions at least by the early 18th century. Schopen cites Niebuhr as reporting that qat bundles were available daily to the nobles during the months of May, June and July (1977:53). Much more important information regarding early use comes from the Qanun Sanaa (Statute of Sanaa). This document, penned in 1819, includes laws on qat going back to 1748 (Serjeant and al-Akwa 1983:189, 233—34). It shows that by the late 18th century qat sellers were a regularly accepted and regulated part of the market scene in Sanaa, and that the drug was relatively cheaper in relation to income than it is today (*Ibid*.:189). This also throws doubt on the assumption that the drug was restricted to the upper classes, even apart from the probability that from the beginning ordinary Yemenis chewed it in the areas where it was grown.

Later in the nineteenth century, in 1836—1837, Paul Emile Botta, a medical doctor in the service of Muhammed Ali, Viceroy of Egypt, made detailed comments on qat after a trip through Yemen and other parts of the Middle East. Sponsored by the Museum of Natural History in Paris, Botta collected specimens of many plants which were relatively unknown at the time. He apparently chewed qat frequently during his stay in Yemen and took a special interest in it from a botanical point of view.

What is most interesting in this present context is the fact that though he never reached Sanaa, Botta explored the Jabel Sabr massif above Taiz, something which Forsskal and Niebuhr had been prevented from doing. He reported that qat plantations there were more extensive than any other type of cultivation (Mancioli and Parrinello 1962:127, Krikorian 1983:10). This, along with the evidence we have cited, seems to conclusively show that the use of the drug must have been nearly universal in the southern part of Yemen as early as the beginning of the 19th century. Such great quantities of the drug could not possibly have been consumed by the relatively small groups of nobles and esoteric Sufi groups alone, and there was apparently as yet no export trade. The interpretation we have given of Niebuhr's statement indicating common use in the Taiz area is further supported.

During the 19th century travelers across the Yemeni region, or stopping at the Port of Mocha continued to remark on the use of qat in their memoirs. These occasionally provide bits of illuminating information on customs of use, in addition to their typical expression of dislike and prejudice. For example, an American sailor, in the course of a description of how an Arab merchant of Mocha returns to his home after 10:00 A.M. to rest and smoke during the heat of the day, includes the following:

> After the heat is contented with smoking, *Kaht* is passed round and eagerly devoured by the ruminating guests. The name of this choice and expensive luxury is given to the tender leaves of a tree resembling in appearance and taste the foliage of the apple tree. It is brought to Mocha from the inland towns three or four day's journey distant, in a tolerable condition of freshness, secured by the mode of packing. So delicious is it thought, that the day would be of little event which did not expend three or four dollars from the coffers of a rich Arab on the single item of *Kaht*. While thus smoking or chewing, Arabs expectorate but little, although to do so would be thought no breach of politeness (1854:234—235).

Thus, in Mocha, a coastal town at considerable distance from the nearest producing areas, qat was a luxury item. However, the following statement by Du Couret, describing his travels in the eastern desert on the opposite side of the country, gives evidence of a much more common use, and reports a widespread cultivation of the qat tree.

> During his [the Arab's] journeys he smokes or chews incessantly; smoking tobacco mixed with the leaves and skins of hemp, and chewing betel, which he calls *kaad*, a plant which grows

abundantly all through Arabia, especially in Yemen and which possesses the intoxicating quality of hemp (1860:22).

In 1871 Fulgenic Fresnel, the French consul in Jeddah also mentioned that:

In Yemen they consume Khat . . . a substance which produces a long and mild insomnia, and whose effect takes the place of sleep and replaces it advantageously for whoever wished to feel alert. The fact is that the inhabitants of Yemen only sleep but three or four hours out of twenty-four so that the length of their daily activity corresponds with ours in a relationship of 5 to 4 . . . (cited from Krikorian 1983:10).

Again, from this account it can be inferred that the use of qat was widespread in Yemen during the 19th century. But widespread use by this time is even more evident in the account of Albert Deflers, who in 1887 traveled from Hodeida to Sanaa, and visited such areas as Kawkaban, Amran, Taiz and the coastal townships Zabid and Beit al Faqih. He reports:

Although it is generally ignored in the Hedjaz and even in Jeddah, the use of khat has become by contrast a custom, nearly a need for the inhabitants of Yemen and Hadramaut where there is enormous consumption. At vigils for the dead, at feasts and ceremonies celebrating births, circumcisions or marriages, khat is always distributed to the guests. Numerous caravans loaded with this merchandise which is nearly as precious as tea arrive daily from the interior to the coast and the sole city of Aden receives each year more than 1000 camel loads (Deflers 1889:12, quoted from Krikorian, 1983:22).

Thus, as we approach the modern period the evidence becomes much more abundant. At some point, probably by the middle of the nineteenth century, the Yemenis began exporting qat to Aden, and perhaps to Saudi Arabia and other places as well. The trade was well established by 1900 A.D., as attested by Zwemmer, whose book *Arabia: The Cradle of Islam*, appeared in that year:

While waiting at Taiz I had an opportunity to study Yemen town life and the system of government, as well as to learn about the cultivation of coffee and kaat, the two chief products of this part of Yemen. Taiz is the center of the kaat-culture for all Yemen, and coffee comes here on its way to Hodeida or Aden. Amid all the wealth of vegetation and fruitage every plant seems familiar to the tourists save kaat. It is a shrub whose very name is unknown outside of Yemen. While there it is known and used by every mother's son as well as by the mothers themselves. Driving from Aden to Sheik Othman, one just learns the *name*. Why are those red flags hoisted near the police stations, at intervals on the road, and why are they hauled down as soon as the camels pass? Oh, they are taking loads of kaat for the Aden market, and the flags are to prevent cheating at the customs. Over 2,000 camel loads come into Aden every year, and each load passes through English territory by "block signal" system, for it is highly taxed on its use. Step into any kahwa (coffee house) in any part of Yemen shortly before sunset and you will see the Arabs each with a bundle of green twigs in his lap, chewing at the leaves of kaat (1900:62).

This comment as well as the earlier one by Deflers documents a thriving, increasingly heavy trade, indicating again that the taste for the drug was widespread, not only in North Yemen, but in areas such as the Tihama and the Port of Aden to which it had to be transported some distance. The estimated magnitude of the trade (1000 camel loads in 1887, 2000 loads in 1900) implies that it had been going on for a considerable period, particularly since it takes time to develop a market and to provide the economic apparatus of supply.

In Zwemmer's comment, too, is the earliest reference I could find on the use of qat among women. The silence of the earlier sources on this matter is not proof that women did not use it prior to the late nineteenth century, but presumably it was mainly a male pastime up until then.

An interesting sidelight to our description of the history of qat use in Yemen is that this drug even became a minor ingredient in European pharmacopia early in the 20th century. In Lyons, France, around 1910, a pharmacist was reportedly selling a patent medicine for nervous disorders made from dry qat leaves imported from Ethiopia and Jibouti. Apparently, events of World War I cut off this supply so that the medicine had no chance to become popular in France (Azais and Chambard 1931:13).

The people of London also were able to experience at least the mild effects of dried qat in 1917 when M. Martindale, a pharmacist of that city, produced a series of products based upon qat he obtained from Aden. Among his products were tonics called "catha-cocoa milk," "khat milk," "glycerine phosphate," and another medicine in which qat was combined with effervescent phenolphthalene, "slightly laxative and tonic." He also put out a tonic pill based on qat. These products enjoyed a minor success up until 1936 when worsening political conditions in the Red Sea area again cut off supplies. Apparently, no harmful effects of these products were ever reported (Mancioli and Parrinello 1972:149 citing Exell, in League of Nations document U.C. 1617, 1936). These were the only instances of the European use of qat for medical purposes which I was able to unearth. There may well have been others.

There is scant evidence pertaining to the history of the use of qat by subgroups in Yemen, yet its use is well documented among Yemeni Jews today in Yemen and in Israel (Goitein 1954, Brauer 1954), and there seems no reason to believe that they would not have used qat from a very early period, particularly since they do not have the proscriptions against alcohol that the Muslims have. A good piece of evidence that the Jews did indeed use qat quite early comes from the report that a poetic play featuring a dialogue between coffee and qat is still performed in Arabic by the Yemeni Jews in Israel (Rodinson 1977:82). Since the author of this play, Sholem bin Joseph al-Shabezi, was born in 1619, at least an early 17th century use by Jews in Yemen can be argued.

There seems little question that the use of qat was widespread in Yemen by at least the early 19th century, but for the early part of the 20th century there is no doubt whatever. Wyman Bury, a physician who spent a considerable amount of time in many parts of the countryside of Yemen just prior to World War I wrote:

Unfortunately, all but the poorest classes are addicted to the qat habit, more or less; the degree of addiction being proportionate to the amount procurable (1915:152).

And:

It permeates every class that can afford it, and many that cannot, for sometimes a man will starve himself and his family to get it. Women do not often succumb to the vice, and when they do are worse than men, for they have less self-restraint, and it makes them very irritable (*Ibid.*:152).

Sometimes, even at the present time, Yemenis claiming authority on their own history will say that the Bedouin of Yemen and, indeed everyone outside of the major cities, has always disdained the drug. However, individuals making this claim are often acculturated young men who having gone abroad to study or work, now deplore the use of the drug among their countrymen. Such may be the source of Wenner's statement that ". . . the tribesmen scorn it" (1967:26).[8]

It is certainly true that the use of qat has been spreading rapidly into areas where it was unknown or, more likely, unavailable. The introduction of many automobiles and trucks into the country and the construction of roads facilitating rapid transport has certainly given a big impetus to the merchandising of qat. These changes have made it possible for tribesmen, even as far removed from the areas of cultivation and as distant as the *Jauf*, to consume it two or three times a week. Also, we found relatively young qat plantations (between 10 and 20 years old), in the vicinity of Beida, well out in the eastern desert of the country.

Any blanket statement, however, that the tribesmen of Yemen did not use qat until recently must be severely qualified. In all things Yemeni one must beware of generalizations. Harold Jacobs, a British Colonel who spent some time in Yemen just after World War I, was captured by the Quhra tribe who occupied a strategic position on the trail between the Tihama town of Bajil and Sanaa. The statement that Jacobs reported one of the Quhra Shaykhs illustrates the tribal and individual independence which has been so important in Yemeni history, and it also shows that, at least among this group of tribesmen, the use of qat was a valued and common practice:

Who is the Imam? We are Quhra, tribal people. God give us freedom, and we are numerous. We have more grain than we need. Our houses are secure. We get our qat from Jabel Rayma by special arrangement. We want nothing more (quoted by Stookey 1979:175 from Salim 1963:250).

As we move towards our own time, most accounts unhesitatingly claim that qat chewing is universal in Yemen. For example, Amin Rihani, an American of Arabic descent who made a prolonged trip through Yemen in the late 1920s says:

> It is planted in cuttings, is cultivated in supper Yemen at a height of from 2000 to 7000 feet, like the coffee tree, and is a product for home consumption as important as wheat or corn. There are varieties of it as in coffee, the best being the Bukhar, which grows in the district to which it is attributed.
>
> I first tasted ghat in Aden at the house of the Resident Qadi, who introduced it to me in these words: 'This is our sovereign habit o philosophe, and it is one of the bounties of Allah. We chew it, and through it we recover our strength. We obtain a little keif too: not the keif which wine affords, but a keif of the spirit — a bodily repose — a spiritual satisfaction, which otherwise we do not feel, except of course through religion. Al Ghat is our food and our coffee. We all indulge in it.

Rihani goes on to claim universality for the habit in Yemen: "The Yemeni can go for several days without food, but not a single day without ghat. Men, women and children, they all use it" (*Ibid.*:46).

This must be regarded as an exaggeration, since qat use is even now not universal in Yemen. However, Rihani's observations generally have the ring of truth about them, and the statement can be taken as evidence of a very wide use, even among women.

Van der Meulen, a missionary who spent time in South Arabia in 1931, also called qat-use the "national habit" of Yemen and described how he observed it on a wide scale in the Tihama city of Hodeida at that time (1961:117) Since then almost without exception, travelers have spoken of it as universal in the country and as a negative influence (e.g., Helfritz 1936:184—185, Farrago 1938:61. Ingrams 1970:113, Shaffer 1952:240).

Of course no amount of travelers' reports can be taken as definitive evidence. Not only are they generally not systematic observers, but they notoriously borrow from their predecessors.[9] Looking at the situation at the present day, it is clear that the use of qat is increasing. Important conditions bringing this about are modern transportation, an inflow of money from outside the country, and new plantations of the drug in many areas. Such increases obviously mean that it was less widespread in the past, but this conclusion must be taken with caution.

It is well-known in Yemen that among certain tribes, particularly those of the eastern and northeastern areas, qat chewing was regarded as *eib* (shameful) for both men and women until recently. This proscription was not at all uniform in those areas, however, and there were some villages and tribes where it was only shameful for women. These patterns have largely broken down, and some of these same areas now even grow qat both for themselves and for the market. There are still some regions where chewing is rare except for weddings and holidays. This seems to be because they are still largely isolated from sources of supply.

On the other hand, many of the northern "tribal" areas such as Jabel

Razih, Mahabisha and Hajja are now among the extremely large growing areas for qat. Without further research we do not know how far back in time this cultivation goes, but the extensiveness of it suggests at least a moderate historical depth.

There are still no good figures on the extensiveness of qat use. Our own study did not have the resources to do this kind of work, since it would necessarily have involved mounting a massive survey in a country in which such research is completely foreign to people's thinking, and where the masses are illiterate. When the first national census was planned for 1975, I perceived an opportunity to partially solve this problem and obtained permission from some high government sources to add some questions about qat use to the census interviews. However, when it actually came time to make this input I was put off with vague bureaucratic delays until it was too late. I am not certain what the reasons for this were, but I assume it may have had something to do with the image it would present to the world when the inevitably high figures on "drug-use" were published. Whatever the reason, this was a great opportunity lost, since it would have cost nothing to gather this important information, and it was not necessary to publish it. The best data available on distribution of use in the country comes from a study by two Italian doctors, Mancioli and Parrinello, who served in the hospital in Taiz for nearly 12 years between 1955 and 1967. They had the good sense to perceive the opportunity for a contribution here, and they gathered data on qat use from 27,410 patients (15,051 males and 12,359 females) who passed through their clinic.

It has been pointed out by Chelhod (1972) that there is probably some bias in this sample due to its having been selected from individuals who were ill, and they all might have been at least partially ill from their qat habits. This is true, and until we have a truly representative sample of the population, nothing definitive can be said about frequency. However, the frequencies of use given by Mancioli and Parrinello actually seem low according to our observations and the observations of nearly all visitors to Yemen. It should also be noted that if there is a bias in these figures it is toward under-representation. Thus, the report of Mançioli and Parrinello may well have been substantially accurate for at least this one large area. Since 70% of their patients came from outside the Taiz region, and their clinic was in Taiz, their sample seems to be a fairly good representation of people south of Sanaa. Of the people who passed through their clinic in that 12-year period, 90.26% of the males and 58.55% of the females over the age of 12 chewed qat, but only 60.26% of the males and 34.91% of the females were classified as "habitual" chewers. The rest only chewed on special occasions such as weddings, funerals or holidays, and could not really be called "users" in any important sense.

As mentioned, in the 1970s, the proportion of individuals who could be classified as habitual users appeared to us to the somewhat larger than this.

We had real difficulties in obtaining sufficient samples of non-users and light users in every area in which we worked. This would seem to indicate that a higher percentage of people have moved into the category of regular or habitual users since the middle sixties, but it also provides tentative general substantiation to the figures of Mancioli and Parrinello.

My conservative estimate is that perhaps 50 to 60 percent of women and 80 to 85 percent of the men in North Yemen now chew qat more than once per week. This is only somewhat better than an educated guess, but it corresponds fairly closely to other estimates. Hughes, 1973, places the proportions of chewers at 80% for urban men and 90% for qat growing villages. He also estimates that 30 to 50 percent of women use it regularly in areas of high use (1973:40). Hess estimated 90% for men and 60% for women (1978:741).

NOTES

1. Three excellent reviews of the history of qat are El-Mahi 1962, Rodinson 1977 and Krikorian 1983.
2. Interested readers may consult Rodinson and his sources for fuller speculations on this.
3. This date is even accepted without reservation by Stookey (1978:158).
4. An example of the continuing power of this dogma is Krikorian's recent statement that "In Harrar province of Ethiopia one view held is that khat originated in Yemen. *This is wrong since the center of origin is Ethiopia . . .*" (1983:21) [italics added].
5. Manuscript copies for us were made by Abdullah al-Hibshi from his personal copy.
6. See Serjeant 1983 pp. 173—174 for a fine translation of much of Ibn Hajar Haythemi's document.
7. E.g., "The spread of qat cultivation seems to have been slow, with advances and retreats, in a constant competition with that of coffee. Consumption passed from Sufi circles to 'distinguished city millieus'. Only fairly recently did it reach the middle and poor classes of the cities. In the villages it was consumed only when the sale price was so low as not to be prohibitive, and during festivities" (Rodinson 1977:79).
8. Weir (1985:81—82) cites several other sources which support the hypothesis of widespread early use. However, she chooses to discount this evidence and accepts the prevailing dogma.
9. One of the most obvious examples of such borrowing is to be found in Helfritz 1936, who often plagiarizes Rihani almost word for word.

CHAPTER IV

A SOCIAL INSTITUTION

> *Women's Song*
> Long live qat,
> which makes us kind, and
> makes us stay peacefully at home
> with our friends and families.[1]

Children are discouraged from the use of qat before the age of 12, but this rule is not strictly adhered to. Children in qat growing areas and those of poor families of cities and towns often begin occasional chewing at much younger ages than do those of the elite. Poorer children can be seen picking up the remains discarded from adult sessions, or from the streets around the qat markets, and I have observed children of not more than 5 years old being offered a few sprigs from their grandfathers' robtas in sessions on Jabel Sabr. The common feeling is that qat is too strong for small children but that small amounts occasionally will not harm them. Younger teenage boys and girls gradually begin to attend the qat sessions of parents and relatives, and are thus gently introduced to the pleasures of chewing. In times of famine and among the very poor, qat may sometimes be given to children in the morning to reduce hunger.

Qat is an eminently social drug and the favored way to use it is with a group of like-minded people. There are many occasions on which it is enjoyed by solitary individuals, but this is rarely by choice. Merchants sitting alone in their tiny stalls in the market chew and smoke their water pipes to avoid boredom as they wait for customers in the afternoon. They want to be in a mood similar to that of their qat-chewing customers. The taxi or truck driver chews as he drives. He wishes to remain alert, particularly if he has to make a trip out of town over the hazardous mountain roads of North Yemen. The stonecutter chews as he sits chipping away at the large stone blocks which are favored for the construction of the tall houses of Sanaa. "I can cut only two to three stones in the morning, but I can finish eight to ten in the afternoon," one of them proclaimed to me. The farmer chews to maintain his energy as he pursues his arduous tasks. Yemenis who must extend their labor into afternoons chew in order to enhance their speed and efficiency and to stave off fatigue and drowsiness.

Some old Qadis chew alone in the afternoon, or perhaps one or two friends drop over to chat, but the great proportion of qat chewing is done in larger groups of the same sex during a specified time set aside exclusively for that purpose. The afternoon session, called the *majlis al-qat* (literally, "the council of qat"), the *matka* (arm rest), or the *maqayyal* (from "sitting"), is definitely the preferred way to partake of qat's pleasures.

Considerable amounts of thought and effort are devoted to this substance. On the days an individual attends a session, time must be set aside to go to the market, for qat must be chewed while fresh. In all large towns of Yemen an important section of the general market area is exclusively devoted to the sale of qat. In other more remote areas where there are weekly markets, numbers of qat merchants arrive to set up their stalls, while in places even more distant from any markets itinerant merchants pass on regular routes, their pick-up trucks or motorcycles loaded with the leafy bundles.

Though richer people send a servant to the market, and older boys may be sent by their fathers to purchase the afternoon supplies, most men select their own qat. They relish the hustle and bustle of the market and the give-and-take of bargaining, but more importantly, they prefer to make their own choices of the particular bunch of leaves which suits them from the varying daily array. Large cities like Sanaa, Hodeida and Taiz feature a number of markets, and within each is found a large selection of varieties, qualities and prices, which fluctuate daily and by season. In towns of any size, like Sada, Hajja, Dhamar, Zabid, Ibb and Turba, several types of qat are nearly always found, but even in smaller and more remote places an expensive and a cheaper type usually are sold.

It is surprisingly easy to purchase a poor robta of qat. Even though it might appear lush and abundant, the bundle may not have many good tender leaves. One can be fooled by a robta whose leaves turn out to be overly astringent, or one which is "weak." Poor quality may be due to the fact that the qat is from a rainfed area of "strong" qat, because it came from the lower parts of the tree, because it has been overly long reaching the market, or because the season was not a good one in a particular area. Perhaps it is a day or two old having been held over due to a failure to sell it the day before. A careful buyer must take all such variable conditions into account, and men pride themselves on their abilities to select a good robta from what is available.

Certain kinds of qat have a reputation for being the finest, and these are considerably more expensive. The cheaper varieties have a reputation for being "strong," producing more of the negative side effects such as sleeplessness, poor sexual performance, confusion of thought or irritability. It is easy to make an expensive mistake, spoiling a whole afternoon.

Most kinds of qat are readily distinguishable by the size and type of bunch. For example, in Sanaa the most expensive types, from Wadi Dahr or Dula, come in slender, leafy bunches (*marbata*) which may be 24 to 30 inches long, while the cheapest variety often is *sawti*, sold in small five-to-six inch packets (robtas) of prepicked leaves, which have been brought from great distances wrapped in special banana leaf containers called *qarn*. The varieties intermediate in quality, perhaps from Bani Hushaysh or Haraz during certain seasons, are also readily distinguishable.

The following citation from Stevenson is an excellent description of the bargaining process for qat encountered in many parts of Yemen:

'Amrani men always bargain for gat. No one pays the price asked except when the supply is limited. Buyers are suspicious of gat sellers as they are of butchers, but for reasons not related to status. Sure they are being robbed, customers strive to get the best deal. A man may even show his purchases to friends announcing the cost as somewhat lower than it was.

"What have you got?" asks a man muscling through the crowd around a gat seller. "Give me a look. Where is this gat from?"

Picking up a wrapped bundle, a buyer carefully opens the covering to see how much gat is actually under the many layers of protective, non-gat, leaves. He is particularly careful to note the number of tender young leaves since these make for the best chewing.

"How much is it?" he asks.

"Forty," comes the reply.

"What's your final price?" he queries.

"Thirty-five, and I'm only making two riyals," responds the seller.

"Thirty," offers the customer, but the vendor simply takes back the gat.

Later, the customer finds some other gat to his liking or comes back to the first seller. If demand is heavy by then, the price may have gone up.

"Give me long branches of gat," shouts a man.

"Here's some locally grown," says the vendor and hands long stalks to the customer.

"Where's it from?"

"From Dha'wan."

"How much?"

"Fifty."

"Forty."

"Forty-five," says the sellers. "That's my final price."

"Okay, but give me something for cigarettes."

They settle for forty-two riyals as the loudspeakers on the mosques begin to announce the noon prayer (1985: 15—16).

Preparation of one's body for the session is a very important part of the culture of qat chewing in Yemen. This tradition is particularly strong in Sanaa, where the "notables" have long been the style-setting elite. They have provided the model for the institution of qat-use which is imitated in varying degrees throughout most of the country.

In the days prior to the revolution elite Sananis often ran considerable distances, or took long walks in the late morning to dehydrate their bodies. After the exercise they went to a Turkish bath to spend an hour or so steaming themselves. Imam Yahya, the King of Yemen during the first half of the 20th century, accompanied by many of the wealthy Sayyids is said to actually have made a daily run up Jabel Nuqum, the mountain rising about 600 meters above Sanaa. In many villages near Ibb there was a custom of *dawra* (trip) which was either to run out into the fields or to make a trip to the baths to heat the body sufficiently. The powerful thirst created by some dehydrating practices must then be slaked by quantities of cool, sweet water while chewing. In general, qat is considered *yabis* (dry).[2] By soothing the dry astringent effects of the leaves, water enhances the pleasures of chewing. The intensification of thirst makes the qat even more sweet and refreshing.

The custom of eating a large hot meal, often containing several peppery dishes, before chewing is similarly justified, but this practice has the added advantage of mitigating some of the potentially negative gastrointestinal after-effects of qat as well. During Ramadan, fasting during the day is said to intensify the pleasurable effects of qat when it is finally taken in the evening.

With the recent spread of qat use the customs of exercising and bathing before chewing have not been preserved except by a few of the traditional elite. Everywhere, however, attempts are made to eat a substantial hot meal before the qat session. More than 95% of those answering an interview question concerning their eating habits claimed that they take a large meal before they chew.

The Sanani version of the preferable meal is rather standard. It includes *shafout* (a flat, porous bread soaked in soured milk), *sohawag*, a salad made of chopped tomatoes, hot peppers and onions, *bint a'sahn* (a sweet cake with honey), *lahma*, meat that has been boiled tender (mutton or beef), *maraq* (a hot broth or gravy made from the meat sauce), and *helba* (a green soup made from fenugreek seeds). Potatoes and other boiled vegetables may be added and are sometimes put into the bowl with the helba. Local bread tops off the meal, and sometimes a thick yellow pudding called *mahalabaya* is served as dessert.

For feasts, several other dishes may be added to this well salted basic meal, and among the poor people several of the ingredients may be left out; particularly, the amount of meat may be very small or absent. As a preparation for qat chewing, however, the maraq gravy and the helba are considered essential. There seems to be considerable traditional wisdom behind the belief that this greasy carbohydrate meal nullifies at least some part of the potentially negative side effects of the qat.

The extensive set of beliefs and practices regarding the preparations which are desirable and even necessary for qat chewing give additional evidence of how qat permeates Yemeni thinking. The concerns with qat are not confined to the time of chewing alone, but the drug engages a great deal of waking consciousness, not only in the hours of preparation and anticipation, but in the continuing experiences of effects after the three to four hour session.

The noon meal, which is the main Yemeni daily repast, is eaten anywhere between 12:00 and 2:00 P.M., and since qat chewing preempts most of the afternoon for such a large percentage of the population, many businesses close for the afternoon. On many jobs, such as those in the government ministeries and business offices, the day is concluded by 1:00 P.M. Most offices do not open again until around 9:00 A.M. the following morning. Some shops open again in the evening, but among many social segments of the cities and towns, the Yemeni work day is finished by early afternoon. Farmer's hours are more flexible and they can usually find time in the afternoon to gather with friends. If not, they may chew while continuing work. In qat growing areas the availability and cheap prices of the drug allow people to gather in evening sessions as well, particularly in harvest seasons.

QAT SESSIONS – THE SANANI MODEL

There are many sources of difference in the styles of Yemeni qat sessions: sex, interest, socioeconomic class, rural vs. urban residence, area of the country, particular social occasion, etc. I describe here what may be called the "Sanani model," since the elite class of Sayyids and Qadis in Sanaa has set the national standard of what a qat session should be. Though there is considerable variation in practice throughout the country, even in remote areas of the south attempts are made to emulate the style of the urban elite session.

The setting for qat chewing is regarded as very important, and at least some attempt usually is made to achieve the cultural ideal. Even Yemeni architecture reflects the importance of the qat institution, and a special room in the house is specifically set aside for enjoyment of the qat session. In Sanaa each of the great houses of the old city has its *muffraj* on a top floor. These penthouse rooms look out over the mosques and buildings of the ancient city, and many include a view of Jabel Nuqum, the mountain which looms behind Sanaa.

Outside of the older section such penthouse muffrajes are more rare, and particularly in *Bir-al-Azab*, another affluent part of the city, the wealthier houses often have a garden muffraj. These ground level rooms have windows facing on a green garden, often with a stone fountain shooting up jets of water. Poorer people cannot afford a special room solely for the pleasures of qat, and so for several hours in the afternoon they temporarily set aside the best room in the house for chewing. However, to the degree possible, every chewing area reflects an attempt to approach the spirit of the model established by the Sanani notables.

This model, which undoubtedly owes some of its features to the long sojourns of previous Turkish overlords, emulates ancient oriental ideal places of peaceful relaxation. It is a place where the cares and problems of daily existence can be forgotten during a period of pleasurable conversation and comradeship. In Yemen this concept includes the added feature that the facilitation of pleasure is enhanced by the drug qat.

The muffrajes of the elite families in Sanaa are some five to seven stories above the level of the street, and since each stone step is more than a foot high, one becomes quite breathless climbing the steep spiral staircases.

These pleasant rooms are usually long and narrow with high ceilings. The narrow width, usually 3 or 4 meters, is determined by the length of the log beams which provide the support for the ceiling and roof. These beams are plastered and whitewashed to blend into the walls of the room itself. Set deeply into the two-foot-thick walls on at least two sides of the room are tall windows with wooden shutters which extend down to within two or two-and-a-half feet above the floor. Above each there is another half-rounded double window with panes of multi-colored glass, or light-filtering alabaster.

The white walls and corners of the room are graced by delicately molded built-in plaster shelves carved with arabesque and flower motifs. On the floor around the walls of the long oblong room are colorful, comfortable mattress-like cushions, upon which the guests recline while chewing. These are backed with softer finer cushions, and each sitting place is marked on either side by hard movable bolsters (matkas) which serve as arm rests.

The center of the floor is covered with Persian or Bedouin rugs and upon these, or sometimes on a low table, are one or two large shining brass trays. On these rest one or more of the tall gleaming water pipes which are so much a part of the traditional qat session. These *mada'as*, as they are called in Yemen, have large intricately cut hookah bases imported from India. The three-feet-tall aluminum stems engraved with elaborate filigree designs, and the long hoses with their silver-studded wooden mouthpieces are mostly made in Yemen. These hoses are usually encased in colorful crocheted or knitted sheaths made by women of the household. Sometimes they sew the coverings from brightly colored cloth instead of knitting them.

The brass trays also hold engraved brass incensors which may be lit and passed among the guests during the session, and a number of brass or aluminum spitoons. On the muffraj walls between colorful velvet tapestries from Syria or Turkey are hung pictures of the owner of the house and his family. The tapestries depict romantic scenes of people, deer, lions and tigers in exotic settings of mountains, trees and water. The family photographs frequently include various members against the familiar background of Mecca where they may have made the pilgrimage, or occasionally in the setting of a European or Middle Eastern city where one the family may have traveled for school or business. Japanese calendars, pictures cut from magazines, or beautifully calligraphed sayings from the Qur'an are also placed here and there on the wall. At the end of the muffraj, extra cushions and bolsters are piled for use during occasions when there may be many more guests.

It is obvious to any visitor that the whole purpose of the muffraj is the creation of an environment facilitating pleasure, relaxation and human companionship. Even in the muffrajes of country Shaykhs, whose houses may be far from the road among the mountain peaks, a traveler may find similar graceful and pleasurable rooms. This comfortable setting, which cannot help but remind one of storybook tales of oriental potentates, is the preferred environment for chewing qat.[3] Because of the public nature of qat sessions, and the association with the fine living of the elite, the relative elegance of any muffraj reflects the wealth and status aspirations of the host. Recent increases in affluence resulting from migrant labor or successful business are usually reflected in the relative opulence of muffraj decorations and accoutrements.

Having purchased one's qat, finished the large meal, perhaps taken care of some family business and rested a bit, the time for moving towards a qat session approaches. In Sanaa people usually begin chewing around 2:30 P.M., but in the countryside they may not start until after the afternoon prayer, often after 3:00 P.M. There are many variations.

Even though all preparations have been made there is still the question of where one is going to chew, and much discussion often precedes the choosing of a location. Since qat is generally chewed in groups, obviously many people rarely use it in their own homes. Certain houses are known as gathering places for particular interest groups on particular days. Dorsky's description of this situation in Amran reflects the situation in Sanaa and Taiz as well: "Although most men chew regularly in the same places, there is considerable morning and after lunch discussion in the *suq* as to where each man will go. At least some of the time these are real discussions, as men do occasionally switch allegiances. A particular home will attract large numbers every day for months, only to fade gradually or abruptly in popularity, often for no obvious reasons" (1986:69). In country villages choices are much more limited, though even there, there are often some alternatives for chewing, and usually one can find chewing companions apart from the central session of the Shaykh.

Male qat sessions are theoretically open to anyone, and this ideal is pretty well adhered to in the smaller towns and villages as well as the poorer neighborhoods of Sanaa. People bring their own qat and water flasks, while the host generally provides a place for the gathering, perhaps along with a water pipe or two. However, even though there certainly is a degree of fluidity and democracy, the majority of sessions are primarily confined to like-minded people or friends and acquaintances. In the larger cities and towns, the rough and ready tribesmen, tradesman or Suq people are rarely encountered in the sessions of notables and scholars, or *vice versa*.

This pattern appears to be a change from the past where traditional sessions included people with a greater range of status positions, as is still the case in most of the village sessions of the countryside. As money has been displacing criterion of descent as the measure of status, and as education has increased, the tendency to gather with peers in qat sessions has increased. Though for lower status individuals some purpose occasionally may be served by submitting oneself to the humbling servility of the patron — client pattern of more traditional sessions, in the changing world of the present this is less often necessary. More options for selecting a session have become available and people tend to choose the less stressful and more convivial company of those similar to themselves in status and interests.

In Sanaa, a number of houses attract important political figures every week, and there are others where people may drop in on a daily session with such notables if they wish. Qadis and scholars of Islam also tend to gather together, as do businessmen, merchants, soldiers, bureaucrats of various levels, young intellectuals who were educated abroad, groups of friends of various professions, or individuals from the same area of the country. For example, in Sanaa there are regular sessions for people from Amran, Haraz, Taiz, Hujjariyya, etc. A common interest, regional affiliation, or simply friendship can provide the basis for a qat gathering. Though there are exceptions, the range of social status tends to be similar, particularly in the sessions of the larger towns and cities.

Some guests may arrive at the session as early as 1:30 P.M., but no matter how empty the room may be each person is careful to choose a seat appropriate to his relative status, and relationships within the group. The generally understood arrangement is for the host, his closest friends and any older or more important guests to occupy the seats against the interior wall, and away from the door. They face the windows, and later, as the sun is setting are in the best positions to contemplate the beauty of the changing landscape outside. They are also more protected from any drafts which might come in through window cracks or from the door, an important consideration, for it is believed to be easy to contract a cold while chewing. Custom prescribes that the windows and the door of the muffraj be kept tightly closed during a session, and this often creates a dense atmosphere of smoke and heat.

Particularly on a Friday, ordinary sessions may be attended by as many as thirty or forty or more men, though in many qat gatherings only four or five people are present. For large weddings, funerals or other special events, such as a session honoring a political figure, a hundred or more may jam into a large room. Sometimes several crowded rooms are set aside for chewing. In this type of session the host provides much of the qat, though many participants also bring their own.

In mixed sessions, older important individuals are ranged with backs to the wall, while younger men of good family and intermediately ranked older men sit facing them with their backs to the windows. Around the lower end of the room, near the door, may be grouped poorer men of the neighborhood, one or two servants of the household, or some boys aged 12 to 14 avidly listening to the conversation of their elders. Those close to the door participate marginally in the main discussions, and are expected to bring glowing coals for the mada'a, to pass the incensor, or perform whatever tasks or errands are desired by the host.

This pattern is found, particularly in the houses of the elite, in Sanaa, Taiz, Hodeida, and the larger towns such as Sada, Ibb, Dhamar, Beida, Turba and Zabid as well as in the sessions of many local village Shaykhs and *Amils* (e.g., Gerholm 1977:178—185). In qat sessions of the poor, or in those of the increasingly common special interest groups, whose members are mostly of similar rank, such status-determined seating patterns may be absent or at least they are much less formal. The host of these sessions generally sits in a good, but by no means always the best place, and people find any spot they can. Visitors from out of town or special guests may be ceremonially "forced" to sit in the culturally favored positions.

When a person enters a qat session he salutes the group: "As-salam 'alaykum" (Peace be with you). The answer "*Hay Allah mun ja*" ("God greets who comes") is a standard greeting pattern of the Zaydis of Sanaa. The replies may be "*Ma'nashi*" ("Nothing bothers us") or "*Kayf halkum*" ("How are you all?") are also common. The host may then gesture to a place near himself, or if the person is of lesser importance, others may squeeze against those next to them to make a place for him. The newcomer then places his bundle of qat, which usually has been wrapped in a sheet of blue or green semi-transparent plastic, and his thermos bottle of cool water on the floor in front of his place. Hanging his outer coat and perhaps his janbiyya or his rifle and bandolier on the wall above, he carefully seats himself.

If he is a young bureaucrat who works in an office, he may take out a futa, the Indonesian-style skirt worn by most Yemeni men, and wrap it around himself, dropping his western-style pants from under the skirt before hanging them on the wall. Yemenis find their futas more comfortable than trousers for the long afternoon of sitting. The guest then makes himself comfortable, reclining against the firm back cushion, usually resting his left forearm on a matka (movable arm rest). One leg is curled back on the seating cushion, while the other is perpendicular to the floor. Though there is no rule about this, the majority of men lean to their left and keep their quid of qat in the left cheek. Since the chewer's position is relatively fixed for the session, his choice of place may be next to an individual with whom he has business. He knows that several hours later, during the quiet moments, there will be an opportunity to talk over mutual affairs in subdued tones.

Qat is used in a number of symbolic ways to reinforce status considerations. The quality and quantity of the bundle in front of a person is some indication of financial standing, but if a person attempts to assert status by using an amount and quality of qat beyond his known means he may be laughed at behind his back. On the other hand men of known wealth do not bring cheap qat, for this would be demeaning.

The host or others may take an especially nice sprig of qat from his bundle and ceremoniously throw it like a spear to some person across the room. In some cases this generosity may be an expression of *noblesse oblige*, but often it simply serves as a gesture of friendship and esteem between equals.

The symbolic importance of qat is especially indicated at weddings or other special events, where the family's generosity and prestige are often judged by the value of the qat provided to the guests. Similarly, when a high official holds an important meeting, people speak about the worth of the qat consumed at it. When President al-Hamdi met with the Shaykhs and notables of Ibb on an occasion in 1973, the common people marveled that he had spent more than one thousand rials on qat for the occasion (Messick, personal communication).

When preliminaries are over and most of the guests seated the session begins in earnest. Each chewer opens his packet of qat, and picking a branch from the robta, runs his hand expertly over the leaves, carefully inspecting the quality. Taking two or three of the small tender leaves from the top of the branch between his fingers, he then swiftly cleans off any dust which may remain on them, tucks them into one side of his mouth and begins to chew. Immediately more leaves are picked, rubbed and placed in the mouth. Each man's eyes and hands are in constant motion and the conversation begins to flow freely.

The Yemeni word for chewing qat is *khazzin*, meaning "to store," and this is an appropriate term, for the leaves are never swallowed. They are simply formed into a ball (*takhzina*) which is "stored" in one cheek. The session itself may also be referred to as a takhzin, which in this instance might be best translated as a "chew." Unlike qat chewing practices in East Africa where small branches and leaves may be swallowed after mastication, the Yemenis ingest only the juice. When the quid of packed leaves in the cheek grows too uncomfortable, part of it is discretely expectorated into one of the spitoons which are placed for the use of every 2 or 3 chewers. Such discomfort is usually not experienced until near the end of the session, by which time everyone's cheeks are bulging incredibly.

Older men whose teeth are gone may take a cloth package from their pocket and carefully unwrap a small wooden mortar which they use to pound the leaves into a powder. Tribesmen from the country or older chewers also may place a small chunk of crystallized sugar or a clove in the cheek along with the qat. Such means of slightly altering the taste are not now as common as they as once appear to have been. Most people seem to relish the slightly bitter and astringent quality of the leaves alone.

When a shoot has been stripped of its most tender leaves, it is thrown out onto the rug in the front of the chewer, and as the afternoon wears on, the mountain of still leafy branches in the center of the room may reach the height of a foot or more. The Yemenis say that it increases their enjoyment to look upon a large pile of qat branches as they chew.

Cool water is sipped from time to time to enhance the pleasure of chewing, and many men carry their own wide-necked Chinese-made thermos bottles to a session. The thermos, with a dipper, is placed in front of them on the floor, along with the brass or aluminum spittoon which the host has provided. In times gone by water was provided in clay jars or glass bottles, but, except for some poor and remote country areas, these have been almost entirely supplanted by thermos bottles. Some people do not bring their own water, so containers are generally shared between every three of four chewers.

If a chewer desires water which is out of his reach he simply says "*Sah*" (health). The person nearest the thermos then passes a dipper full of water to him, replying "*Sah, wa'afiyya*" (health and well-being). After refreshing himself, the drinker returns the dipper saying "*Sahakum Allah wa a'fakum*" (plural of the above). The proper way to show pleasure and appreciation is to drink with a loud slurping noise, and towards the end of the session, when the chewers become mute, sounds of drinking and the gurgling of the water pipes may be the only sounds heard in the muffraj.

Water quenches the thirst produced by the astringent qat, but the enjoyment of the water, in its own right, is an important part of the enjoyment of the occasion. I spoke earlier of how salty and peppery food are eaten and of the exercises and Turkish baths taken to heighten the chewing experience. The Yemenis say that the thirstier one is, the more enjoyable the qat, but conversely, the better the qat is, and the better one has prepared for chewing, the better the water tastes as well.

The water of Yemen is naturally sweet, and though the astringency of qat is enough to enhance this sweetness considerably, the custom of holding the water container over burning incense before filling it produces an even more agreeable flavor. If there has been no opportunity to prepare the container by this incensing process a few drops of perfume may be added. In Taiz and the Hujjariyya area of the southern part of the country, tea, coca cola, and other soft drinks are increasingly being substituted for water in the qat sessions, but Sanani purists believe that such beverages spoil the taste of the qat.

The other ingredient crucial to the enjoyment of the qat chewing occasion is tobacco, and the mada'a, or large water pipe, is almost always a part of the session. This elaborately incised metal and coconut shell base filled with water sits on the brass tray, while the wooden mouthpiece attached to the brightly colored hose is passed between a group of smokers. Each smoker draws several draughts through the bubbling water before passing it on. The tobacco is often a strong local variety grown on the Tihama plain, and the first few puffs often produce dizziness, particularly in the novice. After one has become accustomed to the pipe it is easy to understand why the water-filtered smoke is regarded as another ingredient in the agreeable relaxation aimed for in the qat session.

One of the tasks of one of the servants of a wealthy house, or of the older boys, is to keep the tall pipes properly lit, and rarely are they allowed to go out while a session is in progress. The smoker who is not getting full satisfaction says a word or makes a gesture, and a new clay cone (*burri*) with fresh hot coals and damp tobacco is immediately brought in to replace the spent one. The Yemenis generally do not use hashish in their water pipes; the combined effects of the strong tobacco smoke, along with those of the qat being chewed are enough for most of them.

There is an etiquette to using the mada'a. It is understood that several others are eagerly anticipating their turns for the mouthpiece, so one does not monopolize it for too long. When passing the hose to the next in turn the mouthpiece should be held so its opening points back towards the passer. The receiver should be able to grasp the upper part of the hose, and then to turn the mouthpiece towards himself at will.[4] Nowadays, however, many men smoke cigarettes. They are too impatient to wait out the long intervals sometimes necessary for their turns at the mada'a, and point out that this is a much more sanitary way to receive the benefits of smoking while chewing qat.

What do people talk about in a qat session? Virtually anything and everything of interest to the Yemeni people can serve as a topic of conversation, but in many sessions there is an understood topic of discourse according to whether the group is based upon a particular interest, or whether a certain occasion is being observed. However, before discussing this, the general temporal pattern of the sessions should be mentioned; it is a pattern which is structured significantly by the physiological effects of the drug.

The first stage of a qat session is usually very lively, involving everyone in the muffraj. The enlivening effects of the drug do not begin to manifest themselves for the first half-hour or so, but they are anticipated by the users and soon after commencing to chew the sound level increases; the conversation becomes increasingly animated.

News and gossip are passed and jokes are told. A well-known storyteller may set the whole group laughing or hold it spellbound with an account of recent adventure. Poetry may be read or recited. In sessions organized for weddings or other festive occasions an *oud* (a large lutelike instrument) player or other musician provides music, or men may dance a janbiyya dance to recorded music from cassette players or radios. Spirited arguments may occur, but never did we see any violence in a qat session.

Many sessions have a serious intent, and as the alertness producing effects of the qat begin to manifest themselves the talk may begin to focus upon a single topic. The group then will dwell upon this theme for several minutes. On occasion this will continue for an hour or more before the interest turns to another subject. Sessions are often meetings of special interest groups and in these the topic may be confidential or secret, such as political action or a business transaction. Sometimes those present at a session wrestle through a complex set of intellectual or legal intricacies concerning some local dispute, or argue a theological question in great depth. For example, the talk may concern a current world event, a set of historical incidents, or perhaps even some happening which occurred during the Prophet Muhammad's time.

I do not wish to imply that much trivial conversation does not occur in qat sessions, but only want to emphasize the degree to which high mental concentration and focus upon a single topic are often collectively achieved. For at least two hours this intense conversational interaction continues, and the attainment of such a high level of sustained group communion and collective concentration does appear to be related to the effects of the drug, as Yemenis believe.[5]

It should be emphasized here that most of the business and politics of Yemen take place in qat sessions. The session is not simply a place for playfulness and educational discussion; economic and political deals frequently are struck, and many other kinds of decisions are arrived at. In Sanaa and Taiz aspiring and established political leaders hold regular sessions on particular days of the week to which they attempt to attract important personages. Younger officials, aspirants to power, and those now out of the political limelight must decide, particularly on Thursdays and Fridays, which session holds the most interest or promise for them. If they guess correctly they can experience an exciting and stimulating afternoon; mistakes can lead to four hours of boredom and futility, which can be exacerbated by the drug.

Because of the implicit openess rule of the qat session, public accessibility of political information in Yemen is probably unparalleled in any other country. Some exclusion does take place through the processes of mutual interest, social class norms, as well as the sheer limiting size of the muffraj, yet direct access to higher political figures is available to younger politically motivated individuals.

The qat session also provides the means to business success. The business families of Sanaa, Taiz and Hodeida, still largely Taizis or Adenis, have their own regular sessions, and a Zaydi from the North is rarely found chewing with them. As with political sessions these too serve as information centers. Business and trade are discussed and opportunities for profitable contacts are provided.

The older Qadis and Sayyids have their own sessions, where they discuss theological questions, the fine points of tribal law, or historical events. Young soldiers' sessions may revolve around women and current politics, but they too sometimes dwell on religion or food prices. Butchers, laborers and poorer people of various menial occupations in particular neighborhoods, all have their own regular sessions in which important social business is carried out in the convivial atmosphere of qat chewing.

After two hours of intense conversation the noise level gradually falls, and by the time another hour has passed, the most audible sounds are the quiet gurgling noises of the water pipes. The sun is beginning to set and it is a time for contemplation and reflection, "*sa'at Sulayman*," ("Solomon's hour") as the Yemenis call it. Someone in the room rises to push back the curtains, allowing the privileged guests to gaze out over the minarets of the city, or perhaps to be soothed by the rising spray of a garden fountain. They may contemplate the changing shadows of mountains and fields, but whether the household is a poor hovel with no muffraj, or a majestic Sanani mansion, the late stages of the qat session are a time when the guests gradually withdraw into private reflections and hushed conversations. This quietude clearly is encouraged by effects of the drug, but it is also a matter of custom, and of the natural fatigue which follows excitement and effort.

However, when the topic is exciting to all participants, animated discussion may continue uninteruptedly for up to five hours. On such occasions, though some individuals lapse into silence, there is no general "introverted" phase at all. In the common pattern, however, the chewers prefer to be left alone during the final hour, and this wish is usually not violated, except occasionally by boorish foreigners.

The subjective feeling-state during this later stage cannot legitimately be called "depression" as many writers have rather carelessly stated; it is rather a period of preoccupied rumination. Darkness is falling and many low-voiced, dyadic conversations may be observed in the long room. Some individuals sit quietly, their glowing eyes reflective of the seething thoughts within. Interruption of these preoccupations may be irritating. There is certainly some fatigue from the hours of animated talk, but the chewer does not feel less stimulated; there is rather a turning inward of racing ideas and plans which may be too rapid to be shared. After the third hour of the session, most of the men now sit quietly, staring ahead with eyes glowing, or murmuring in low tones to a neighbor. Though the mood is often one of muted sadness or of failure, this has been overstressed; the late phase is one of intense concentration and mental focus, whether of a positive or negative tone.

There is no rigid rule about departing the session, but after three to four hours of chewing men usually begin to rise, don their outer garments, and with a quiet "Salam alaykum," step through the door, grope for their shoes in the hallway and depart. The leaving is scarcely noticed by those remaining.

A few guests may linger on for another half-hour, perhaps sharing the remains of an extra-large bundle of qat with a neighbor, but at last the host signals the ending phase by lighting a kerosene lamp, or if the session is in town, he switches on an electric light. He may order a tray of glasses of qisher or tea for the few guests who have stayed. But when the servant or young son comes into the muffraj and begins cleaning up the branches and leaves littering the center of the room, even the remaining lingerers know that it is definitely time to depart. They too exit the muffraj, slip on their shoes, descend the stairs, and quietly walk into the darkness. Perhaps they move towards the mosque, the market or the house of a friend or neighbor, where companions may gather for a post-session meeting. The women, who around 6:00 P.M. have often just returned from their own afternoon gatherings, do not usually expect them home for at least another hour.

The course of the qat session is depicted in Diagram 1.

RITES OF PASSAGE

Qat chewing is an integral part of all rites of passage as well as the regular Islamic feast days in Yemen, and on these occasions even most of the "non-chewers" are induced to participate. For example, qat is brought to the luncheon celebration for an infant son's circumsion ceremony, and for a marriage it is a part of each stage of the festivities. At such events the host is expected to provide qat for the guests, though in events of poorer families

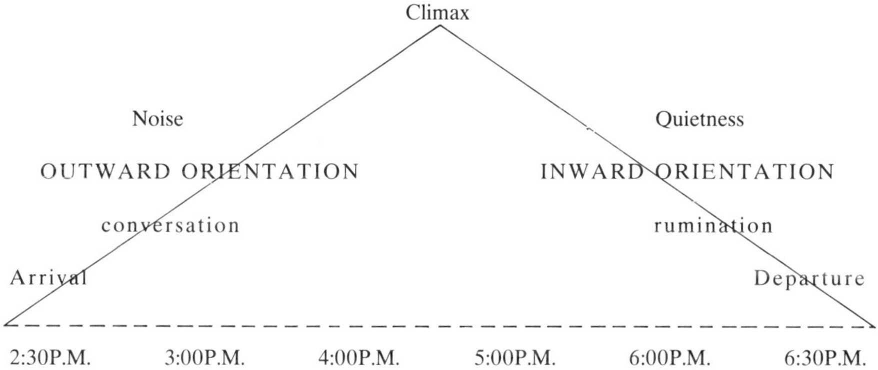

Diagram 1. Intensity of sound and Frequency of interaction.

many may bring some of their own to supplement the symbolic amount supplied.

A qat session is the setting in which the engagement negotiations for the brideprice are made. On the wedding evening there are innumerable rituals, and in the afternoon the men all gather at the groom's house to chew qat. Particularly in weddings the groom's father is responsible for seeing to it that a generous supply of qat is available for the guests. The groom always sits in an honored position in the session and is given special deference. Though he has numerous jokes directed at him people do not speak directly to him, honoring his liminal status. Local musicians play, and while the men join in janbiyya dances, explosions of hundreds of fire-crackers and the sharp blasts of rifles being discharged are heard throughout the neighborhood or village. Heaps of used qat branches on the floor attest to the generosity of the host family on these happy occasions.

The next day, which is the official wedding day itself, the bride is bedecked and prepared at the house of her family. Family guests are also found here, and in the evening a celebration is held at this house too. However, *no* qat is in evidence at the bride's family house because the tone of the group which is about to lose a daughter should be much more subdued. At the house of the groom, on the other hand, the major wedding events and parties go on all day and into the night. After the large feast in the early evening provided by the groom's family at their house the men and women separate into different rooms for chewing qat, joking and dancing. The groom's father is responsible for providing qat of high quality for the women's sessions as well as those of the men. Despite this, many people bring bundles of their own, especially if the area is one where qat is grown. Late at night, after the parties, the bride is brought on horse or donkey in a procession to the groom's house, where she is received with drums, frenzied bursts of firecrackers, explosive gun shots and joy cries.

Similar celebrations take place on the first, third and seventh day following the wedding day and there is an informal qat session each time. The groom begins chewing with his friends, but soon, amidst a barrage of jokes, he leaves to chew alone with his wife. According to custom, she is supposed to hold the robta for both of them, plucking the most tender leaves and placing them gently in his mouth. The twentieth day marks the end of the celebrations and is the scene of more feasting, dancing and qat chewing sessions (see Schopen 1978:150—158, and Dorsky 1986:98—132, for detailed accounts of Yemeni weddings).

Mourning ceremonies and episodes of serious illness are also occasions in which qat chewing has a prominent role. Serious sickness calls for a gathering of the family with a *Fagi*, or Quranic specialist, who prays and exhorts the family from time to time. Meanwhile those present chew qat to intensify their concentration on God. Sometimes an animal is sacrificed near the end of the session.

When someone dies, a qat session is held on the afternoon following the burial. The mourners supply qat for the family of the deceased as well as bringing their own. The session is in special honor of the dead person and goes on for the whole night. Qat sessions are also held on the next few days, but these are more informal and have the purpose of giving social support to the bereaved. People gather "to share the grief."

The periods of the major Islamic holidays, the Small Feast (*Id'al Saghir*), the Big Feast (*Id al-Adha*) and the Prophet's birthday, the *Moulid al-Nabbi* are also occasions for extended qat sessions. On each of these family holidays, as well as for the entire month of Ramadan, people make every attempt to return to their villages; large amounts of qat are chewed, and an abundance of food is provided for all.

THE VILLAGE SESSION

As described, in Sanaa, Taiz, Hodeida, Ibb, Dhamar, and a few other large towns the trend is toward qat sessions among the likeminded or those of a similar social position. In small villages, on the other hand, there are generally only one or two important sessions on any given day, and they are more traditional in style. Often the major session is situated either in the home of the local Shaykh or Amil, who presides over it in a public building in the center. There are always some men who do not come to the principal session on any given day, preferring to chew with a small group of friends, or even alone at home. However, the major village session is usually crowded and the seating arrangement there is often a close approximation of the social hierarchy in the area.

Gerholm provides a good example of the operation of such village sessions in his description of the town of Manakha, in the Haraz region. He describes how the men of wealth and prestige bring their own mada'as, tobacco, thermos bottles, and more and better qat than do their neighbors. The seating pattern is a clear indication of status. The Shaykh sits in the center of the muffraj looking out of the windows flanked by his peers, while the villagers are seated in descending order around the room with their backs to the windows or toward the door. He describes how those in the prestigeful area of the muffraj are quieter, more dignified and are accorded service and deference by those in the lower part. The elite of Manakha occasionally dispense qat, as well as the mada'a mouthpiece to those at the lower end, and sometimes direct jokes towards them.

Those in the poorer section entertain their social superiors with jokes and coarse risque burlesques. The higher status people, on the other hand, ritualistically pass the finest branches of qat among themselves and by whispering, exclude the others from their conversations. As Gerholm summarizes the local "status drama": "Whispering and ceremonial qat exchanges at the upper end of the room dramatize the special standing of these men to those sitting at the lower end. And conversely, shouts and fights among the servants (the lowest of the low status individuals present) establishes *their* status beyond all the doubt, in the eyes of the elite" (1977:183).

In some areas I have seen qat used to symbolize status, just as is depicted in older accounts. Here all the village men bring their bundles of qat and deposit them in front of the Shaykh, making a large mound. At his discretion, he dispenses them during the afternoon. For example, he may pick particularly tender shoots and majestically hurl them to other members of the elite, while he flips the mediocre or poor shoots to others later, at his whim.

The following graphic description from the late 1920s still holds for many country qat sessions in Yemen:

> I must explain, in justice to the Ameer (sic) the presence of straw and grass on the floor of his *majlis*. We arrived about sunset when he and his guests had finished eating the *qhat*, which is brought from the hills, a day's distance from Mawia, wrapped in green grass or foliage and bound with straw or reed back to keep it fresh. These bundles are brought into the *majlis* and placed before the Ameer, who distributes them among his *qhat* party. The proper way to do this is not to offer a bunch to your guest, but to throw it at him. "He never threw a bunch of *qhat* at anyone" says a Yemeni of a miser.
>
> With this the *qhat* eating begins. Everyone opens his bundle, picks the leaves from the twigs for chewing, and throws the grass wrappings and binders on the floor (Rihani, 1930:35).

Such village sessions serve as forums for discussion of local problems and for the settlement of disputes as well as for diversion and entertainment. Local gossips spread the news of what has happened to various durra or qat fields, of what the "local development association" is doing, the cost of food, or the prices of qat and coffee. The contents of letters from relatives outside the village, the actions of various well known Shaykhs, plans for upcoming weddings, and bits of foreign news heard earlier on the radio, all find their way into the conversation.

The village qat session is the primary mechanism for the distribution of information in the countryside of Yemen, but it has the added functions of an arena where some of that information is further processed by the group and sometimes acted upon; where opinions are formed and leadership is exercised.

In one session in Hujjariyya which I attended, the Amil held forth in the large muffraj of the municipal building of the village. Dressed in a colorful Adeni futa, his head wrapped in a large turban of purple silk and with a large and glittering "*sayfani*" janbiyya (one with a rhineocerous horn handle) resting on his stomach, the corpulent Amil looked the part of a powerful Turkish Sultan.

The long muffraj was packed with more than 40 men. Only the Amil, his secretary and another 3 notables of the area shared the one large water pipe on the brass tray in front of them, and sipped from two large Chinese thermos bottles of water. The men were mostly peasants dressed in worn and sometimes soiled futas. Each had his bundle of qat in front of him, and a number of clay jars of water and two large mada'as were being shared by the group.

The most important matter of the afternoon was a land dispute. It seems that one farmer in the area had expanded his cropping area into some land which had been unused for some time. Now, those claiming to be the traditional owners came to present their case to the Amil.

At the lower end of the muffraj, two peasants in worn and tattered muslin shirts and old cotton futa' skirts waited patiently with a veiled woman to be called. After some moments the Amil was ready to hear their case and he beckoned imperiously. The two men did not rise but began laboriously advancing on their knees. It took more than a minute for them to traverse the entire length of the muffraj. When they reached a point directly in front of the Amil they paused, took their janbiyyas from their girdles and presented them to him handle first. He nodded to his secretary, an impressive person in equally fine robes, and leaned condescendingly forward to receive the two knives. The valuable janbiyyas were pledges that the litigants would abide by the official's decision. With this done the Amil asked for the evidence in the case, and each man told his story.

From somewhere in his voluminous garments the claimant to original ownership of the land triumphantly drew out a ragged and yellow paper scroll. It was a document of title to the land recounting the previous sales transactions and stamped with an official Turkish seal. The Amil gave this to his secretary for an appraisal of its authenticity, and it was passed around to various older men, each of whom commented on it. The Amil then called for other opinions or evidence. Several men offered bits of information or opinion and the Amil after a few moments deliberation rendered a judgment in favor of the man with the document. The petitioners then retreated on their knees to their places in the muffraj and the session continued in a more convivial vein.

The impression left by many writers on Yemen is that the qat session is a place where most Yemenis go to spend every afternoon idly wasting time, chatting and joking in a drugged delirium. This misconception must be dispelled. Of course, there *is* much relaxed euphoria in the qat session, and many of them are primarily recreational. However, it must be emphasized that the stimulant properties of qat are more often than not harnessed to the serious business of life. There are many "qat parties" to be sure, but if used in a generic sense, as it often is, the word "party" is very misleading.

Even Gerholm, in his fine analysis of the Manakha qat session as a "status drama" underplays the important social content and the socio-political functions which these groupings possess. In the qat sessions of the city the social functions may sometimes be attenuated or specialized, but everywhere the purposes of business, politics or communication are often the main *raison d'etre*. In fact, it is not too much to claim that the politics of North Yemen are worked out in qat sessions, and it is therefore interesting to speculate that the chemicals in qat have played a regular role in Yemeni decision making and political life for a number of centuries.

Weir has certainly not underplayed the role of qat sessions in her recent book, but her interpretation of this role is questionable. She makes interesting assertion that qat "parties" contrast in form and function with other group events in Yemen, i.e., with the gatherings of residential kin and political units:

> The groups of people who assemble at qat parties do not form and represent any enduring social-structural entity which extends reliability into the future, even if they can be seen to have achieved a certain longevity retrospectively. They are essentially ephemeral; they have no names. They are also free associations of people assembled by choice. There is no obligation to attend as a consequence of some ascribed affiliations, however, you do not belong unless you have such an affiliation. And qat parties are individualistic, hierarchical and competitive, not egalitarian and cooperative (1985:142).

By such a sharp contrast certain aspects of the qat session appear to be highlighted. However, according to my experience the distinction is not all that clear. In the first place, as I have described, qat sessions are integral to nearly all events put on by family, tribe or community. Through attendance at ordinary qat sessions is largely voluntary, the usual kin and community obligations do apply to these events.

Second, Weir has overemphasized and overgeneralized the "competitive" aspects of qat sessions. In very few of the sessions I attended did I see any evidence of competition. If some competitors in daily life brought their concerns into the session this did not indicate a competitive *quality* to the sessions as a general defining characteristic. In my experience a strong sense of *cooperation* was much more common than a competitive element. Additionally, while I have noted that social hierarchy is certainly displayed in the seating patterns and other aspects of many qat sessions, this feature as well as their traditional formality is undergoing change as more and more people opt to chew with peers most of the time. For instance as Varisco remarks, referring to the rural community of Al-Ahjur, "As an institution the *qat* chew can be used by individuals as a forum to affirm or break down social barriers. Ethnographic research in Al-Ahjur indicates that in this tribal area there is no fixed hierarchy of seating at a chew based on status. Seating depends on a variety of factors, including the formality of the occasion, the number of people present, the wishes of the host and the time of arrival" (1986:9). This is a good description of the situation in many parts of Yemen. Furthermore, hierarchy generally, is largely incompatible with competition; people tend to know their position in a hierarchical system, and competition is structurally inhibited.

Thus, Weir's attempt to sharply set off the qat session from other Yemeni institutions seems to me incorrect. Instead, as we have seen, these sessions are integral to all other Yemeni institutions. Traditionally, the mixed session bringing together people of differing status and power, has served as one vehicle for integrating these other institutions. The recent increases in wealth and other social changes have reduced the importance of many of the traditional socio-political categories. One result has been a trend towards more egalitarian sessions. The self-selective feature of attendance has enabled these excellent natural arenas for social, political, and economic intercourse to adapt to changing circumstances.

THE FEMALE SESSION: THE TAFRITA

Yemen is a male dominated and sex-segregated society, and it is true that men are the major consumers of this drug, yet probably more than 50% of the women of Yemen also chew qat regularly. As is the case with the male session, it is the women of Sanaa who have developed the most elaborated and institutionalized form of the female qat session in the country. It is called the *tafrita*.

After lunch the streets of Sanaa become more quiet as shops and businesses begin to close. By about 2:00 P.M. the only people on the streets are men or veiled women moving towards one or another house for a qat session. Their destinations are revealed by the clearly recognizable bunches of leafy branches wrapped in protective red or blue sheet plastic which they carry in their arms.

If men are chewing at a given house, women seek another meeting place. Thus, they too often also have access to a full-fledged muffraj with its cushions, carpets, and brass trays holding incensors and waterpipes. Some houses have another sitting room or a lower floor called the *diwan*, which serves for tafritas, and at other times for small gatherings of friends of either sex. Tafritas are always held if there is a birth or marriage, but they are also the principal regular leisuretime events in Sanani women's lives, and they are eagerly attended.

When the women arrive at the muffraj, they remove their stereotypical black or blue and red outer cloaks (*sharshaf*) and leave these with their shoes at the door. Their previously concealed personal styles are now revealed in a profusion of bright velvets and gleaming gold and silver brocades; if they are from the poorer segment of society there is an array of colorful cottons and synthetic fabrics. The tafrita is also an occasion on which women can display their treasured gold jewelry and strings of coral beads, and every woman also wears a brightly colored scarf of muslin or similar material over her hair. Those that are married indicate their status by a brocade band around their foreheads.

Men's sessions are often quite crowded, but women's tafritas are even more thickly packed. Often so many women crown together thay they form two or more rows in the narrow room. One row may have their backs to the cushions and wall, while the others sit out in front to them on the rugs. They may even fill the entire central space, making it difficult to pass back and forth with the usual tea, qisher, candy and popcorn. Many women have learned to love the waterpipe and they pass the decorated hoses back and forth around the room. Unlike the male sessions, very few cigarettes are in evidence.

The overall impression on coming into a group of women at a tafrita is that it is more informal and light than a typical men's session. Carla Makhlouf captures the feeling well: "Upon entering a woman's majlis, one is taken by the glimmer of all the colours and brocades, by the chatter and music, the pungent smell of tobacco, the heavy scent of incense, the sweet fragrance of perfume, and the hot damp atmosphere of the room" (1979:23).

Qat is much less central to these afternoon female parties than it is to the male sessions, in which chewing is integral to the activities. Often only about forty to sixty per cent of the women chew in any given session, and frequently two or three women will share a robta, whereas for men it is standard for each man to chew at least one bunch of qat. Many of the women drink only tea or qisher, and most of them nibble on the nuts, candy and popcorn as these are regularly passed around. Such edibles are not part of men's sessions, for they would interfere with serious chewing.

In the earlier phases of the tafrita the women joke, tell stories, and bring out new riddles for the others to guess. Many of their jokes are at the expense of males, who are satirized as making burlesque fools of themselves. Women may put on their father's or husbands' robes to play the role of some pretentious man known to all, or perhaps make fun of well-known classical Arabic love poems (Makhlouf, 1979:45—46).

As I have described, in some men's qat sessions a musician entertains, or one or two men get up to dance a janbiyya dance in the tiny available space in the muffraj. Since there is much less serious talk, less qat, and primarily an entertainment focus, women's sessions almost always feature music and dancing. Sometimes professional female singers attend and entertain the group, accompanying themselves on tambourines, but much more often a cassette player provides taped music by one of the famous local oud players, or by popular Egyptian and Lebanese singers. As the afternoon entertainment goes on, a number of women are stimulated to dance, and others clear the trays and picked qat branches from a small area to accommodate them. These subtle quietly swaying dances are not as flamboyant as are the male janbiyya dances, but they are just as complex (see Adra, 1982).

Earlier, I pointed out that in many male qat sessions status differences are pronounced and dramatized. In the female tafrita on the other hand, social distinctions are minimized. As Makhlouf aptly puts it: "The social conditions of *tafrita* are such that they seem to stress nearness and community rather than discordance. Since it is common for over fifty women to be sitting on the floor of a room of three by six meters, perspiring and smoking together, one obvious result is that status difference will appear to be less relevant" (1979:26).

The women's tafrita does not follow the male pattern of rising euphoria and intensifying conversation, with a denouement of introversion and quietness. Its form is much less dictated by the psychophysiological effects of qat; nor do you find the more formally structured session around a particular topic. Women's sessions are much more uniform in their basic preoccupations with visiting and entertainment than are men's. Qat is peripheral rather than central.[6] The evening call to prayer is the signal for the festivities to end, and women feel pressure to return to their homes. Men have more freedom to linger on or to visit the market, the mosque, or the home of a friend before returning.

If the qat session is central to male society, the tafrita is even more important to female society. Sanani women's lives are generally so circumscribed that their only activities, apart from the social activity of an occasional wedding, funeral or feast day, are household duties, a rare visit to the market, and the afternoon tafrita. Even though there is a relatively general lack of recreational and entertainment possibilities in the culture, besides their own houses and qat sessions, males still have the outlets of the market and the mosque in addition to their workplaces. Largely secluded within the confines of their own homes and those of close relatives and friends, women are much more restricted. The tafrita provides a welcome outlet for personal expression and expansive sociability, and thus it takes on special intensity.

CONCLUSION

It should be evident by now, why it is justifiable to speak of the "institutionalization"' of qat use in North Yemeni society. The use of this drug is legal, its use is nearly universal in the country, and the patterns of use are surrounded by custom and etiquette. The qat session provides the social framework for politics, business, scholarship and entertainment. Its social importance is shown by the fact that houses are designed to accommodate its use, and the timing of daily activities is structured by its use characteristics. Qat is an important part of all markets and of nearly all household budgets. As we shall see, it is a dominant feature of the economic system of Yemen. Though alcohol and other drugs certainly play important roles in other societies, it is probably safe to say that no other society is so influenced by the use of a drug as is North Yemen by the use of qat. The general question this raises is whether, or to what degree this may be harmful for the Yemeni people. Can we speak of massive "drug abuse," or have the Yemenis come to a workable accommodation with a mind altering substance? Let us explore further.

NOTES

1. Recorded by Claudia Fayein (1957).
2. The way some Yemenis express this is by the phrase *yabis batin*, "it dries the stomach" (Messick, personal communication).
3. I am describing here the male qat sessions. Further on the female version will be discussed.
4. In Lebanon and other parts of the Middle East a man often carries his own small plastic mouthpiece which fits onto the larger wooden ones, but this practice had not reached Yemen at the time of our stay there.
5. In order to strengthen her argument regarding the symbolic and social importance of qat, Weir equates the effects of qat with those of coffee and tea, and generally attempts to minimize its pharmacological effects (1985:42, 149). It should be evident from much of the discussion here that while these effects are not as overwhelming as traveler's reports would lead one to believe, they are one very significant determinant of qat session behavior, and of the Yemenis generally high valuation of the drug. This will be further demonstrated in Chapters 5, 7, and 9 of this book.
6. This is especially the case in many towns and villages. "Women too visit in the afternoons, but extremely few of them chew *gat*. Whereas in Sanaa and in most villages in the Amran area it is quite acceptable for women to chew *gat* and to smoke the *mada'a*, this is not the case for 'Amran women themselves. Most women and men of 'Amran believe it is wrong for 'Amran women to chew, but tolerate the *gat* use of Sana'anias and villagers" (Dorsky 1981:56).

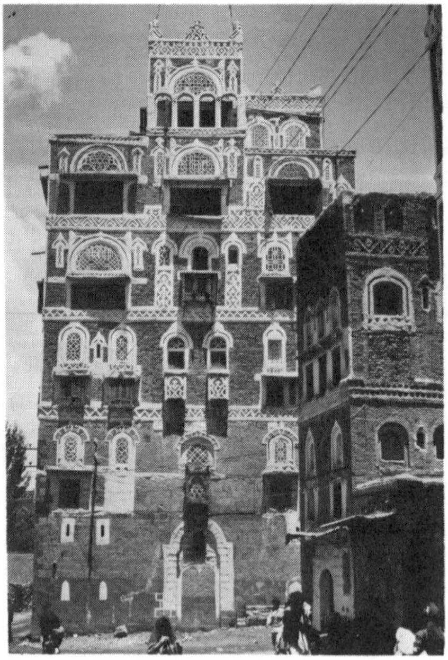

Photo credit John Neuhart

House in old city of Sanaa — top floor is muffraj

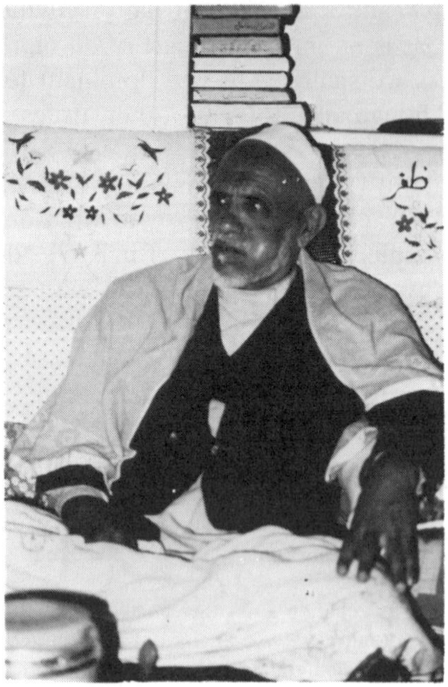

Qadi chewing qat at home

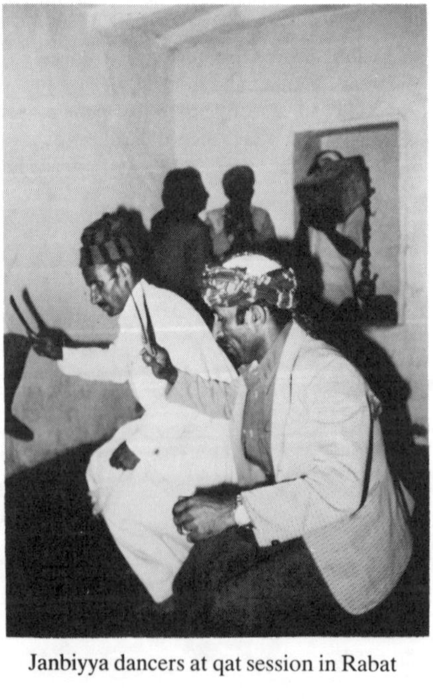

Janbiyya dancers at qat session in Rabat

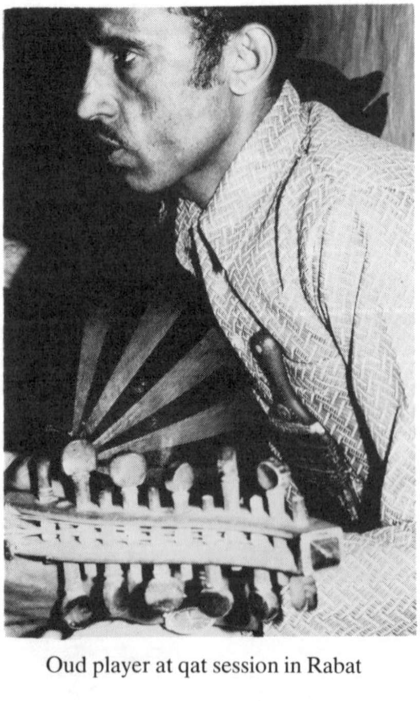

Oud player at qat session in Rabat

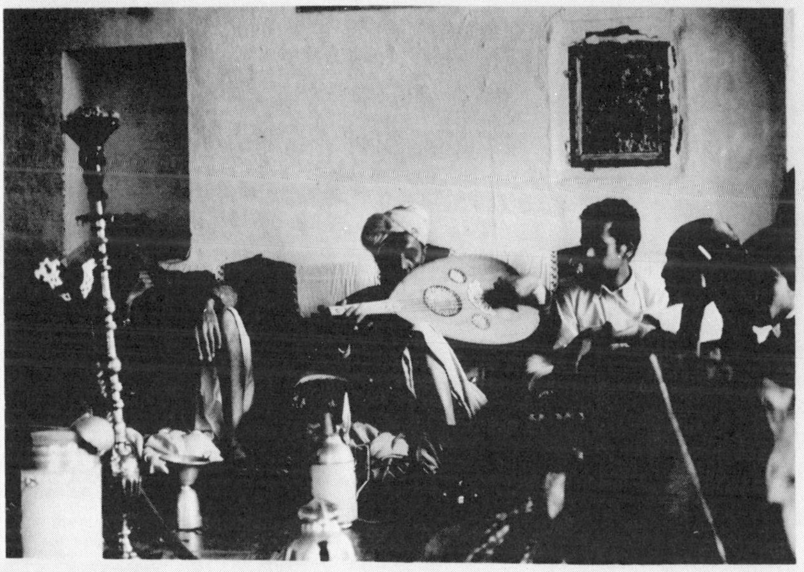

Photo credit John Neuhart

Qat session with oud player in Ibb

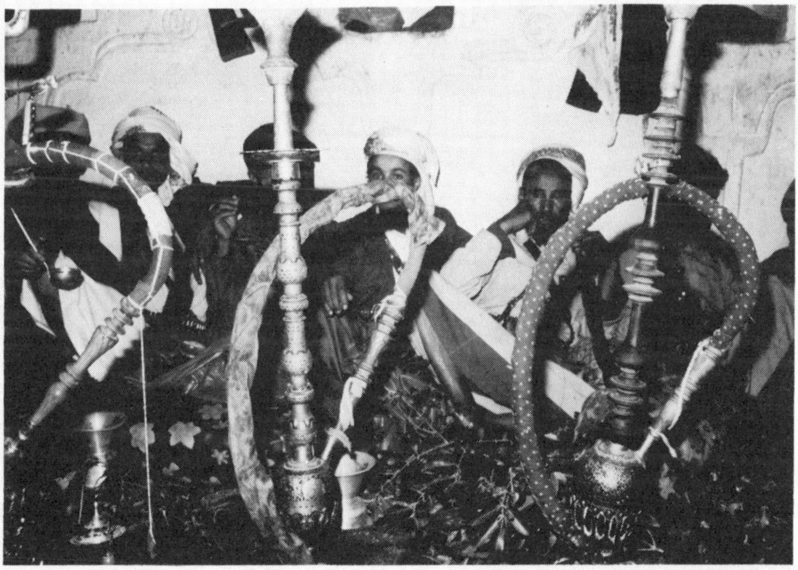

Photo credit John Neuhart

Wedding in Bani Hushaysh (near Sanaa)

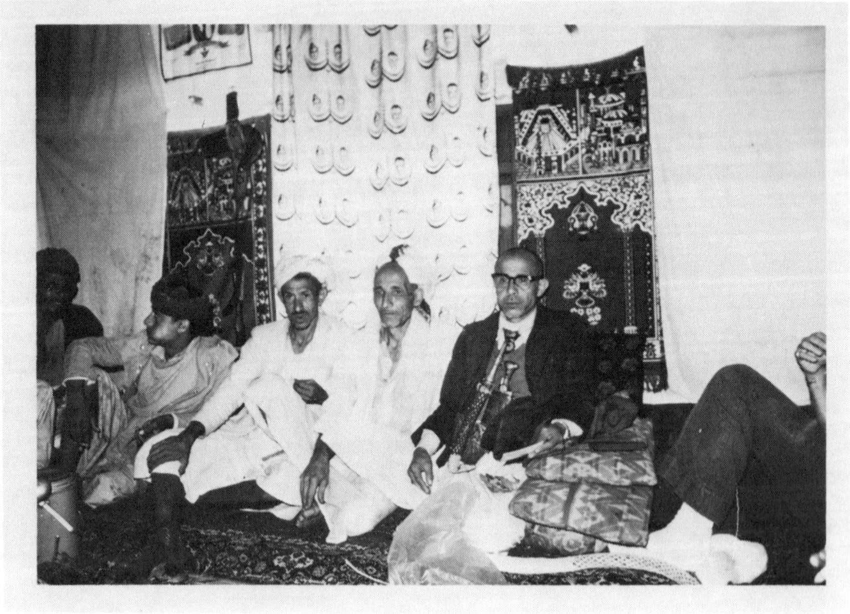

Village session in Shemran (near Manakha)

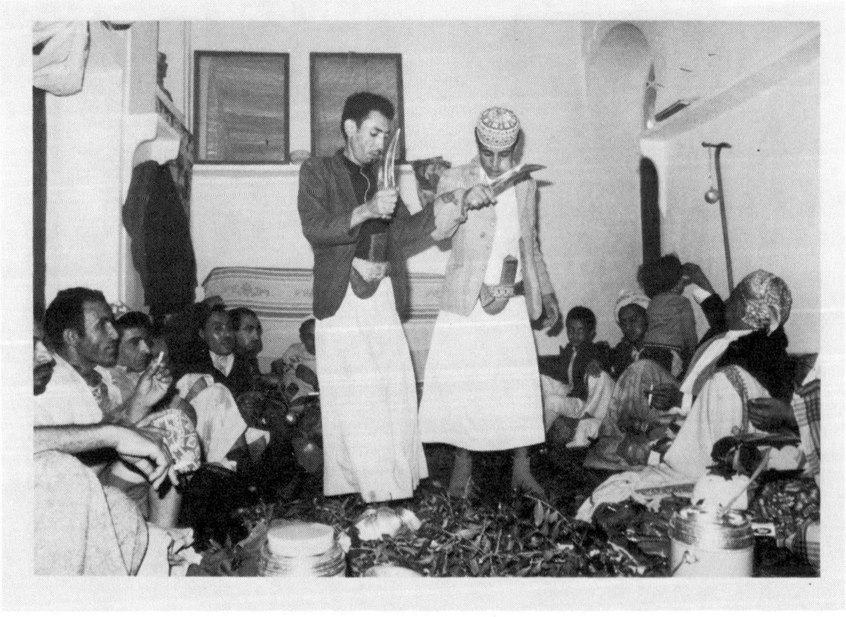

Window makers' session in Sanaa

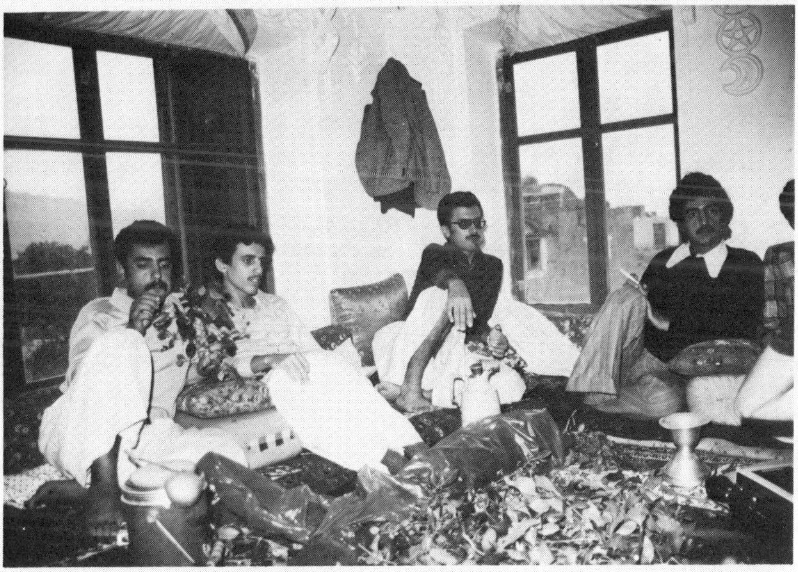

Educated young men's session in Sanaa

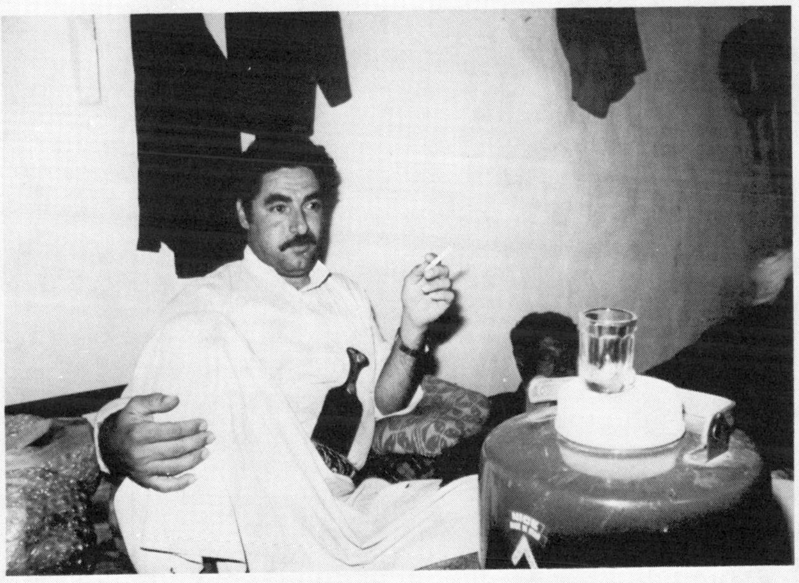

Young Shaykh chewing at Bani Hushaysh

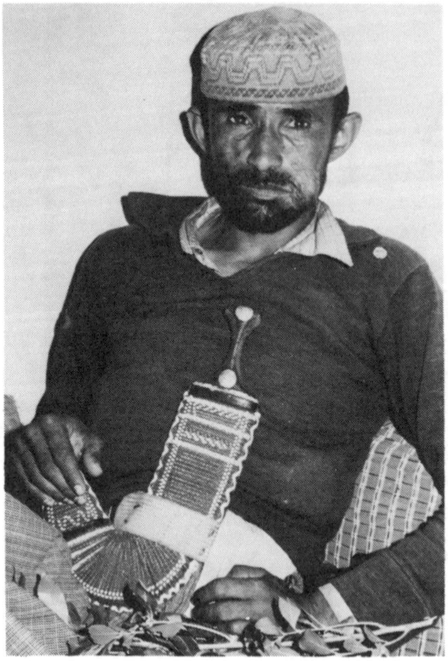

Tribesmen at qat session in Medinet al-Abid (near Utmah)

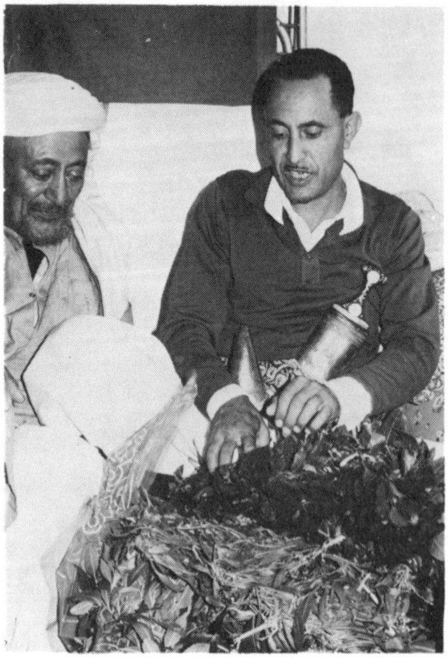

Shaykh dividing qat for group in Medinet al-Abid

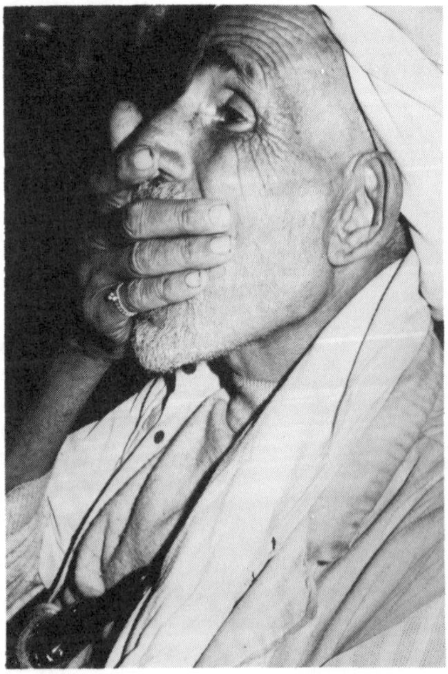

Old man chewing ground qat in Medinet al-Abid

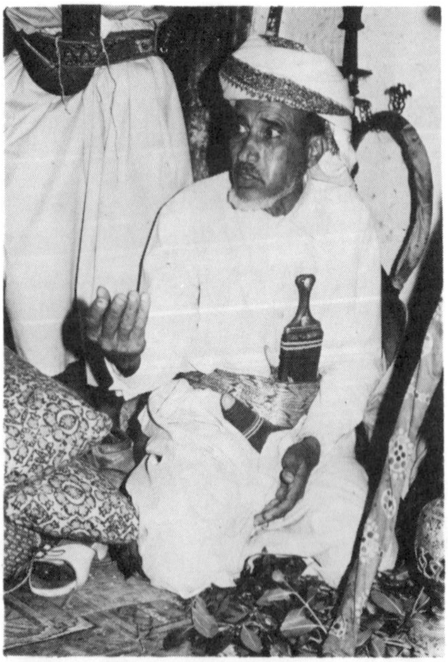

Pleading case before Shaykh in qat session at Medinet al-Abid

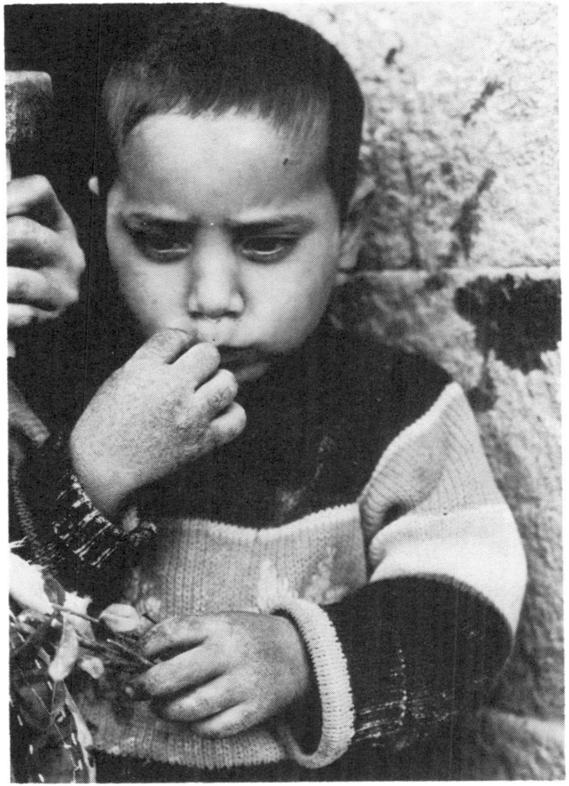

Photo credit John Neuhart

Boy chewing qat picked up from street in Sanaa

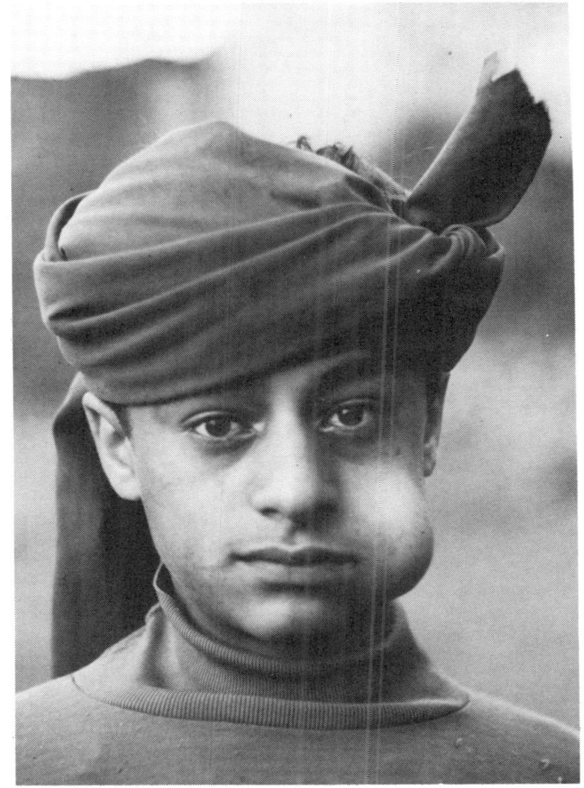

Chewing in Manakha

CHAPTER V

THE QAT EXPERIENCE

> Qat brings joy to the spirit.
> It illuminates the heart and
> frees the chest of sadness —
> It becomes the comrade of happiness.
> Do not say it is bitter
> if you cannot have it,
> as did the fox of the grapes
> that did not fall into his jaws.
>
> Abdul Hadi of Taiz
> (16th century Sufi buried
> in Taiz mosque)

By this time perhaps the reader is convinced that qat is central to Yemeni life. I now want to demonstrate this further by examining the phenomenology of qat use in Yemen, the subjective experiences associated with the drug and the meanings attached to its use. Exploration of the subjective aspects of qat use should illustrate how cultural beliefs and norms interact with psycho-physiological effects in creating and sustaining qat experiences, and provide more understanding of why people use, and occasionally abuse this drug.

Poetry has always been an important mode of expression, communication and commentary in Yemen, and like the example above, most qat poetry has been in praise of the drug. Nevertheless, an ambivalence about it has always been present in Yemeni attitudes. Since its introduction hundreds of years ago, Islamic scholars and judges have been divided on the question of whether or not qat should be placed in the category of haram (forbidden) substances, along with alcohol, hashish, etc. As we noted earlier, some have argued that analogous to wine it has consciousness-altering properties, and since it is on the basis of such properties that alcohol was forbidden by the prophet, qat too should be forbidden. However, the prevailing legal ruling in Yemen has usually been the more strict interpretation; that since it was not explicitly mentioned in the Qur'an it should not be forbidden.[1]

The 35th Imam, al Mutawakkil 'ala Allah Yahyya Sharaf al-Din, who ruled Yemen from 1506—1558, wrote a long poem on the virtues of qat. He used the image of a precious emerald, spoke of it as a shield against sensual desire, and said that it brings peace to the soul, joy to the heart, drawing the user closer to Allah. His son, Abdullah Ibn al-Imam Sharaf ad-Din who died in 1565 is one of the famous poets of Yemeni history. Using similar images, he too wrote a poem praising qat.

Emerald image
it sweetens my heart
making my state of mind and
my days so pleasant.
Qat is everything that one could
wish for; it brings good and
drives evil away.
The good-in-heart have written
the name of Allah in its leaves.
Qat unveils the mystery of Allah.[2]

There is a long tradition of such laudatory poetry in Yemen, but as I mentioned, there is also a long history of uneasiness about the drug. The clear cut negative symptoms which can occur from chewing, particularly of some types of qat, have been experienced by nearly everyone, and the sacrifice of money on it, particularly the poor in the larger towns has long been widely recognized as a problem. Even though the majority of Yemenis are not ashamed of chewing and proudly encourage the foreigner to participate, there never has been a unanimous acceptance of the custom.

Illustrative of the general ambivalence, which recurrently has become an issue of public debate, is the story of Amin Rihani, an American of Lebanese descent who traveled through Yemen with his companion Constantine Yanni in the early 1930s. They chewed qat everywhere, and met people from all strata of Yemeni society. The people of Yemen at the time were still very isolated from contact with the outside world, and these two travelers, who both spoke Arabic, made a tremendous impression wherever they went. Rihani later wrote a popular travel book, *Arabian Peak and Desert*, about Yemen, and the accuracy of much he described is well supported by numerous customs which persist in the same forms to this day.

Many older people in Yemen still remember the names of Rihani and Constantine. Some of the events which happened to them are still recounted, and the house they occupied in the *Bir al-Azhab* section of Sanaa is well known. The best remembered event conerning the two travellers is a poetry contest about the virtues and evils of qat which Imam Yahya, then in the middle stages of his reign in Yemen, engaged in with Constantine Yanni, the young Turkish officer. Because it concerned an issue of great salience in the country, this contest has achieved legendary status.

Constantine had a gift for classical Arabic poetry and one day he composed the following poem and sent it to the Imam:

What is it good for? Tell me.
Does anyone have an answer?
I tried it, and what I learned
requires many words to explain.

Even more than with alcohol
the youth's body becomes
inflamed and trembling.

It weakens the sexual powers
There is no doubt about that!
Qat gives no benefits at all,
only pain and hardship.
It annihilates the mind
and tires the heart and nerves.
The eyelid wilts, the eye clouds
The stomach is upset, and constipation
makes one rude.
The head becomes heavy, it aches
and spins.
Even the joints are affected.
Surely, qat brings closer the
threshold of death.

This poem was so good and provocative that the Imam, famed for both his poetic ability and his love of qat, was moved to write the following answer:

Qat is admirable
according to the Friends of the Prophet.
The sheep, pursued by wolves
discovered it,
tasted it, and found it pleasant.
Saliva flowed.
The shepherd then gathered it until
his pack was full,
He went around praising it
and he was right.
The people believed him.
They tasted it and liked it too.
It gives clarity of sight for the
eyes.
With it weakness fades away.
Like a melting emerald
on beautiful teeth,
What could be better to moisten
the mouth?
Is it treacherous, as it was said to be?
It cures loved ones
relaxing the weary soul.
It is a source of energy.

Thought is sharpened to a
fearful and burning brilliance.
For the scholar who sits to read
it chases away sleep.
As for Constantine, what he
said is a mirage.
Aren't there also those who overindulge
in food and drink?
Excess in anything brings disgrace
and sorrow
even to the virtuous ones.
As for your citation Constantine,
there is our reply, offered
in a veil of modesty,
for my dust cannot match your pearls.
Hide Yahya's creation, for in
concealment there is pious merit.[3]

These poems stimulated much discussion and imitative poetry at the time and they are passed down in the oral poetry tradition which still exists in Yemen. I heard them recited, not always completely accurately to be sure, in several remote villages, and also at Kawkaban near Sanaa and Beni Youseff near Taiz. Each time I heard people forcefully repeat these poems I was impressed by the living emotional energy evoked by these now distant events.

Common people and leaders derive special pleasure from Imam Yahya's poem, since to them it clearly justifies the use of qat while at the same time they assert the pride of identity of the Yemeni against the foreigner. The arousal of so much emotion over this story is further evidence of the cultural and psychological ambivalence which exists about the drug: questions about which there is no doubt do not arouse such an impassioned defense. In order to appreciate this ambivalence, let us proceed to look more closely at some aspects of the qat experience and the cultural concepts and beliefs relating to it.

THE KAYF

The state of well being which the qat user attempts to reach is called al *kayf* (mood) or *taradi*.[4] However, because of variables such as the grade of qat, and the amount chewed, the kayf is not always achieved. A term coming from the same Arabic root allied to kayf which describes the state reached by oneself or another is *mukayyif*. Other words used to describe this euphoric mood are *nashwa, mintashi* and *murtah* (Messick, B: personal communication). All of these refer to pleasant and comfortable aspects of mood, to the desired state.

If qat is chewed rapidly over an extended period of time a second stage of the kayf is reached which is referred to as *khedra* or being "drugged." The *sa'at al khedra*, which describes the waning period of the qat session, literally means "the hour of being drugged." During this period a chewer may say "*ana mukhadr*," "I am under the influence of qat" (literally, I am drugged). The next morning a person may exclaim "*ams wa ga'atli khedra ya latif!*" which roughly translated is "Oh my God I reached a great "drugged state" (or kayf) yesterday!" This might be better rendered as "I reached the sought after altered state experience," since the word "drugged", which has primarily a negative connotation in English, is not what is meant by the broader Arabic term. In any case, this is the sought-for state, one produced most surely and effectively by the expensive types of qat.

When the ordinary kayf has been superseded by a confused state, however, as it occasionally is with overindulgence, the person may substitute *khudr shadida!* in the above phrase, meaning "Oh my god I was really strongly drugged (out of it) yesterday." If this had been the case, he may go on to describe negative effects such as confused speech, gloomy thoughts, hallucinations, or fantastic manic fantasies of unrealizable projects.

All of these phrases and expressions referring to later stages of qat experience are based on the word *khadar* whose meaning is much broader than the word "numb" in English. Qat chewing does not usually produce numbness in the English sense of the term. Although a few Yemenis have mentioned that their feet or other extremities get cold after prolonged chewing, this is rare. The "numbing" or "drugging" in this instance refers more to a shutting out from perception of all but a narrow range of perceived reality, to a higher focused concentration which "numbs" one to many other impinging stimuli.

These comments should not obscure the fact that the kayf refers to a euphoric optimistic state in which everything seems possible. The individual's subjective experience during the first two hours of a session is one of heightened attention and increased mental excitement, a feeling of euphoric confidence, and a sense of being at the peak of one's mental powers. During the kayf many different happenings may be apprehended simultaneously. One may be speaking to one person while simultaneously attending a conversation some distance away. At the same time, attention can be devoted to noting the quality of qat in one's hand, or noting the interesting features of various people in the room. While it is true that we all have the power occasionally to have such multiple experiences under ordinary circumstances, the awareness-heightening qualities of the qat enhance them considerably.

The principal qualities of experience which informants identified for us as constituting the kayf were increases in alertness, ability to concentrate, the flow of ideas, contentment, confidence and friendliness. Some people say they experience all of these, while others only identify two of three of them as resulting from qat. In the kayf condition it is easy even for reticent and inhibited people to speak up on issues, and to act in a relatively extroverted manner.

An accurate approximation to the ideal of the desired state may be to describe it as a mild hypomania, which after a time transforms into meditative concentration. The early combination of the rapid flight of ideas with an increased sense of grandiosity and of self worth almost always makes the experience rewarding enough to compensate most chewers for the negative aftermath effects which sometimes occur. The following quotation concerning a visit to Imam Ahmad by a missionary in 1931 describes the qualities of the later stages of kayf:

> The qat began to work and he started to speak without restraint. He told me that he had good, private sources. . . . The audience lasted more than an hour. Only during the latter part did the *qat* seem to have got the better of his Herculean body. His great round eyes showed an enlarging of the pupils, his looks became wild and his words streamed over me like a waterfall. His two concillors seemed to have reached the same state (Van der Meulen, D. 1961:142).

With extremely heavy use there may come a point when the amount of the active ingredients in the system produces too much excitation. A person's speech becomes disjointed, his mind leaps ahead of his tongue, and words tumble out in a manic jumble. Another euphoric qat chewer may follow the meaning of this jumble, or may feel that he does, but non-chewing observers often claim it is total gibberish.[5]

Such confusional states can and do occur, but it is important to note that they are definitely not the rule. Swanson, a long time observer of the Yemen scene, notes that: "The strength of the substance should not be overrated, however. One could probably becomes as intoxicated drinking large quantities of strong coffee as one would at an afternoon qat session" (1979:40). This understates the case somewhat, but it underscores the point that often *no one* in a qat session exhibits *any* of the confusion described above. Still, I have seen sessions, particularly of poor workers chewing large amounts of cheap, "strong" qat, in which *all* the chewers together exhibited this somewhat euphorically confused speech.

A feature of the qat experience which is admitted by all chewers is the encouragement of self-confidence, sometimes to the point of grandiosity. The shy individual may be encouraged to speak and sometimes finds torrent of words flowing from his mouth. Imagination and even creativity may be unleashed. Critics of qat point out that the grand plans are often "castles in the air" and frequently come to nought. Often they are simply forgotten by the following day. Again, this phenomenon should not be overemphasized, since chewers having such experiences often compensate by careful review the following day. Certainly many important and rational decisions are taken during qat sessions, and even many serious government policies are made.

Much joking goes on during the euphoric phase of a qat session, and there are customs which provide a great deal of amusement for the group. One of the more institutionalized of these games is called "*ghusan al salam*" (branch of peace). If a person finds a sprig of qat in his bunch which is definitely bifurcated into 2 branches, he may take it and throw it at some other individual saying "*ghusan al salam Ali* (or whatever the perons's name is) *al salam alaykem.*" The thrower then leaps up and runs out of the muffraj. If the target of the throw is not able to jump up and catch the thrower he must provide him as well as the others present with a lunch at some future time. However, if the recipient of the qat *does* catch the thrower, he, with the assistance of other, pours water on him and generally ridicules and abuses him. This custom has now largely died out in the cities but still persists in country areas like Jabel Rayma (Charles Swagman, personal communication).[6]

As the later "introvert" phase of the qat session approaches, people withdraw psychologically, focusing their attention upon their own seething thoughts. This phase may be quite pleasurable for many people. Thomas Gerholm describes his experience of this phase and those of his informants in Manakha: "Each one is deep in his own thoughts, often quite pleasant ones: qat does not make one take a bleak view of the future" (1977:178). Whether the direction of the thought will be optimistic, pessimistic or objectively neutral, however, seems to depend upon variables of setting, chance conversation, physical condition, recent life events, personality factors, and the amount of qat chewed. At this stage the drug mainly creates a disposition to obsess. The preoccupation may take any direction; the mood may be somber or optimistic according to circumstances.

One often-experienced effect of this interesting preoccupied phase is a sense of detachment from the surroundings while still being entirely aware of them. This mood strikes some non-chewing observers as one in which the chewer does not care what others want or think. For example, it is often said that many of the shopkeepers in the central suq of Sanaa will not bargain during the later afternoon hours. They simply shrug or reply with an irritated rejection to any attempt to make them change their prices. Under ordinary conditions they actively and good-naturedly enter into the bargaining process. In my view the unspoken rule that one does not disturb the group by chattering during the "Solomon's hour" of the qat session is based upon the chewer's desire to concentrate upon the rapid flow of thoughts which is engaging his total attention. Distractions are irritating.

After participating in many qat sessions, it once dawned on me that I had never witnessed any kind of fight or overtly aggressive behavior at one of them. This is, of course, much different than the situation with alcohol to which we are accustomed in the West, so I inquired into it and observed further. In answer to direct questions the unanimous answer was that fighting is out of the question at qat sessions and never occurs. In order to probe further into whether the drug stimulates or encourages aggressive behavior, I asked whether fighters going into battle were given qat by their commanders.

The universal reply was that this is never done; according to all informants the drug makes the user less aggressive, inclining instead to passivity and rumination.

Arguments, verbal duels and hostile sarcasm occurred in the early stages of some sessions, but they were always under control. It is reported that some men, feeling agitated and depressed after heavy chewing, go home and abuse their wives and families. The few who do this often blame it on the qat. However, a more common opinion is that qat is not the cause of such behavior and that it only triggers traits or moods which characterize the individual under any circumstances.

It is surprising that in qat sessions people can sit for periods of three to seven hours for the most part without becoming agitated or engaging in much physical movement. They may be rather tightly packed in against one another and still manage to be quite comfortable for the whole time. This seemed remarkable to me because the literature on amphetamines and other stimulants, as well as some of the articles on the use of qat (miraa, chat etc.) in East Africa, had led me to expect that the drug would produce jitteriness and impulses to move around nervously.

It is true that the hands and the mouth of the user generally are continually in motion for two or three hours, but this and conversation are the principal activities during qat sessions. There is very little standing up or movement around the muffraj, unless the mood is for dancing. People adjust their leg positions from time to time, and lean forward to drink water or to handle the long hose of the mada'a but overall there is surprisingly little movement. Motion becomes ever more diminished as the "introvert" phase of the session develops.

One physiological change which assists this ability to sit for long periods is that urination and defecation are inhibited. Qat tends to constrict the muscular vessels, reducing their normal functioning, and this is reinforced by the lack of movement which is called for by the norms of chewing. My own experience leads me to accept the Yemenis' claim that "qat quiets the body as it quickens the mind."

During our early participant observation in qat sessions we tried to find out what the feeling of kayf which the Yemenis described was like to them. As indicated earlier, several dimensions of the experience were mentioned again and again, so these were incorporated into the final interview form which was administered to the sample of men and women in our socio-medical study. The six pleasurable dimensions of the kayf experience were: contentment, ability to concentrate, increased flow of ideas, increased alertness, increased confidence, and increased friendliness. Additionally, it was fairly frequently mentioned that some distortion of perception could occur with unaccustomed or heavy use, so this was also included as a possible dimension of the kayf. Figure 1 presents a tabulation of the answers to this question broken down by sex. It is interesting to note that 14% of the users

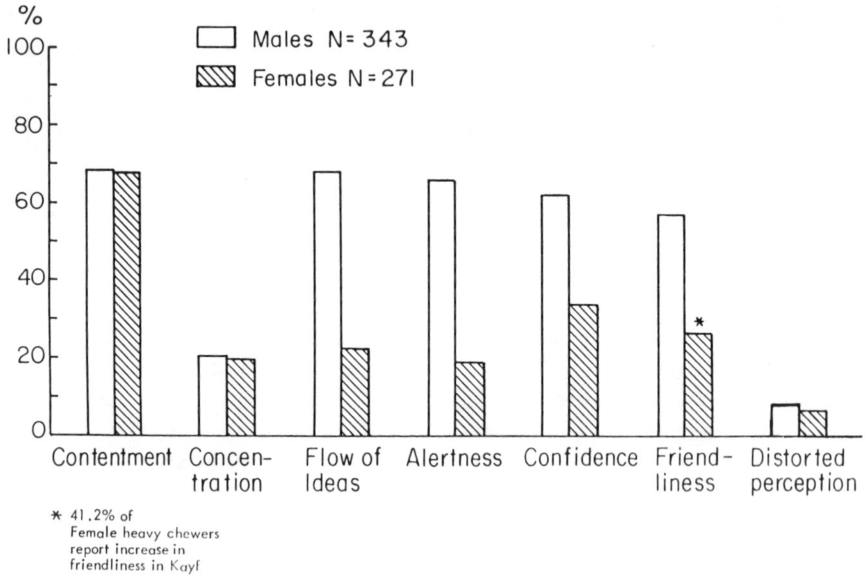

Fig. 1. Dimensions of kayf reported by qat users.

reported that they did not experience *any* of the pleasant effects commonly held to result from chewing. This finding is not so surprising, however when it is noted that these tended to be primarily female light users. The reverse of this is that 86% of users reported at least one of the common kayf effects.

The first observation to be made regarding this figure is that there is a high degree of agreement between male and female chewers on the contentment dimension, as about 70% of both sexes reported regularly experiencing this. However, almost equal percentages of male users also reported frequent experiences of increases in the flow of ideas, alertness, confidence and friendliness. Females reported such experiences much more infrequently. Only one-fifth of chewers of each sex reported that qat usually or always enhances their abilities to concentrate. As we would expect, those reporting frequent distortions of perception while chewing qat were very few. It should be noted that there are no statistically significant differences between heavy chewers and light chewers on any of these dimensions except "friendliness" among women. There the increase from 25.5% among light chewers to 41.2% among heavy chewers is statistically significant.

How can we account for these sex differences? In the first place we could say that "contentment", in a sense, is nearly synonomous with kayf itself, and is the basic experience associated with chewing by both sexes. Next we might hazard the idea that Yemeni women do not value experiences such as increased flow of ideas, alertness and confidence as much as do men, and do not see any need to enhance these. Men see such qualities as important to business and trading transactions, and value intelligent conversation, competitive argument, good memory of historical and current events, poetry, etc., whereas women do not. Their conversations have traditionally been more oriented around family, children and neighborhood gossip, rather than intellectual acuteness. Thus it seems logical that they should not have paid as much attention as men to those dimensions of the qat experience which enhance cognition. They are much more attuned to the mood enhancing qualities of the drug, i.e., contentment, and increases in confidence and friendliness.

It might be pointed out too that women have only fairly recently participated in qat use on a large scale. Our respondents probably do not have as much experience with the drug, and in this society, where the lives and recreational patterns of the two sexes are so highly segregated, they may well have a much less or clearly articulated set of ideas concerning it.

Finally, it could be thought that women actually chew less qat and thus have less qat induced experiences because they get less cathinone into their systems. I tend to doubt this explanation because we were so careful to classify our chewers correctly, and because some of the medical data to be presented later shows that women are subject to more qat related disease effects. Nevertheless, this possibility cannot be ruled out. My own opinion is that the answer may lie in a combination of the factors I have adduced.

It was mentioned in an earlier chapter that Yemenis believe that the use of qat gives them energy to work. Our interview data on that point indicates that this belief is very strong (See Figure 2).

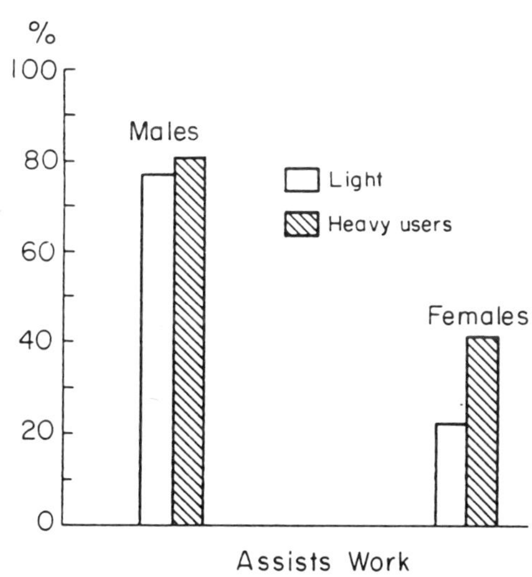

Fig. 2. Qat and work.

again we have a significant sex difference, and much of the same ; applies. Women's household tasks are varied, and are not regarded ing the amount of sustained concentration which men's work does. Men tend to see qat as maintaining alertness and energy needed for work, whether it be for the mental tasks of the clerk or the hand-eye coordination of stone cutting, construction or mechanics. If there is a choice as to the male or female of the household having access to the relatively expensive stimulant, there is little question as to who gets it. Female tasks are not *regarded* as particularly taxing of mind or body, or even as "work" in the male sense of that term.

THE OTHER SIDE OF THE COIN

Although people generally extoll qat for its kayf and its beneficial qualities, it is clearly recognized that regular negative behavioral and experiential effects may be produced as well. These occur when the amount of the drug ingested is excessive, when the kind of qat chewed is of inferior quality, or for both reasons. In each local qat-producing area there are cheaper "stronger" varieties, known to produce more of the bad side-effects associated with the drug: nervousness, sleeplessness, impotence, and nightmares. Also, any kind of qat, picked too early to taken in excess can produce the confusion described, and even hallucinations, but the inferior grades produce these much more quickly and reliably.

It is said that some of these inferior types of qat will not kayf, which means that when chewing these types most people do not experience the euphoria and reverie which are most desired. Such unwelcome effects do not deter the poor from purchasing the qat they can afford, since most of it does kayf, and because they feel (often correctly) that they will only chew enough leaves to produce an agreeable effect, but not enough to push them over the edge into a confused state.

In addition to bad "types" of qualities of qat, there are believed to be occasional "bad trees," even within a stand of the best types. There sometimes may be just a "bad harvest" from an otherwise fine tree as well. In these instances, where people experience inexplicable negative consequences, a supernatural explanation may be given to account for them. For example, in the hamlet of Shemran, high among the peaks of Haraz, it was explained that qat planted inadvertently on graves or on old graveyards produces hallucinations. However, when such a tree is discovered, the sickness-producing effects of its leaves may be neutralized by sacrificing a goat and, with the appropriate incantations, spattering its blood on the tree. Such beliefs are restricted to certain local areas, but all Yemenis know that some kinds and quantities of the plant can surely take one beyond the normal "manic" state to produce confusion and then a number of bad after-effects.

There are a number of variables which, in Yemeni eyes, influence the quality of qat, and also, therefore, its price. The main variables are: are color, season, picking time within the season, the part of the tree from which it is picked and regularity of watering (i.e. whether rain-fed or irrigated from springs). "Good" quality qat has three main attributes: (1) it tastes good (not too bitter), (2) it creates a kayf and (3) it does not produce bad after-effects such as anxiety, spermatorrhea (loss of semen), impotence, etc.

"Bad" quality qat, on the other hand, produces all or some of these negative effects. There are, of course, many intermediate qualities and, according to variables such as season, part of tree etc., a blend of "good" and "bad" features is often found. For example, in Kusmah on Jabel Raymah the "white" *asili* ("root" or "original") qat is said to be more mentally stimulating, i.e., to produce pleasant thoughts and a good kayf, while the "red" *habashi* qat is said to be stronger and more physically stimulating. It is regarded as better for the hard work of climbing up and down mountains, etc. (Charles Swagman: personal communication).

Particularly in areas where qat cultivation and use are a relatively new phenomenon, buyers are often not so discriminating, and in many markets there are only an expensive "good" type of qat (which also may simply be called baladi (country), and an inexpensive one. The experienced buyer, however, generally takes account of all or most of the possible influences on quality in making his selection.

In general, the *abiyad* or "white" (light green) or *azraq* (blue) qat (more grayish) is considered better than the *ahmar* "red" (reddish stems and veins on leaves) varieties, though this is not always the case. In certain seasons and areas the red may be better.

Some discriminations depend on the distance it comes, For example, in big markets like the one in Sanaa, one can often find qat from many distant areas. If it is from far away as from Taiz, it might simply be called "*taizi*" in Sanaa, but if you were to buy the same qat in Taiz you would know whether it was "*mabarrah*" i.e., the best "trimmed" qat from the first cutting of the season or whether it was "*habashi*" a poor type from Jabel Habashi, etc. In the large markets of Sanaa and Taiz, which are located in qat growing regions, the most varieties and grades of qat are found. In the Tihama on the other hand, where all qat is brought from a considerable distance, general area designations such as raymi, shami, and harrazi are often all that is found, and there are fewer varieties.

An entire book could be devoted solely to detailing the varieties of qat in Yemen, and in another section of this one I present some examples to illustrate complexities involved in choosing qat. In many ways the situation is analogous to that of wine in the West, though discrimination is not so refined and elaborate. A great many people are not aware of all the subtleties, but some, particularly the more wealthy, are quite concerned with them. Without doubt some qats are much better than others in taste and effects, but as with wine, the differences may not be quite as pronounced as the "connoisseurs" would lead us to believe. It is clear that good and expensive qat does not produce as many bad side effects as do the cheaper grades, yet in sufficient amounts or in susceptible individuals, some of such effects can result from the finest plants.

CHEWING TO EXCESS

I have spoken at some length about euphoric and introvert stages of kayf. Now I want to discuss the character of the confused state that sometimes occurs, and the effects which follow the session. Much as we in the West laugh at stories of drunkards or drunkeness, the Yemenis enjoy funny anecdotes of disoriented qat chewers. One story in particular I heard in six different widely separated regions of Yemen. It is typically recounted when the topic of possible hallucinations or altered states of consciousness and their associations with qat use is brought up.

A man who was chewing qat at a session was asked by his companions to go out of the muffraj and replenish the coals of the mada'a. he got up and went out, but instead of going to the kitchen area to get the coals, he went out of the house and kept walking. Finally, after some wandering, he came to the next village, whereupon he walked into the kitchen of a similar looking house and said to the woman: "I need coals to replenish the mada'a."

This tale always invokes much laughter, and though people are well aware of its apocryphal nature they agree that such an incident probably has happened more than once; it certainly is well within the bounds of possibility. Many such accounts of disorientation were told to us in qat sessions. For example, the joke is told of the man who tried to warm his hands by a fire several kilometers away, and another of the man who tried to swim in an empty cistern. In one session in Sanaa, I was told the following story illustrating misperceptions of time and space.

A father and son left a qat session in the evening and wanted to deliver some money to a house about a mile away in Beni Hushaysh. It was a time of troubles and there was danger of being shot by tribal enemies. They were very afraid and they crept around carefully for about three hours. They heard many shouts in the distance and finally went back home unsuccessful in their mission. The next day they followed their own tracks and discovered they had been wandering around not more than a few meters from their own house the entire time.

Many men claim that because it aids concentration and reflection qat chewing often creates a religious mood in which they feel much closer to Allah than on other occasions. They therefore feel that it is good to take it before the evening prayer. However, sometimes strong qat produces ludicrous behavior in the mosque.

A Sanani man with a great reputation for piety did not ordinarily chew qat. However, on one occasion he was sitting with a group in the muffraj and his friends forced him to chew. When he went to perform the evening prayer in the mosque he was completely out of time with the group. When they all knelt, for example, he stood up, and when they were raising their heads from the mat, he was putting his head down. He was the laughing stock.

Another man, after chewing, took his mada'a with him, and stopped at the mosque. He set the pipe by the ritual washing pool and went in to pray. When he came out after the prayer it was darker and thinking the mada'a was some jinn or supernatural being, he sneaked up behind it and struck it a great blow. If fell over, breaking, and only then did he realize that it was only his own waterpipe.

A man left a qat session in the darkening of the evening and was walking down a side street of Sanaa. He saw a large shadowy shape which terrified him because he *knew* it was a jinn. In a shaking voice he said: "*Bismillah*! If you are a jinn, please identify yourself and tell me what you want." He was surprised when the being answered, asking him the same thing! The two friends then embraced in great relief.

Some of the younger, educated Yemenis said that many of the supernatural experiences which people in Yemen recount are simply results of qat disorientation. Many of these young men told stories of being confused in their work after chewing. One of these, who worked as a clerk in a government office, told how he once went back to the office after a session to finish some typing. It was supposed to be in Arabic but the sat down by mistake at an English typewriter and typed two pages of gibberish before he came to his senses.

The most common hallucinatory experience mentioned by qat users is the feeling that hundreds of insects are crawling all over one's body. This was reported in all parts of Yemen, and it is always said to result from chewing too much of cheap strong varieties of qat. Examples of qat which can more readily produce hallucinatory experiences are *sharoo* and *maqtari* in the south near Turba, *sharabi* from Sharab near Taiz, *jashani* from Dhi Sufal near Ibb, and *sawti* and *harami* from North of Sanaa.

It must be emphasized again that "inferior" types of qat certainly do not always produce such sensations; most people who chew cheap qat control their intake and do not experience them often. I only wish to mention that such potential for disquieting psychological experience exists if one over-indulges. In an attempt to probe this aspect of the qat experience we asked participants in this study about specific hallucinatory experiences they might have had. Again, the questions were based upon comments users made to us in qat sessions regarding such experiences. Figure 3 expresses the answers to these questions.

About 35% of the male users reported experiencing at least one of these hallucinatory effects frequenty and about 25% of the female users so reported. There were no differences among heavy and light chewers in the score. Again we find the males reporting more of the qat effects. In terms of our participant observations in sessions and our own experiences, the amounts of reported hallucinations, particularly for males, seem on the high side. However, it must be noted that Yemenis do not regard such experiences

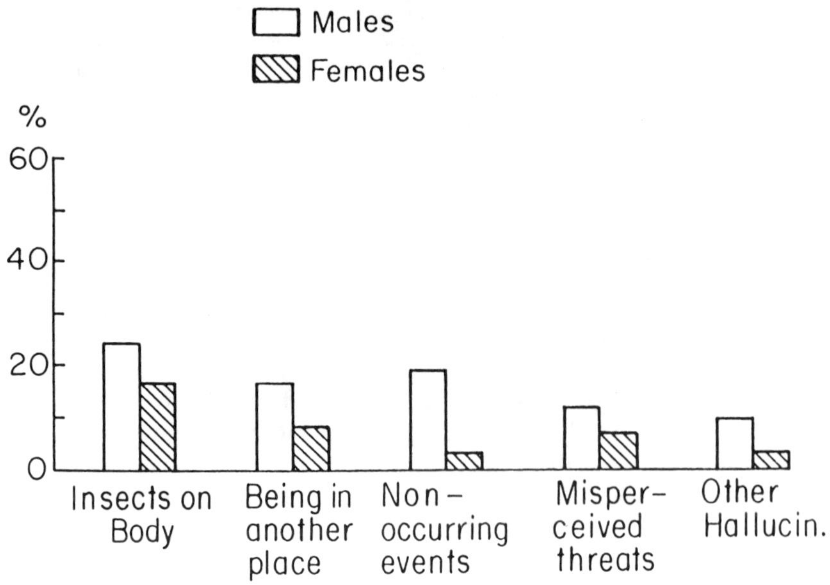

Fig. 3. Hallucinations.

in the same way we do. To them, they are expected occasionally and often the chewer knows, even while in the state, that it is an effect of qat. Yemenis have no fear of being pushed over the edge of sanity by such an experience.

One point which should be stressed in discussing the occasional confused states or hallucinations associated with qat use is that they are temporary. I was not able to identify even one case of a permanent psychosis which could be attributed to qat. This speaks not only for the limitations on the ingestion of cathinone which are created by customs of use, but also perhaps reflects the less behavior-disrupting character of that substance in comparison with true amphetamines (see Chapter VII).

Since qat produces alertness and confidence, it is chewed by many of the pupils at high schools, and at the University of Sanaa. It is believed to assist with long hours of study especially in preparing for examinations. One story I was told concerned a student from the Sudan at Sanaa University to whom qat was a new experience:

> He soon discovered that a robta of qat assisted him with his studies, and began to chew large amounts every day beginning in the morning. However, after a few weeks he became completely disoriented. He did not know what country he was in and wandered around like a mad person. His friends captured him, put him in bed and did not allow him to chew any qat. After about three days he returned to normal functioning.

NEGATIVE AFTERMATHS

Qat rarely produces confusion or hallucinations, but at the end of a session the chewer must often begin to cope with a series of other different effects which are largely negative, though not so severe. These vary considerably among individuals, and according to type of qat and amounts chewed. After leaving the session the user is still in a state of mental agitation in spite of his quiet mood. As mentioned earlier, some men go to the mosque after chewing. Others return home, and after taking a light meal or perhaps just some milk or qishr (for qat generally reduces appetite), they may do some work for several hours. Many Yemenis scholars and writers say that this is a time when they can work single-mindedly for many hours, and this was my own experience, provided that I had not taken too much qat. When I discussed this with Yemeni scholars they would agree, but usually laughed and commented that on the very next day one must carefully examine what was written the night before. As was mentioned earlier, grandiose fantasies have a tendency to creep in, and these must be edited, but frequently intellectual work may be completed which under normal conditions of laziness and inhibition simply might not have been done at all.

A mildly depressed mood is a common experience for qat chewers near the end of a session, or afterward for an hour or two. A Yemeni diplomat expressed his feeling to me that at the end of a session he often feels that somehow he has lost a battle. He obsesses on the time that has been wasted and is overcome by an aversion to going home. Judith Obermeyer, a member of our research team, when she identified herself as a psychologist, was asked by the young men working in the medical clinic in Zabid why they frequently felt worthless and as failures after they chew qat. Another informant at a qat session in Sanaa told me that during the final phase of a qat session he inevitably feels like he is covered with garbage.

These examples certainly should not be taken as the universal norm, since undoubtedly personality factors play a part, along with the variations caused by "strong" varieties of qat, or by whether or not the individual ate a large meal before chewing, etc. My own experience was that there were times that I was quite depressed after chewing, while at other times I was simply reflective and quiet. My worst experience, which included irritability and mild paranoia along with depression, came after a long session at a wedding celebration in Sanaa. I had chewed two fairly small robtas of inexpensive harazi qat. My notes read:

> I returned home at 7:15 as the last few people were leaving. I then had the worst feeling I have had so far after a session. I was agitated. I ate a meal of potato pancakes and drank two gin and lemon drinks, but nothing helped. I was irritable to those in the house. My thoughts turned to my work and I had the feeling that I am accomplishing nothing. I am not doing what I like to do or what I do best. I am snowed under with bureaucratic nonsense and the study is not going well. Nobody can be depended on. I went to sleep after listening to some songs

on Radio Kuwait but awoke about 3:00 A.M. and then slept fitfully until morning, sweating profusely.

What I want to stress here is that this experience was unusual for me. I was chewing on the average of three times per week and this was the most extreme experience of agitated depression I had. It also was related to certain reality factors. The study *was* somewhat bogged down. We had lost a couple of important assistants; some of the researchers were not performing as expected, etc. My own natural cycle of high and low moods was probably involved as well, and the kind of qat I chewed was certainly not the best. In my estimation, what the drug did in this instance was to intensify my latent, already depressive mood.

During that afternoon's session, which was a part of the wedding of a Yemeni friend, I had been totally engaged in attempting to document the event, while at the same time carrying on conversations with friends. As the evening came on and the celebration drew to a conclusion the combination of fatigue and the cathinone in my system potentiated the negative thoughts of my work, etc. which arose during the quiet phase of the qat session.

I experienced a range of states at the ends of sessions — from a simple reflectiveness to agitation or sadness. It is true that all of these states tended to be on the somber end of the mood scale, but rarely did they verge on what could be called truly "depressive" in any exact or clinical definition of that term. On the other hand, I observed a number of individuals who did appear to be almost clinically depressed after qat sessions. Knowing some of them under other more ordinary circumstances led to the inference that their personalities tended to fall towards the pessimistic or even depressive side.

What we can say about this "introverted" part of the qat session is that generally the chewer feels a physical fatigue following three or four hours of concentration, talkativeness and euphoria, and that this leads to a slowing down of verbal and other behaviors. However, the tendency to focus, or even to obsess on a single theme or idea is enhanced. Since these obsessive ideas frequently concern real-life problems, the ruminations, intensified by the qat, often have a depressive cast which reflects reality. Since one does not *always* experience a negative mood, and since the longer euphoric stage of the session is so rewarding, the occasionally depressive aftermath, even when coupled with other unwanted effects of sleeplessness, occasional temporary impotence problems, etc., is not so punishing as to offset the rewards, in people's eyes.

Yemenis are well aware that their confidence increases, sometimes to megalomaniac proportions, as part of the reward of the qat kayf. Most of them accordingly are very prudent and cautious about important decisions arrived at during qat sessions. These are often abandoned the following morning unless they have been finalized in some irrevocable manner, or they may be recognized as being rational and wise.

It does occasionally happen that a questionable decision is made which is difficult to revoke. An example illustrating this was recounted by a man I knew well. During a qat session in which people were discussing the problems of marriage, the husband of this man's female cousin made a sudden resolve to divorce her. He not only declared the Muslim divorce oath three times in the public forum of the session, but then called for a piece of paper and wrote her a letter with the news, even stipulating that he would pay nothing for child support should she take the baby with her. During this some of the men remonstrated with him, but they could see that because of his condition they could do nothing to deter him.

When I discussed this case in another qat session, all those present agreed that this somewhat passive man had probably wanted to do this for some time, and that the qat probably bolstered his courage. They cited other instances where qat enabled normally reticent or fearful persons to act, but also said that most of such behavior could be changed and excused on the grounds of qat effects.

One such was the case of a policeman, known to be especially good and pious, who was caught burglarizing a store. Under ordinary conditions Islamic law dictates that this offense could result in the loss of a hand. However, his defense was that he had chewed an immense amount of poor grade qat during the afternoon just prior to the robbery attempt. Many witnesses attested to this, and the judge, allowing it to be a legitimate extenuating circumstance, spared his hand, and sentenced him only to a few days in jail.

It is said too that some men, still agitated by the qat, inevitably quarrel with their wives and other family members after returning home. However, many do not react in this way, so it is difficult to ascertain whether and how much of such behavior is actually a result of qat, or simply stems from a quarrelsome disposition, and/or any frustrating conditions which might be present.

To explore the question of the frequently reported negative effects felt by many chewers at the end of the session and afterwards we included a number of specific questions in the sociomedical survey to tap these experiences. From the exploratory phase of the study we came up with the following seven negative dimensions: sadness, failure, hopelessness, fears, people are evil, nervousness, and losing ambition or frustration. Figure 4 indicates how the respondents replied to direct questions about this experience. It is notable that only 63.5% of male users and 61.7% of female users reported at least one such negative effect, and that there were no significant differences between reports of heavy and light users.

We again see here that males and females differ on a number of the dimensions. Women in general report very few negative late session effects, while men, though reporting considerably more, are still surprisingly low, especially in view of what people tell you on an informal level. Could the sex

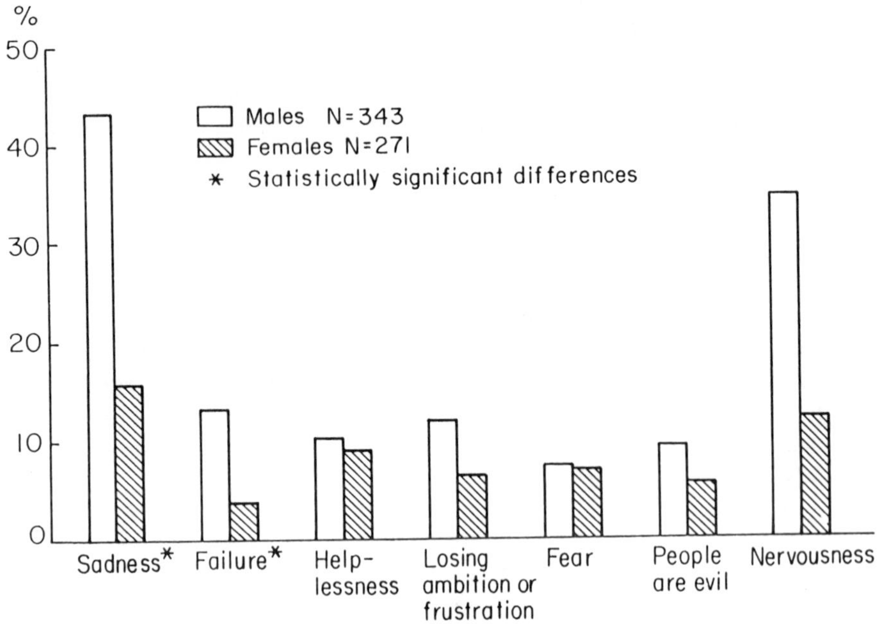

Fig. 4. Negative aftermaths (late session).

differences be due to factors such as we addressed in discussing the positive dimensions of kayf? My own view is that people experience such negative effects much less frequently than they do the positive ones — a situation which is one factor accounting for continued use. This is borne out by the fact that both questions asked whether effects were experienced usually or always or seldom or never. The figures represent the "usually" or "always" answers.

It is interesting though, to group these answers into fewer dimensions. It seemed to me on examining this data that "sadness," "failures," "hopelessness," and "losing ambition" could be grouped into one dimension called the "depressive dimension"; that "fear," and "people are evil" could be grouped in a "paranoid dimension" and nervousness and frustration could be called a "tension dimension." The results of this are shown in Figure 5.

This indicates that over 50% of chewers report that they frequently experience some kind of mild depressive reaction as a late session response to chewing, and that about 10% report often experiencing a mildly paranoid reaction On the tension dimension males report significantly more such experiences. It is interesting that females report more depressive experiences than do males, a fact in line with the repeated findings in the West that women generally tend to be more susceptible to depression than do men. On the other hand, the tension dimension, reflecting nervous agitation and

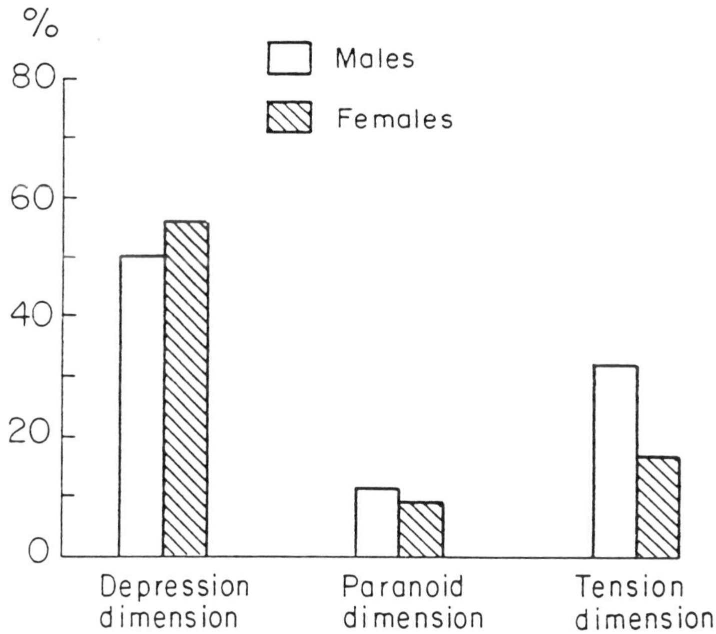

Fig. 5. Negative aftermath dimensions.

frustration is significantly more common among males, perhaps indicating a kind of agitated depressive phase which may be caused by greater ambitions or by greater felt responsibilities.

We should not leave the question of the late session effects of qat chewing without noting that people also report positive effects, and experience of these is another reason that the unquestionably negative reinforcements do not lead people to abandon the use of the drug. The major positive effects reported were "drawing one close to Allah", "increasing the desire to work," and "increasing general understanding" (e.g., of "life" or one's problems). We included questions regarding these in our interview schedule and the results are shown in Figure 6.

Contemplating this figure makes it more apparent why the reports of negative aftermaths are not high, and again, why chewers are not motivated to quit chewing. It is because the possibility of having a good later experience is nearly the same as having a bad one. In fact, according to reports of individuals in this study, it is slightly better. Of course, there is a possibility that one may, on any given occasion of chewing, experience both good and bad aftermaths. For example, I, myself, have on occasion experienced a depressed nervousness late in the session and for a time thereafter. This then gave way to a desire to work accompanied also by a feeling of "increased understanding." Thus, by presenting these feelings in numerical form I do not

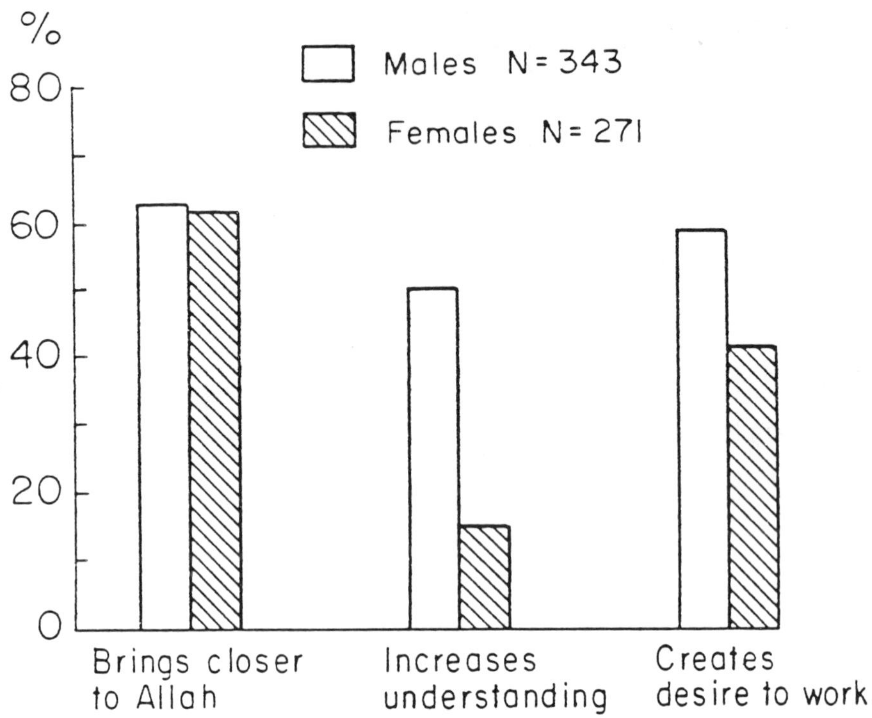

Fig. 6. Postive aftermaths (late session).

want to oversimplify the actual, often complex situations of mixed feelings or of the short phases in which differing feelings, both positive and negative, may follow one another.

The one further point I wish to make with regard to Figure 6 is to take note once more of the male-female differences. Here again, I suggest that Yemeni women do not value abstract "understanding" in the same way men do, and perhaps the concept had little meaning for them. Also, since many fewer of them associate qat with work, it is not strange that they tend not to attribute to the qat their later increases in desires to work.

Yemenis consider the inhibition of sleep which often follows the use of the drug to be a more universal negative effect. Daily heavy chewers claim *not* to experience this, but all others, and that includes the majority of Yemenis, claim to have a problem with sleep after chewing qat. This is undoubtedly the basis of the custom that most Yemeni business offices, including those of the government, do not get into operation until after 9:00 A.M. Even then a great many people seem to have difficulties in functioning adequately at first. In our survey chewers reported that they slept an average 6.6 hours per night after chewing. Non-chewers reported 7.8 hours per night. However, only 42% of the chewers reported fitful sleep after chewing.

The insomnia feature of the drug is also directly related to the rise in alcohol use in the country. We were somewhat unprepared for this, but soon found that in Yemen qat use and alcohol use are often linked. Though alcohol is strictly prohibited in Yemen, some groups, and in particular the young men of more affluent families, rendezvous to drink at another house after a qat session. A bottle of Scotch whiskey is brought out and each man drinks several water glasses filled with one-third whiskey and two-thirds water. It is believed that three such drinks are sufficient to counteract the effects of the qat; somber moods are dissipated permitting early sleep, allowing sexual activity, and stimulating an appetite for food. In rural villages and among the city poor the same purposes are sometimes served by a powerful alcoholic beverage called *baladi*, which certain families distill from grapes, grain and other ingredients.

SEX

I have earlier alluded to the effects on the sexual life which are associated with qat use. There seems little doubt that sexual experience is affected, but the issue is not as straightforward as that of effects on sleep. The reports are more varied. Some claim it takes away desire, while others report that it produces a draining of sexual fluids from the penis, and in this way produces eventual impotence at an earlier age than would be expected.

As opposed to the usual negative report, there is a minority opinion in Yemen that qat both stimulates sexual desire and enhances ability to perform. Particularly, it is claimed that an erection may be sustained for a longer period than under normal circumstances. One explanation for the existence of such diverse opinions on sexual effects is that any particular result depends to some degree upon the kind of qat which is chewed; some stimulate, while others inhibit sexual desire and performance. The finest most expensive types are claimed to have no negative effects on sexual performance, while the cheap varieties reputedly produce negative side effects. As with the question of sleep, however, heavy regular users generally claimed that their sex lives were not affected.

My own experience was that desire was usually enhanced and length of performance increased, but there was also less difficulty in refraining. Due to the constriction of vessels produced by the qat, ejaculation was sometimes painful, but on other occasions more pleasurable than usual. Again, it appears that many variables of health, food intake during the day, personality, mood, and beliefs operate in conjunction with the pharmacological effects of the qat to produce a given result.

In our interview schedule we asked about both positive and negative effects on sexual experience (see Figure 7).

Here, contrary to the nearly unanimous opinion which we elicited in qat sessions and other general conversations, more men claimed positive effects

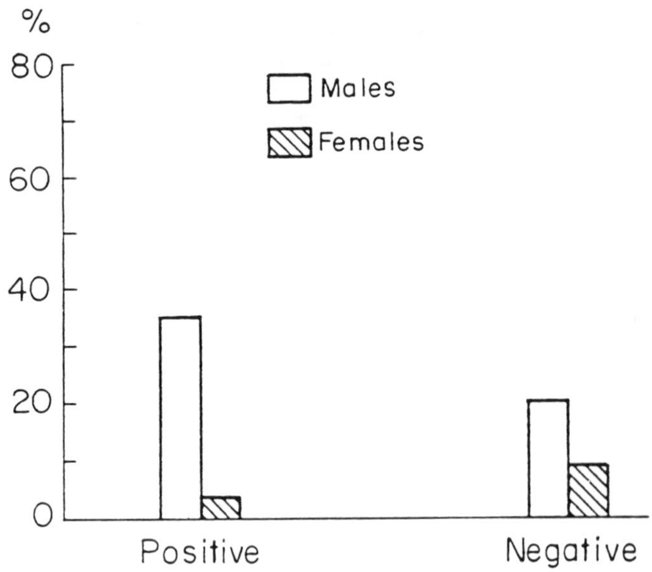

Fig. 7. Reported effects of chewing on sex.

in sexual experience than claimed negative ones. There was also the suggestive finding that only 6.5% of the heavy using males as opposed to nearly 21% of the total reporting male users reported such negative effects on sexual performance. This buttresses the common opinion that heavy users tend to experience less negative side effects than do moderate or irregular users.

ANOREXIA

Another frequently reported result of chewing is "anorexia,"[3] or excessive inhibition of hunger. Some medical authorities have cited this as a cause of malnutrition and gastrointestinal problems in qat chewers (see Chapter IX). People nearly unanimously report that their hunger is diminished after qat, and indeed, a major reason for eating a large meal before chewing is to offset such effects. However, in the opinion of informants, and according to my own experience, hunger inhibition is a temporary condition which is compensated for when the drug effects wear off. Again, Yemenis say that heavy regular users, being accustomed to it, are able to eat as usual.

We may summarize the information in this chapter as follows: The first experiential effects of qat are a gradually developing mild euphoria, i.e., alertness, feelings of contentment, confidence, gregariousness, and the flowing of ideas, called the kayf. Under certain variable conditions such as amount of the drug, food intake, personality and physical condition, this kayf phase occasionally develops into confusion. Ordinarily however, the experience gradually transforms into an "introvert phase" of quiet contemplation in which the stimulation of thought processes continues at a rapid pace while physical and vocal activities diminish. Since this is often accompanied by fatigue, previous problems or pessimistic personality characteristics may transform this phase into a mild temporary lowering of mood.

The post-session effects of qat continue for several hours, and, again depending upon the same variable conditions, many of them are rather negative. Sleep is inhibited, hunger is diminished, sexual desire and performance may positively or negatively be affected and irritability may occur. However, often people experience positive aftermaths such as feeling closer to Allah, more understanding, and a desire to work. When we look at our interview data pertaining to the experiential aspects of qat-use we find consistent male-female differences, with more males generally reporting the experiences. In the eyes of the average chewer the rewarding experiences associated with qat chewing outweigh the unrewarding ones; they are much more regular and predictable.

NOTES

1. This has been translated into folk wisdom, as this anecdote recounted by Scott shows: "When a former British official in the Aden Protectorate was expostulating with an Arab for his too great indulgence, he remarked that the use of the drug would surely have been forbidden, had the prophet ever heard of it. "'No doubt' replied the Arab, but praise be to God, the Prophet never *did* hear of it'" (1942:95).
2. Schopen 1978 contains this as well as a number of other poems about qat. The Arabic originals are included there with his translations into German. This one, like the other English versions here, is my own rendering, an interpretation from several translations I collected.
3. The term "anorexia" connotes a clinical condition of much greater severity than the mild and temporary inhibitions of hunger produced by qat, and in my opinion this term should be dropped unless diagnosed by a physician.
4. The term "kayf" is not restricted to qat experience. It is a more general term for a state of pleasurable well-being. The following ethnocentric quotation from Sir Richard Burton is not in reference to qat but gives the flavor of the wider connotation of the word.

> And this is the Arab's *kayf*. The savoring of animal existence; the passive enjoyment of mere senses; the pleasant languor, the dreamy tranquility, the airy castle-building, which in Asia stand in lieu of the vigorous, intensive, passionate life of Europe. It is the result of a lively, impressible, excitable nature, and exquisite sensibility of nerve; it argues a facility for voluptuousness unknown to northern regions, where happiness is placed in the exertion of mental and physical powers; where *Ernst is das Leben*; where niggard earth commands ceaseless sweat of face, and dump chill air demands perpetual excitement, exercise, or change, or adventure, or dispassion, for want of something better. In the East man wants but rest and shade; upon the banks of a bubbling stream or under the cool shelter of a perfumed tree, he is perfectly happy, smoking a pipe, or sipping a cup of coffee or drinking a glass of sherbet, but above all

things deranging body and mind as little as possible, the trouble of conversations, the displeasures of memory, and the vanity of thought being the most unpleasant interruptions to his *kayf*. No wonder that 'kayf' is a word untranslatable into our mother tongue. (Sir Richard Burton, *Pilgrimage to Al-Medinah and Meccah*. London, 1855, p. 9).

5. Weir is incorrect when she says that there is never any loss of physical or mental control (1985:42).
6. One of Weir's informants described a much more and serious version of ghusan al salam. ". . . if a man finds such a branch among his qat during a party, he gains the right to throw it at a shaykh and demand his daughter in marriage. This demand must be granted if the man escapes from the room before the shaykh can kill him" (1985:156).

CHAPTER VI

THE AGRICULTURE AND ECONOMICS OF QAT

Qat is by far the most important cash crop in North Yemen, even though the entire production is distributed and consumed within the country. Until 1971 qat contributed to the country's balance of trade through exports to Aden (now PDRY). However, since the ban on it in that country instituted in 1971, the popular plant no longer brings in any foreign currency to the Yemen Arab Republic. This is one of the facts martialled by Western economists and some Yemeni government officials in their bitter arguments against the drug. That consumption is totally local is also frequently cited as evidence that qat has little real importance to the economy. The true magnitude of its economic role in the economy has not been understood or appreciated by outside observers.

I want to emphasize the point that qat is uncontestably the dominant factor in the economy of Yemen, despite the fact that statistics on its production and consumption have been omitted from the National Statistical Yearbook almost since it was first published in 1971. The enormous role of qat in the Yemeni economy is shown by the fact that while agriculture as a whole contributed 61.4% of Gross Domestic Product (GDP) of Yemen in 1973—4, the income from the growing and trade of qat was 50% of that total (Ghaibah 1976:4, 28). This means that the qat "industry" contributed roughly 30% of the GDP of Yemen. This overwhelming fact alone should stimulate a great deal more inquiry into the role of this drug in Yemeni economy and society than it has hitherto received.[1]

In spite of the fact that qat must be chewed while it is fresh, even the most remote parts of the Yemen Arab Republic are not entirely without access to it. Excepting only the farthest corners of the Eastern desert, the qat sellers make up a thriving part of all village, town and city markets. A glance at a map of cropping patterns indicates why this can be so (Revri, 1983). Qat is grown in the highland areas above 1200 meters (3,700 feet), that is, all along the central range of the Serat mouintains from the northern border with Saudi Arabia down to the southernmost parts of the country bordering South Yemen (PDRY). The plant is not cultivated on the Tihama plain along the Red Sea, but it is distributed to all points of this region from adjacent mountain production areas. The famous qat regions supplying the Northern Tihama and the port city of Hodeida are Jabel Razih, Mahabisha, Hajja, and Jabel Rayma. The southern part of Tihama is supplied by Rayma, Udain, Dhi Sufal, Jabel Sabr, Sharab, and Jabel Habashi. Qat from these mountain areas also flows eastward to the cities of Sada, Sanaa, Ibb and Taiz.

In the high plains which gradually transform into the great desert areas, qat can be grown at elevations from 2,000 to 2,500 meters. Here, commercially grown qat is found particularly around Rawda, Sanaa, and Amran, as well as Rida and is cultivated as far out into the Eastern desert as Beida. However, because of the periods of cold weather and scarcity of water, only certain microclimates in this eastern region permit it, and qat crops are more uncertain than they are in the mountains.

Qat growing is distributed the length of Yemen, but this should not be misinterpreted, since in every qat region it is mixed in the same fields with other crops. With a few exceptions, the qat trees actually occupy a very small proportion of the available agricultural land.

Reliable information on crop distributions is scarce but the following summary is a fair approximation. The Statistical Yearbook of Yemen last reported figures on qat production in 1972, and in that year it was said to occupy 43,000 hectares, or 2.8% of the cultivated land in the country. In 1976 Dequin estimated it at 8,000 hectares, or 0.6, of the land, while Schopen (1978) estimated 177,800 hectares or 11.75%. Both of these latter figures are so far from the majority of estimates as to be suspect.

Kopp, who made a more careful assessment, estimates 2—3%, (1981), but the most reliable estimate probably was made by Raman Revri. Basing his analysis on Kopp's data supplemented with aerial photographs and "on the spot" sampling in most major qat growing areas, he concluded that approximately 83,764 hectares or 4.4% of the total cropping area of Yemen is given over to qat cultivation. He also pointed out that only 14.1% of the entire country can be cultivated and cautioned that the area covered by qat is not constant and that cultivation seems to be increasing in many areas (1983:8—15).

I will later discuss the question of whether and how qat competes for land with other crops; here I only want to make the point that, according to the best estimates, it probably does not yet occupy more than 5% of the cultivated area of North Yemen. The food cereals, sorghum, millet, barley, wheat and maize occupy from 85% to 90% of the cultivated areas of the country, while the remaining 5% to 10% are planted in fruits, legumes, vegetables, dates, cotton, sesame and tobacco. Coffee at approximately 1.6% of the growing area, and cotton also at 1.6%, are the most important export crops (Revri 1982:14).

This estimate of the extensiveness of qat production should not obscure the fact that in some areas the plant occupies a much higher percentage of the usable land than in others. Its density depends on such factors as microclimate, market availability, and the kinds of other crops grown in the area. A few examples will make this point.

Weir estimates that in 1980, 30% of the cultivable land in Jabel Razih was given over to qat production. This was an increase of some 15% since 1977, when she first visited there (1983:5). In Haraz, another qat producing region, Gerholm reports that in 1973 about 20% of the land was devoted to qat and coffee, with most of it in qat (1977:53). In Sanaa Province 5% of the area is planted with qat (Sergent and Lewcock 1983:18; Revri 1983:113). However, in such small but intensive qat growing Sanani districts as Wadi Dahr and Dula an 80% estimate for qat is conservative.

Swanson has provided us with a fine comparison which illustrates how local climatic variations encourage of inhibit the production of qat. He worked in an area to the North and East of Ibb, an area of high labor migration due to difficult agricultural conditions. Village "A" at between 2,000 and 2,500 meters is within the heaviest rain belt in Yemen, but has only a few fields which are protected enough from frost to allow qat cultivation, and it is the only cash crop. Here, during the planting season and at the end of the dry season, most of the small amount of irrigation water which can be pumped is channeled to Village A's few fields of shrub-type qat.

Village B, at 1,950 meters, is in a dryer zone, and because of its exposure, most of its fields are unpredictably but rather commonly hit with ground frost. "Consequently, qat is only planted in irrigated fields with poor soils. By following this strategy the peasant takes a chance on providing a relatively profitable qat crop on land that would otherwise produce a poor grain crop" (Swanson 1979:46).

Village C is located in a broad high valley (2,000—2,500 meters) in an even dryer zone than Village B. However, because it is protected from the cold winter wind by a ridge of hills, this village has always grown qat, and because water is now regularly available from newly purchased power driven pumps, much more qat can be produced than before. It also produces more than Villages A and B, both of which have better natural rainfall. Swanson speculates that the consequent prosperity of Village C from qat has enabled the men of this village to remain at home rather than having to migrate as do higher proportions of those from Villages A and B (*Ibid.*:75).

The ecological requirements of the qat plant are fairly flexible. For example, it is cultivated in a variety of differing climates and soil conditions in the countries around the Red Sea and throughout East Africa. After examination of the available data on the climates of these regions, Revri concluded that it is most successfully cultivated between the altitudes of 1200 to 2400 meters (3500—8000 feet) above sea level (1983:18). This is not to claim that qat does not grow at both lower and higher elevations; it is grown in house gardens by Yemeni Jews in Israel (personal communications S. D. Goitein, Michelle Safa), and it is found as an ornamental shrub in the states of California and Florida in the U.S.A. However, there is reason to believe that the potencies of the alkaloids may be considerably reduced in qat grown at these lower elevations, and this agrees with the opinions of the farmers in Yemen. They would farm it at lower altitudes if decent quality plants could be produced there.

With such altitude requirements, further limitations on successful qat cultivation are imposed by temperatures, water requirements and soil qualities. Revri's study determined that when the mean average temperature is below 17 degrees C. growth is inhibited, and at least 19 degrees C. is necessary for satisfactory cultivation. Experimental watering as well as weather data showed that below 400 mm of precipitation and above 800 mm per year results in marked retardation of qat growth. The optimum is around 600 mm per year. Local microecological conditions, of course, modify actual pratice, and as Revri points out:

> In the Yemen Arab Republic outside of the Serat Mountain range [where most of the qat is grown] the climate is marginal and qat plants survive only if planted in particularly farmable sites which are frost protected, or where irrigation and adequate means for the retention of water are provided. Especially on the Central Highlands, i.e., the plateau of Sanaa, Rida, irrigation is essential . . . For economical qat production, cultivators in the Central Highlands irrigate either by lift irrigation or by rain harvesting (1983:20).

Other important factors of climate are the relative humidity and the amount of irradiation. In Yemen qat has been shown to tolerate fairly extreme variations of daily atmospheric moisture (between 13% and 85%). However, where the relative humidity, and high temperatures remain constant over considerable periods of time, qat plants are damaged by fungi. This is a major reason why it cannot be cultivated on the Tihama plain, and is a reason for crop damage in some of the more humid Western regions of the Serat mountain chain (*Ibid.*:20).

In terms of irradiation, it appears that equatorial conditions (equal day and night lengths) are most favorable for qat growth, and that daily duration of sunlight may be as low as 6 hours during rainy and dust seasons (*Ibid.*:20).

The soils which will support qat cultivation are immensely varied and even in Yemen this plant is farmed on volcanic soils, sandstone and limestone soils, which vary texturally from loam to clay (*Ibid.*:25—27). These soils also vary considerably in fertility. Revri comments that: "In most cases, qat soils are only moderately fertile. They are generally low in nitrogen (0.05—0.08%) and their total content of bases, together with available phosphorous (P_2O_5) is extremely variable" (*Ibid.*:27). He also cites a number of studies showing variations in the acidity factor, e.g., qat soils may vary from being slightly alkaline, as in Yemen, to highly alkaline ones in other regions (*Ibid.*:27). Two other soil characteristics which are important to the growth and cultivation of this plant are that it is not dependent on soils rich in mineral nitrogen, and that soils upon which it flourishes are very low in concentrations of salt and toxic elements like heavy metals (*Ibid.*:29).

We can generalize then that the qat plant is a very adaptable and hardy one. Even in the climatic zones which seem necessary to produce a level of alkaloids acceptable to chewers it is more adaptable than many other crops, most importantly, coffee. This flexibility, as well as the fact that it takes up little space for the amount of cash yield that it brings, are among the features which make qat so attractive to the Yemeni farmer.

THE CULTIVATION OF QAT

There are some variations in the planting, care, and harvesting of qat, and these primarily relate to differences imposed by differing ecological zones. I cannot discuss them all here, but some contrasting examples will illustrate the general situation.

In the mountain and upland regions of Yemen, qat is planted primarily, along with other crops, on terraces which ascend the steep slopes. However, it is also increasingly being planted in enclosed plots or "orchards" out on the flat high plains along the eastern flanks of the mountains, the region called the Central Highlands. In favored areas where irrigation from natural springs is possible, considerable control can be exercised over the timing of all aspects of qat cultivation. However, even where the amount of rainfall is marginal, the Yemenis have devised ingenious channelling systems to capture rain water and carry it to the qat fields. There are also some places, such as out on the high eastern plains, where modern power pumps have enabled farmers to grow qat where it was not possible before.

Well before actual planting the Yemenis plow or break up the earth by hand with choppers (*mafris* or *magrafa*) in the area where they intend to plant. Sometimes they further prepare the land by sowing beans or legumes in the year prior to planting qat, a practice which is said to have a beneficial effect. The time of planting is also important because the young qat plants must have a fairly continuous supply of moisture during the early months, while a tap root is growing. Therefore, in most areas planting is done just after the beginning of one of the rainy seasons, usually the first "small" one in March through April.

Productive qat cannot be propagated by seeds. It is often said in the literature that cuttings are used for propagation of qat (e.g., Getahun and Krikorian, 1973), but in Yemen cuttings are only occasionally used for this purpose in the Southern Highlands of Hujjariyya. The principal method is to replant suckers, the shoots which have developed around the based of mature plants.

Oftentimes too, the suckers are stripped of leaves before planting. Depending upon soil and other local conditions, qat plants need varying amounts of space between them, but on the average they are given from about 2 to 4 square meters each. Important factors in spacing decisions are frost, (which necessitates closer spacing), fertility, pruning practices and ideas of weed control (densely planted qat needs less weeding). Three or four of these shoots are placed at a 45 degree angle in a hole at a depth of around 8—10 inches. If it is available, some animal dung is usually put into the hole.

Sometimes qat plants are double planted; the spaces between the rows are made half as wide. Then after several years every other tree is removed. The farmers claim that by this method they can increase the relatively low yields of the first few years by as much as 50% to 60% (Revri, 1983:63).

It is important to note that farmers in different parts of Yemen use differing systems of measurement for their fields. In most of the country from Sanaa to the north the unit of measurement is most often called a *libna*, while to the south the term *gasaba* is generally used. However, these units vary in actual size from locality to locality, and an unwary inquirer can become very confused. Furthermore, to calculate the size of these units the traditional measuring unit, the *dhira al Hadi* is still in use. This is said to have been established by Imam Hadi, the first Imam of the Zaydis, who decreed that the distance between his elbow and finger tips was to be the standard for all measurements.

A Sanani libna is one dhira (about 1/2 meter) square, while a libna in Haraz or in the north may be 10 or 16 dhira (approximately 5 or 8 meters square) depending upon local usage. The same situation applies in the South where around Taiz one qasaba equals 10 dhira, though in Iryan one qasaba equals 16 dhira, etc. In the eastern desert around Beida, are found units called *habl* (20 dhira or 10 square meters) or *matrah* (16 dhira). The matrah, equalling 16 dhira, is also found in Utmah. In areas north and east of Ibb the word *shakla* connotes a piece of land approximately 18.5 feet on a side (Swanson 1979:71). Many other terms and local variations exist, and since local profits are calculated according to these units it is obviously very important for researchers to understand the local terminologies.

After the qat shoots have been planted they require considerable care, and they do not begin to yield meaningful harvests for about 3 years. However, there are two major forms of yielding qat plants in Yemen, and they are quite different in many ways. In the mountainous regions which constitute most of the qat growing areas of the country the major form is the slender white tree which may be as much as 100 years old. When they reach about 10 years of age these trees are considered to be producing at their optimum. As one travels through the country, plots and fields of such trees of all ages can be seen.

The other form of qat is the small shrub, which is found mostly in the Eastern plains, in the Wadi Bana, and in areas of the Western mountains overlooking the Tihama. The colder climate marked by frequent frosts in the Eastern regions, does not allow qat trees to develop fully, and the shrubs here only obtain heights of 4 or 5 feet before they must be pruned down to the ground level at intervals of 2 or 3 years. Thus, the shrub form of the qat plant must be considered ecologically marginal, and this is reflected in the fact that none of the "premier" quality qats of Yemen come from these regions.

As I have pointed out repeatedly, Catha edulis is a hardy plant, at least in comparison with coffee and the grains with which it competes on the terraces of Yemen. It does not require fertilizer even though it removes considerable amounts of plant nutrients from the soil. Revri points out that Yemenis are distrustful of mineral fertilizers, feeling that they can harm their crops. Some farmers occasionally fertilize with animal dung or night soil, but he could not find any symptoms of deficiency in the qat plants he studied which could be attributed to the lack of mineral elements in the soil.

> Most likely, due to its extensive root system, qat can draw its nutrients from large volumes of soil and as a result it can perform reasonably well on poor soils, where many other perennial crops fail to do so. Moreover, growth of qat plants, compared with others (e.g., tea, coffee) is extremely slow (1983:66).

Providing sufficient moisture for the qat is the biggest maintenance problem for the Yemeni farmer, although in this respect too, it is less of a problem than for any other major crop. The two rainy seasons, in early spring and later summer usually provide the optimum 600—800 mm of precipitation, and even in marginal regions at least the minimal 200—1000 mm is provided. Where annual precipitation is under 400 mm the farmers employ methods of catching rainwater and conducting it to the plants by furrows, or more recently, by underground pipes. Farmers in the more fortunate areas, with perennial springs and/or wells, (Wadi Dahr, Jabel Sabr, Al Ahjur, etc.) can exercise considerable control over plant growth and can easily protect against unforeseen delays in rain. However, in many areas, such as throughout Hujjariyya in the South, Jabal Rayma in the West, and on the Sanaa plain, newly planted shoots must at first be carefully nurtured by hand carried water to each plant, or transporting it to them on the backs of animals.

For example, one or two *tanakas* (20 liter tins) of water must be brought to each two or three young plants every day or two until there is sufficient rain. In the autumn this must be repeated more sparingly for all plants when they get too dry. In some areas another hand irrigation must be made in February every fourth year, i.e., after a tree has been harvested for 3 years. This time all the leaves are stripped from each tree after the watering, preparing them for another 3 year cycle of growth and harvesting.

As noted earlier, qat is rarely the only crop planted in a given field or on a given terrace. Interplanting is the rule, and almost all Yemeni crops can somewhere be seen interplanted with qat plants. For instance, in the far north at Jabel Razih, qat is interspersed with legumes, peaches, papaya, limes, citrus and bananas (Weir 1983:3). On the Central Highlands, such as at Dula, Wadi Dahr, and Bani Hushaysh, most farmers interplant grapes, quinces, apricots, peaches and pomegranates with the qat. In the mountains and southern uplands, one finds also sorghum, alfalfa, maize and lentils. The Yemenis believe that such mixing helps to inhibit weeds and protects against erosion (Revri 1983:70).

Apart from considerations of water and fertilizer, maintenance of the qat crop requires intensive hoeing for weed control and soil aeration. Each year the young plants must be hoed three or four times, and even when trees are mature they need two hoeings. This must be done assiduously to avoid the immediate stunting and the loss of succulent leaves which result from neglect.

The hoeing of the mature plants is done just after the first heavy showers of each rainy season, that is, sometime in March or April, and in July or August. The immature plants must be hoed in May and October before they enter the dormancy which coincides with the arid periods between rainy seasons. No pruning is done, apart from the harvesting of the leaves, though occasionally old suckers which are not needed for planting are removed.

The other important care and maintenance problem is the control of pests and plant diseases. In the past Yemeni farmers have not paid much attention to protection from these, largely because qat is apparently highly resistant. I heard a story from several farmers of how plagues of locusts periodically decimate virtually all food crops in Yemen and nearby countries, yet qat remains untouched! Some insects particularly tiny green leaf hoppers (identified as *empoasca sp.*) are even considered by the farmers to be completely beneficial. Nevertheless, there are several types of fungi which discolor the leaves in some regions, as well as some yet unidentified insect pests which inhibit growth (Revri 1983:72—73).

These pests have not gone unnoticed by the Yemenis, and in some areas an ancient method of control for them is still in use. For instance, in Wadi Dahr farmers coat the plants with a fine powdery dust called *turab*. Turab is literally a generic word for "dust" in Arabic, but in the Wadi it refers to an especially fine powder which occurs naturally only in certain areas. It must be purchased and transported to the qat gardens and terraces. This dust apparently contains some sulphur (Schopen 1978:74) and this may partially account for whatever effectiveness it has as an insecticide.

In 1975 the turab was dusted over the qat plants two or three times during a season in Wadi Dahr: once in December, before the first irrigation, and once or twice more at later intervals before April. This is an added expense for the Wadi farmer. At that time a pickup truckload of turab cost 140 rials, a price not considered excessive since, that amount would dust about 1500 Sanani libnas of qat, an area of about 1000 square meters.

The resistance to the use of commercial pesticides and fungicides on qat is not entirely due to ignorance, lack of availability, or preference for traditional methods, however. There is a very real fear that such chemicals will be harmful to the users, and thus ultimately damage the lucrative business. This is particularly threatening with a product like qat which goes directly from the fields to the users mouths, with no processing in between. It is thus fortunate that the actual threat posed by pests of various kinds has been relatively small.

As the cultivation of qat has spread, however, the qat plant has encountered more entomological enemies. Especially in Haraz, Hajja, and parts of Ibb and Taiz provinces chemical insecticides are in limited use. Sometimes the farmers are not aware of the exact composition, or of the health consequences of these. However, the potentially negative effects of insecticides are mitigated because the rain sometimes cleans the leaves before marketing, and also, according to agricultural experts I spoke to, the potency life of the DDT in most of the insecticides is only a few weeks. In this case, the poison becomes inactive long before it gets to the chewer. Further ameliorating checks are the customary careful cleaning of each leaf, a part of the ritual of chewing, and the fact that chemically treated qat is often shunned by the buyer because of its moldy or bitter taste. Nevertheless, the long-term effects of this practicc are potentially very harmful to health.

With a crop as valuable and as easily harvested as qat, there is a temptation to thievery, and in the richer qat areas an important aspect of maintenance is protecting the fields. Small stone buildings are frequently erected in central places, and a guard is posted there with a rifle or AK47 machine gun. Farmers usually prefer to guard their own fields and family members often rotate in this activity. Yemeni children as young as nine or ten are trained to fire weapons and sometimes are put in charge of guarding the qat. In many areas the need for guards has created a new full or part-time occupation for men. Of course, part of the pay for this job is an ample supply of qat during and after working hours.

In some regions the theft of qat has been integrated into tribal rivalries, and stealing it from rival tribes is considered a daring and meritorious act. In areas such as Hada, near Dhamar, and parts of Wadi Bana, for example, bringing back a day's supply of qat from a field owned by members of a rival tribe is very risky. All fields are guarded by men and boys who are expert shots, and who shoot to kill. Many raiding youths of these tribes are regularly executed or wounded while attempting to bring back a few robtas of the valuable drug.

In many areas stolen qat is sold in the market, but, as was the case with the Plains Indians, whose glory was counting coup by touching a fallen warrior or stealing a horse, the prestige from a risky death for a bunch of qat is the important thing. It is even said that if a person is killed in a qat field at night it is not required that the killer pay the *diya*, or blood money, to the tribe of family of the victims. The regions where these practices occur are not old qat growing areas. The drug was only introduced recently to the common people here, though the Shaykhs have long used it, and have customarily distributed it to gatherings on special holidays or occasions.

It is still regarded as shameful for women to chew in this eastern region, which is also the region of the tough tribesmen whom Imam Ahmad selected in 1948 to carry out the "siege of Sanaa" during the recent civil war. These tribes were allowed to sack the city. Later, the Imam asked them to restore the confiscated goods but only a small portion of the loot was ever returned to the Sananis. When qat was introduced into this area it was simply incorporated as another element in the local system if raiding for prestige and honor.

As the value of qat has increased, protection of the fields has everywhere become a growing problem. A considerable percentage of the violent deaths in the country result from theft, and, in the absence of efficient police forces, guarding the fields has become one of the significant costs of the qat farmer.

When a qat thief is apprehended in most areas he is punished, but the penalty is usually not severe. For example, in the Sanaa area in the mid-seventies he would be thrown into prison for from 3 days to a week and made to pay a fine of 50 rials. However, if he was shot, as often happens to those stealing at night, he was regarded to have gotten what he deserved and no charges could be brought.

Some farmers of Jabel Sabr have devised their own unique method of deterring thieves from nocturnal stealing. They sometimes spray the poisonous milky juice from the fruit of the local *usr* tree. When the treated qat leaves are chewed the chewer experiences a violent stomach ache and bleeding gums. Since this juice leaves small white spots on the qat leaves, wary buyers shy away from purchasing it and sellers of such marked qat are strongly suspect (Schopen 1979:75).

HARVESTING

The harvesting of qat can begin when the trees or shrubs are 4 or 5 years old. If the plants remain in good condition they may then yield for at least 50 years. The way it is harvested varies considerably according to whether it is of the tree of shrub variety, and according to local conditions, such as rainfall, whether it is perennially irrigated, and threats of frost. Also because harvesting is accomplished by breaking off many branches from the plant, the shock to the plant from picking is considerable. Thus, in most areas of the North every other year is a poor harvest because of this, and trees often must be left to recover for 2 years. In the South picking is more systematically staggered than in the North. For example, on Jabel Sabr the qat trees are allowed to rest for 2 years after their year of harvest.

A very important feature of growing qat, one which makes it very attractive to farmers, is that the harvesting season is so lengthy. No other crop in Yemen can compare in this regard. The greatest amounts of qat are harvested during the latter part of the two rainy seasons, which usually occur in April and May and during July and August. Farmers do not harvest their crop all in one short harvest season, but pick from a few plants at a time. The important point is that the picking goes on for months. In the areas of tree-type qat, rarely is all the ripe qat on a given tree picked on any one day. This is partly because not all branches are ready or ripe simultaneously, and partly because some branches are specifically saved for later harvesting, for example during the beginning of the next rainy season.

It will be remembered that qat must be chewed while fresh, it cannot be stored, and since many producers bring their product to market on any given day, it makes utmost sense to harvest relatively small amounts on any particular day. This means that even the largest growers do not realize the major portions of their profits during any short harvest period; returns are spread over many months.

Usually the picking is done in the morning, for it must reach the market in the freshest possible condition. If the trees are old and tall the picker climbs up into them and breaks off branches on one side, saving the other side for the next harvest. These branches are thrown down to a helper, who divides them into bunches (robtas), amounts appropriate for one session's chewing by one person. Around Sanaa, e.g., Wadi Dahr and Dula, these robtas (also called *marbata*) are from half a meter to 1 meter long, while those from other areas are shorter, varying between 10 to 50 centimeters. As one moves through the markets of larger towns, it is fairly easy to pick out the qat whose quality is within one's price range by the size and shape of the bundles. For example, those from Bani Hushaysh (hushayshi), Haraz (harazi) and Rawda (rawdi) average from 30 to 35 centimeters in length, while bundles coming from the far north, (such as sawti and hajaji) are only 10 to 20 centimeters, and do not include the branches, as the longer varieties do. Moving down the scale from long to shorter bundles, the qualities and prices drop accordingly. However, the prices in each area are determined by season, the part of the tree from which the leaves come, and the reputation of the area. Near the end of the rainy seasons, prices are much lower overall because the market is flooded with rain-fed qat.

A few examples will indicate how some of the variables of quality and price operate. Early in August 1976, near the midpoint of the rainy season, in Sanaa there were three kinds of baladi qat in the market from Wadi Dahr, Dula, and other nearby places such as Bani Hushaysh. The best variety, known as *gifal* (sometimes called ra'is), came from the top parts of the trees. The robtas of gifal were 60 centimeters to one meter long and were priced at around one hundred rials apiece. The second best grade was called *awaradh*, because it was picked from the middle part of the tree. The branches of this quality were around 35 to 50 centimeters and the robtas were priced at twenty-five to fifty rials. The third best type of baladi in the market was *al'afal* or *sufal*, names indicating that it came from the lower part of the tree, that part "nearest the ground." It cost the buyer only eight to fifteen rials per robta, and the robtas were much shorter (around 25 to 50 centimeters).

Of course, these were not the only types in the Sanaa market. There were also some hajaji from Hajja, and even some sellers with taizi from Taiz. Being from more distant regions, among these types the kinds of fine discriminations applied to local varieties were not made. At other times of the year, e.g., in spring, one finds in the Sanaa market the sawti, hoshayshi, harazi, etc., which I spoke of earlier.

One of the oldest qat-producing areas in Yemen is Jabel Sabr, the mountain behind Taiz. Nearly all the early travelers' accounts from Yemen mention the qat from this mountain, even if they neglect to speak of it elsewhere. The people of Jabel Sabr are fortunate to have all-year springs which supply water for irrigation, and they use a carefully staggered system of planting and cutting. Like the farmers of Wadi Dahr and Dula near Sanaa, and others who have perennial irrigation, the Sabris are able to exercise much more control over harvesting and marketing than do the growers in rain-fed areas. As I mentioned earlier the people of the mountain have found that for best results they can harvest their trees only one year out of three. Any Sabri farmer, therefore has his qat orchard divided into three or four sections, one of which is being harvested each year. Also, within the harvest year three "cuttings" are made, during each of three periods of two or three months each.

The first cutting, called *mubarrah*, is made in the period from January to March, and qat of this cutting is called by the same name in the market. The merchants trim off all the lower and coarse leaves, leaving only the upper tender portions on the long branch robtas. Mubarrah is regarded as the most choice cutting, and if it also comes from one of the best areas of soil and water of Jabel Sabr, (e.g., a place called Hadenan), it is called *jiddi* (grandmother) or *hadnani*, and brings the highest prices. In 1975 jiddi was bringing around one hundred rials a robta for that from the upper branches. Hadnani qat can be either "red" or "white" and was regarded as the finest qat of the southern region. Its taste is sweet, its kayf is pleasurable and its side-effects negligible.

Somewhere between March and June, the second or *mathani* cutting is made on Jabel Sabr. It is of lesser quality and the harvest is shorter. Finally, during the summer there is the *mathani-mathani* or third cutting, which is of even poorer quality. It is very cheap because it competes in the market with all the rain-fed qat coming in from the surrounding areas at this time.

Since there are usually a number of grades of qat in the market at any given time, most people feel that they can afford to chew. In the Taiz market on February 18, 1975 (near end of dry season), we found jiddi as well as mubarrah from other areas, and short robtas of awaradh (middle of tree) from Misra. There were also *kalowet* and *gulubi* (hearts), both which are sold in small cheap sacks (mandil) of leaves only, and finally bundles of jashani and sharabi. Both of these are "strong" and cheap varieties from Dhi Sufal and Sharab, respectively.[2]

In the region of the town of Ibb, the best qat comes from Bilad Sharr and Bahrian on the road to Udayn, but *bukhari* from Bukhar is also highly regarded. While, with the exception of bukhari, these varieties do not approach the reputation of qat from al-Wadi in Sanaa, or the hadnani from Taiz, the best types from Ibb are also irrigated from wells and considered quite good. They were bringing up to fifty rials a robta in the seasons August to November at the time of the study. These varieties also go through several cuttings, called *samin, mabruh, mathani*, and *jidda*.

In Ibb during the summer several other lesser types are sold which are reputed not to kayf at all, or rarely. These are *waqash* from nearby Jibla, *subhani* from Subhan, *baladi* from Baadan, *mu'ali* from Naga Ajuma'i, *ja'ashani* from Dhi Sufal, and *jabalayni* from Jabalayn. These inferior grades were all selling from three to fifty rials a robta in the Ibb market at various seasons of the year. While the "white" varieties are generally regarded as the best in the Ibb area, the red from the irrigated region of Bahrian is considered quite good. The reds from Bokhar and Dhi Sufal, on the other hand, are very strong and inferior (Messick: personal communication).

Throughout Yemen the robta usually constitutes the minimum unit which is chewed by an individual at one sitting, but this term certainly does not connote a standardized quantity. In its amount of chewable leaves the robta varies by region and by season. For example in the dry season, when qat is harder to get, the robta tends to diminish in size. In addition to the word robta, a term understood everywhere, there are a number of other terms in use, many of them current only in particular regions. A few examples will suffice to illustrate this local variation.

Up until very recently when synthetic products from the outer world began to enter Yemen, most robtas of qat were wrapped in grasses (*alaf*), millet leaves, or the leaves of fragrant plants called *uthrub* to preserve their freshness. Because of the relatively long trek to market necessitated by animal or foot transportation, the bundles were individually wrapped in the field. This form of native packaging is still found in remote areas of the mountains and in the southern uplands. However, with the advent of automobile and motorcycle transportation and the spread of roads, the robtas of qat are now usually tied in the field, packed into large gunny sacks (*shuqal*) and brought to market. Particularly in the markets of the larger cities and towns, the robtas are displayed openly in the sellers stalls and they are wrapped for the buyer in colored sheet plastic (*mashama blastik*) when the sale has been finalized.

In the Sanaa market as well as in those of other large northern towns, the sawti qat which comes in from late spring through July, is shipped distances of several hundred kilometers, often initially being taken from the fields by foot or donkey to a location where a pickup truck may load it for the trip to the market. The farmers of these northern mountains have devised their own excellent method of preservation and shipping, a method not yet superceded by modern technology. Here, the most succulent qat leaves are carefully removed from their branches and tied in small robtas about 12—15 centimeters long and 8 centimeters thick, and then carefully placed in hollow half banana stems some 60 to 80 centimeters long. These packages are then each closed with another half stem. This makes an 80 centimeter cylinder called a *guruf* in the local are, and *qarn* (horn) in Sanaa. This native container holds from 6 to 12 of these condensed robtas, and preserves them admirably. In the northern region of Jabel Razih, near the Saudi Arabian border, banana stems for this purpose constitute an important secondary crop for some farmers (Weir, 1983).

In other areas another larger container (*barkas*), which holds 10 to 30 robtas, is made of the succulent grasses spoken of earlier. In the Sanani the large expensive bundles coming from Wadi Dahr or Dula are named "marbata" to distinguish them from the smaller robtas from other areas.

The qat sellers of the Taiz area have their own terminology of qat packaging. The shorter robtas are often individually called *zugba* or *kanbala*, while bundles of two or three of these are termed *halqa*. The longer robtas, such as the precious jiddi are termed *aqara* in Taiz while a bundle of such long robtas is called a *hizma*. Small plastic sacks of loose qat leaves, generally of inferior quality, are called mandil.

In Ibb, the word robta is common for the smallest tied unit, but units of 4 of these are sold as *mashbat* (or *marbat*) while in turn four mashbat constitute a *magwat*. Larger sacks or bundles of 2090 mashbat are called a *bandal* (Messick, personal communication), as they are throughout Hujjariyya. On Jabel Rayma and generally in the mountains south and east of Hodeida, the robta is called *zurba*; 2 zurba are a *zawj* or *jamiya*, 4 zurba equal a *dhumuma*, and 8 zurba connstitute 1 *shikla* (Swagman, personal communication).

There are many other local terms in other parts of Yemen. The variety of names, along with the lack of standardization in packaging of qat, again reflects the extreme regional isolation from which North Yemen is only now emerging.

DISTRIBUTION AND PROFITABILITY

We now turn to the difficult questions of profitability and distribution of qat in Yemen. It is necessary to explore some of the vexing questions of motivation. Why do Yemeni farmers continue to expand qat production? Why does the government allow it? How do profits from qat compare with those from other crops? Is qat replacing the famous Yemeni coffee, etc.?

The first and most obvious generalization one can make with regard to such questions is that qat is an extremely profitable product at all levels, to the farmer, the distributor, and the merchant. The taxes upon it constitute an important source of revenue to the government too.

I have mentioned the frequent argument that since qat is no longer exported from Yemen, it is no longer bringing any foreign currency into the country, and if this is the case, its production should be curtailed. This macro-economic argument against qat is made quite separately from the other anti-qat arguments regarding purported negative health effects, and negative impacts on family budgets.

The Yemeni farmers, however, can see no merit in such abstract conceptions. In their view only two main avenues are available for achieving some modicum of financial freedom: migration to the Gulf, Saudi Arabia or America in search of lucrative job opportunities, or growing some qat on their land. It is clear to all that ownership of even a small amount of land in a qat growing area can furnish significant income within the space of a few years. No other crop in Yemen can hope to match the income-producing properties of qat. This has been true for many years, but with the influx of money to the country from emigrees, and from the many international development projects in the country, the use of qat has increased rapidly and it is now used in many more areas than even before. Thus, increasing demand has helped to fuel spiraling prices for the drug as well as stimulating its production.

As far back as 1965—1969, that is at the end of the decade of civil war in the country, the relative net return to the farmer on qat in Hujjariyya was estimated at 10,000 rials per *feddan* (a unit slightly larger than an acre), as opposed to 416 rials per feddan for the main grains of sorghum and millet. This is a difference of 2300% (Yacoub and Akil, 1971). Of course, most qat farmers own far less than a feddan, and a major part of its popularity with small land holders stems from the fact that large amounts of land are not necessary. A plot with a few trees can yield a significant increase in income. Small amounts of the plant can do the same for the small trader, who basically needs very little capital outlay to go into business. Gerholm, points out that in Haraz "... it provides a modest income to a great many townsmen" (1972:10). This is true in many regions of Yemen.

How profitable is qat for the farmer and how does growing it compare with other crops in the provision of income? There is great variability in this matter by season, by area, type of qat, and differing expenses of production, but there are data which allow some reasonable estimates of profitability, particularly in comparison with other crops.

Fears of greater taxation, community jealousy, and other motivations, make it difficult to get accurate figures on just how much revenue given families and individuals derive from growing or trading qat (or, in fact, on any other matter of income). Nevertheless, we do have some ideas from a number of our interviews and from other sources. For example, it was reported to me by what I regard as reliable informants that in 1975, three or four extended families (*bayts*) in Wadi Dahr each sold more than 200,000 rials ($43,956) worth of qat. From all information I collected this would be a very conservative figure.

The actual sales may have been five times that amount. However, this income also would be reduced by costs of production and taxes (together estimated at between 30 and 50%). In addition, profits would be variously divided among the nuclear families making up each bayt. Nevertheless, qat is not the only source of income in the Wadi, and these families must be seen as relatively rich by Yemeni standards.

The cultivable acreage of Wadi Dahr is not extensive. The farms are small, but the area is blessed with sufficient water from springs and pumps, and qat and fruit cultivation are intense. As with farming anywhere, considerable variations in profits occur from year to year; there are occasional frosts or floods, and plots vary in profitability according to age of trees, soil, and local temperatures.

In the Wadi it was estimated that in 1975—6 a 50 meter sq. plot (100 libnas) with trees 10 or more years old yielded a gross of between 1000 and 2000 rials (YR), and a few very old stands of trees could each gross as much as 10,000 rials ($2,198). On the other hand, I was shown one plot of 100 libnas containing 18 trees approximately 20 years old which was said to have yielded only 1500 rials ($329.67) during the preceding year, after production costs and taxes were deducted. Since these trees can be harvested only every second year, the profit would have been approximately 750 rials ($164.83) per year from this plot. The profit per hectare would be 150,000 rials ($32,967).

With such estimates in mind, we can assess the following statement by Obermeyer regarding a qat farmer form Wadi Dahr whom he interviewed in 1972:

> On the basis of a rough estimate of this farmer's land and a tree count, the amount of qat that he says he produces and his angry statement concerning how much qat tax he paid to the government last year (which is assessed as 10% of the estimated profits from his plantation) I calculated his annual income to the amount of $26,000.00! Since this figure seemed incredible to me I checked its plausibility with Yemeni friends and informants as well as with government officers and United Nations experts. Not one person among them was surprised and the U.N. agricultural expert in the Taiz area thought this was probably an accurate calculation (1973:17).

The estimates given earlier show that this conclusion is certainly within the realm of possibility, particularly if we make the reasonable assumption that this was a plantation of 3 or 4 hectares of old qat trees. This would be one of the larger and wealthier families in the Wadi, since most families there are much smaller land holders. For instance, I was also shown a 40 year old plot of 250 libnas which was said to bring in 2000 rials ($440.00)/year, and a 500 libna patch (17.2% of an acre) which brings in only about 1200 rials ($264.00)/year. The production of this plot was said to be lower becuase it also contains a number of apricot and quince trees. Wadi Dahr is rather atypical in that it produces some of the most expensive qat in Yemen, and that its farms are relatively small in area. Some other examples will enhance understanding of the range of the profitability of qat of Yemeni farmers.

Rida is a large village out on the high plains to the east of the city of Dhamar. Abdullah, a relatively wealthy farmer of that region owns about 200 matrahs of land (matrah = 16 dhira, or 64 square meters) but at the time only 500 dhira were under cultivation. He has 200 matrahs in durra, 150 in wheat, 80 in alfalfa, and 70 in qat. He also has a few trees each of peaches, pomegranates, figs, apples and quinces. Abdullah's qat is divided into two plots of 35 matrahs (2240 sq. meters or 22.4% of a hectare) which he alternately harvests every other year. Since rain is unreliable in this region, he

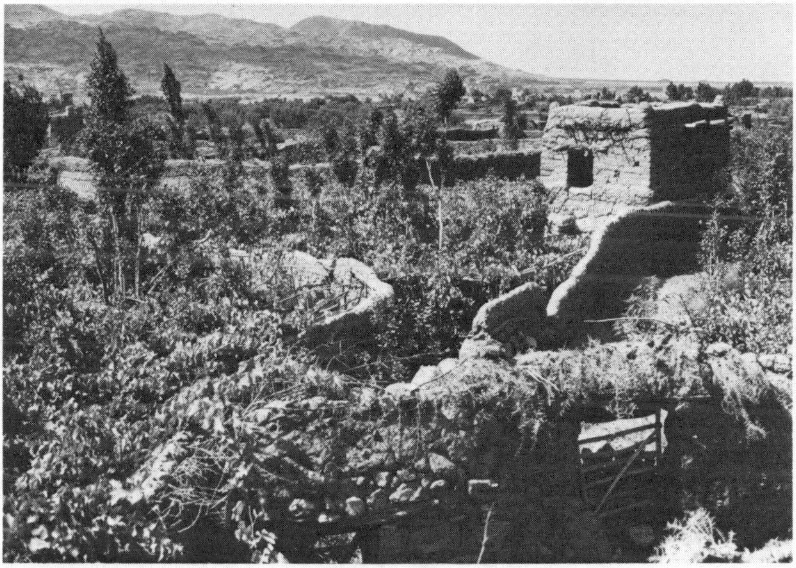

Qat and grape orchard with guard house in Wadi Dahr

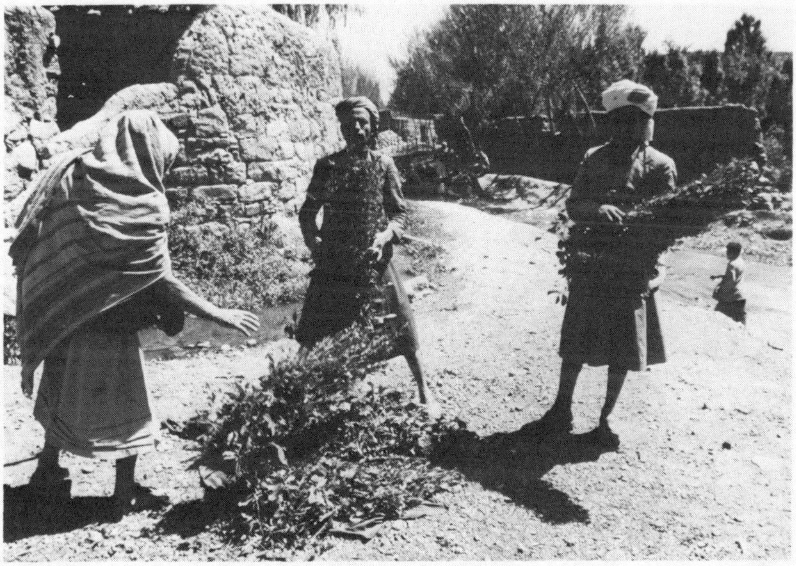

Preparing qat for market in Wadi Dahr

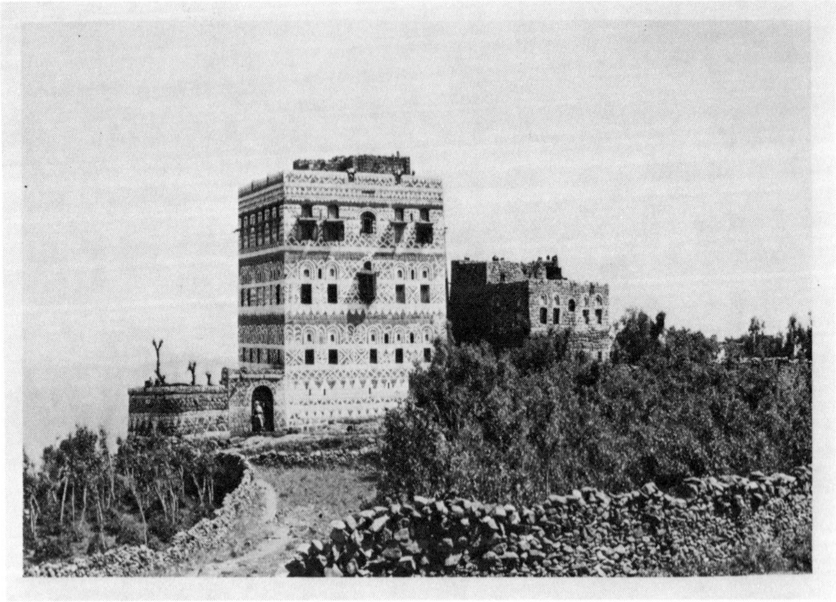

Shaykh's house with qat orchard in Shemran

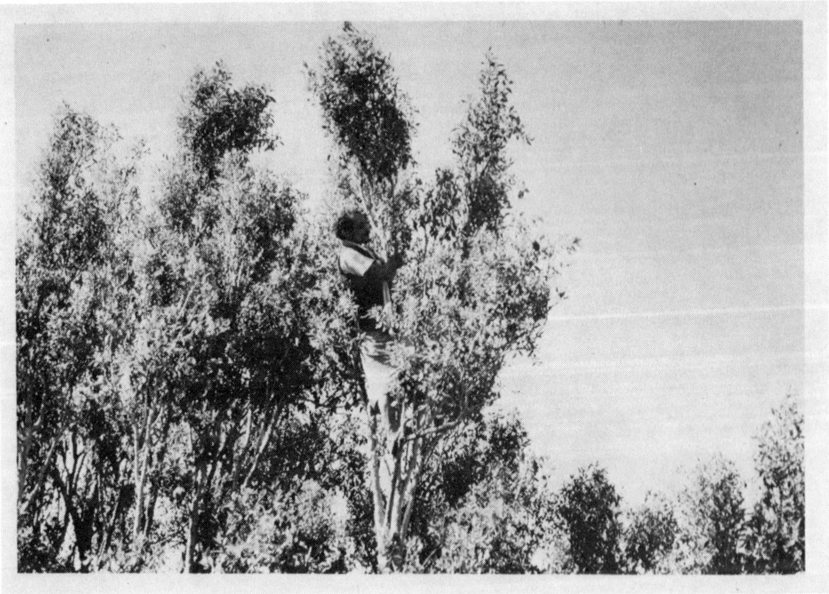

Harvesting qat in Shemran

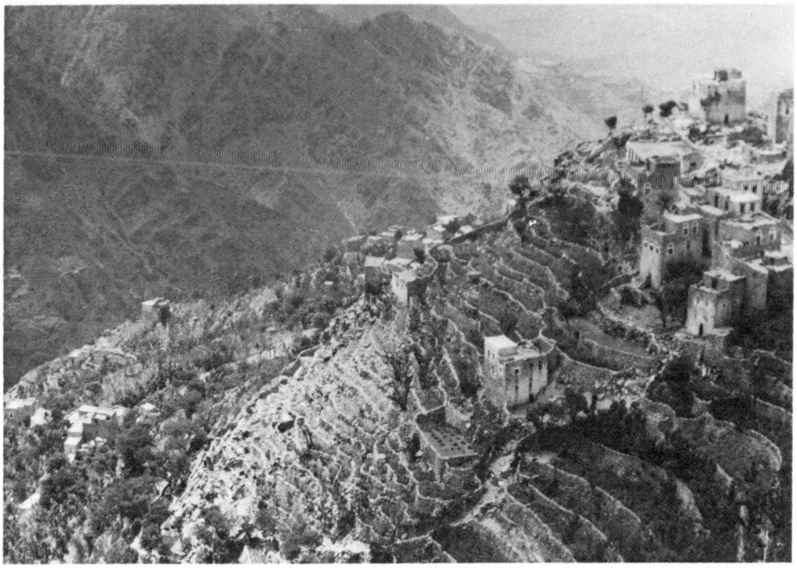

Qat terraces on Jabel Sabr

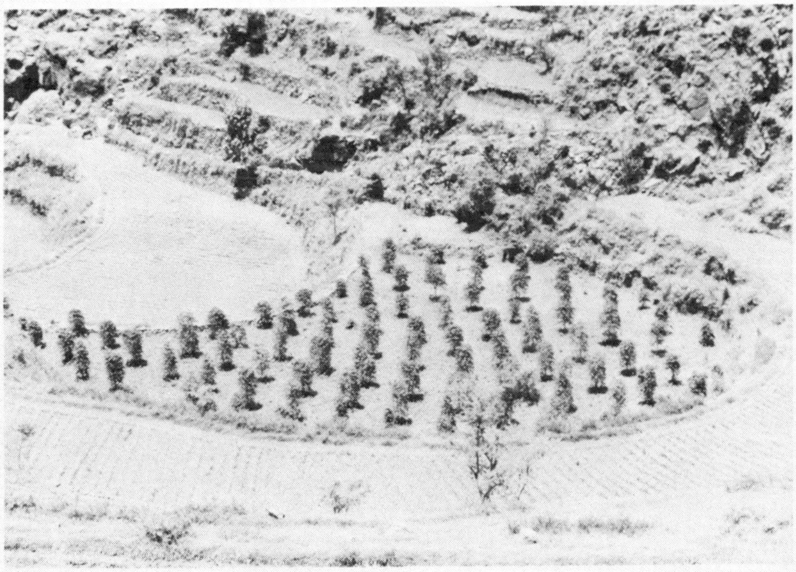

Coffee field in Utmah

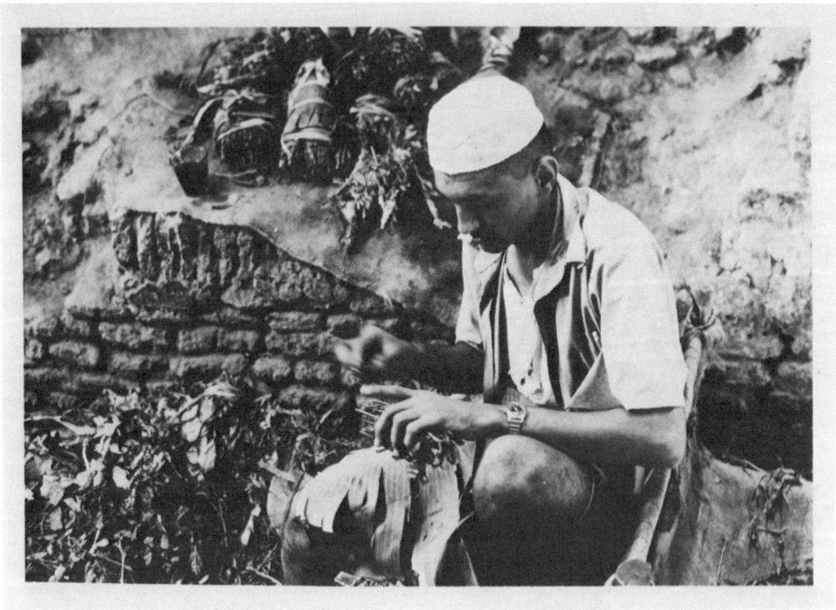

Packing qat for market in Mahabisha

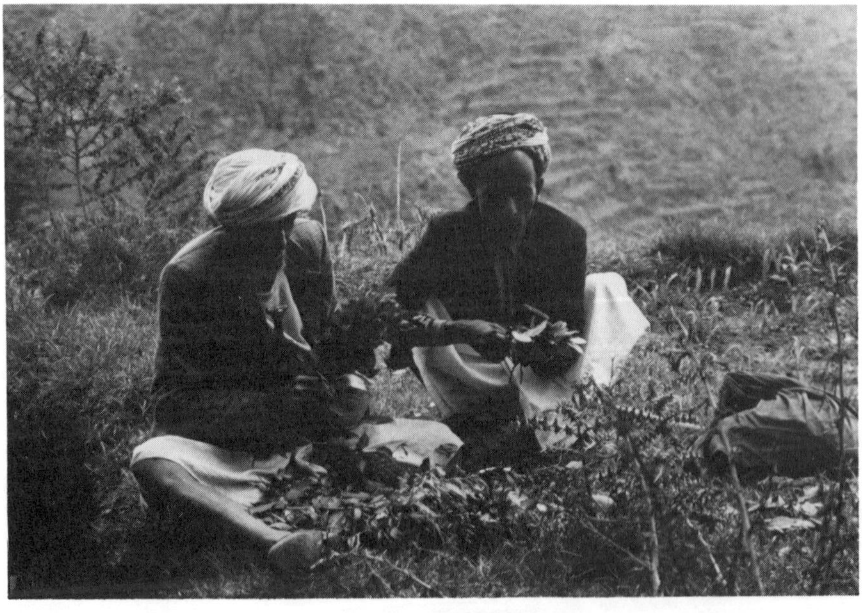

Packing qat for market in Utmah

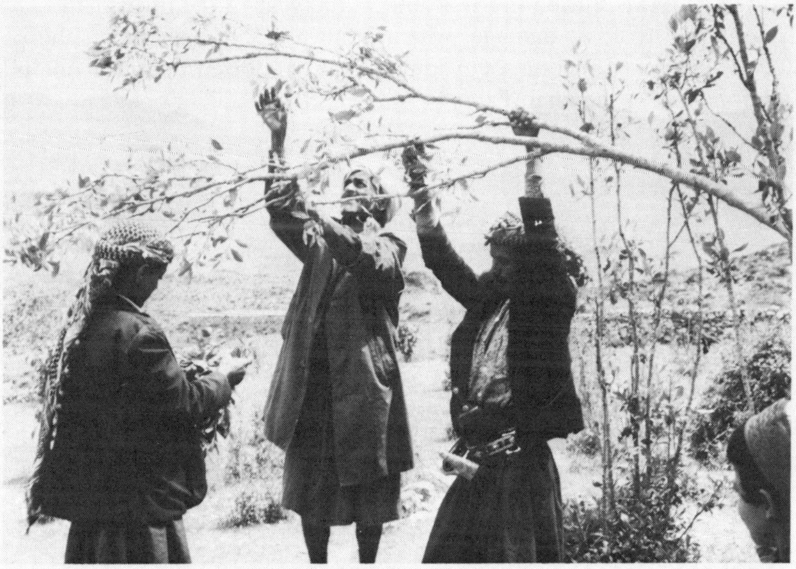

Picking qat near Anis

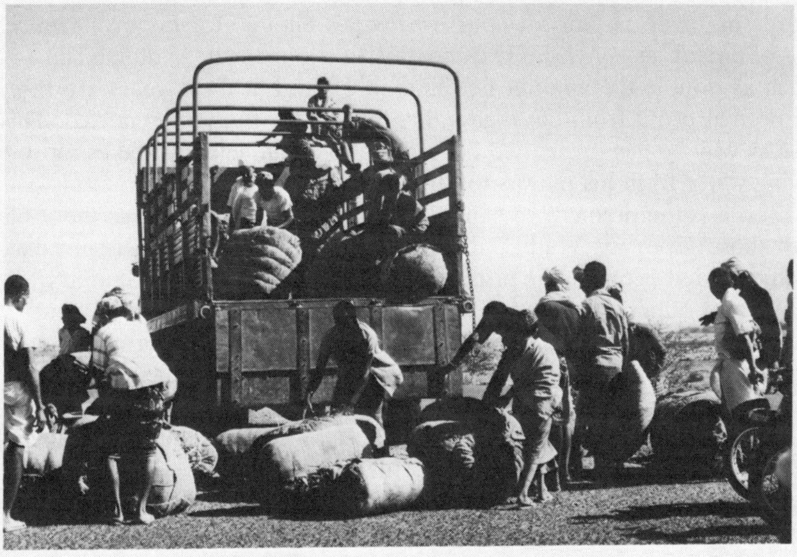

Unloading Sharabi qat at Zabid

provides the water for his crops with motor driven pumps. He usually gets five or six harvests during the year, but in the year of the investigation he got only four due to frost damage, which is always a threat out on the plains. Thus, the costs and income of Abdullah as he reported them for one plot of 35 matrahs was as shown in Table IV.

TABLE IV

1975			
Costs		Income	
Collar trimming	150 YR	1st harvest	500 YR
Cultivating	350 YR	2nd harvest	1,000 YR
Weeding	120 YR	3rd harvest	1,500 YR
Cultivating	200 YR	4th harvest	3,200 YR
Cultivating	200 YR		
Gasoline for pump	280 YR		6,200 YR
Tools	200 YR		
Taxes	200 YR		
Total	1,700 YR		

Profit = 6200 (income) − 1700 (costs) = 4,500 YR

This translates into $989.00 profit for this one of his two 35 matrah plots, or 20,070 Y.R. ($4,411.00) per hectare. If he were to pay taxes at 10%, which is the official rate, his profit would be considerably less. He also guards his own qat and of course provides enough for his own family and that of one of his sons who lives nearby. In a good year Abdullah can earn as much as double the amount he made in 1975, but these years are rare and his normal profit from qat is less than he got for the year reported. This, he says, is why he has diversified his crops. Abdullah actually makes more from selling water from his pumps to other farmers than he does from his qat, but this too is an unpredictable source of income. If one compares these figures with those given for Wadi Dahr, it is evident why the Rida region has not been regarded as one of the prime qat producing regions of the country.[2]

We also obtained some figures from the qat farmers on Jabel Sabr above Taiz. These were generally confirmed by a number of informants and they are consistent with information from other parts of Yemen, indicating the same ranges of exceptionally high profits from the cultivation of qat.

These farmers said that the few richest owners on the mountain owned around 800 qasabas of land. Since the qasaba here is 10 dhira (or 5 sq. meters) this works out to about 4 hectares. These larger farmers are said to have the best and oldest trees, and they generally yield qat which can be sold for 1000 rials per qasaba every three years. Table V tabulates the calculations of earnings on 3 differing sized plots on Jabel Sabr. The informants

TABLE V
Taiz (Jabel Sabr)

	Large Owner	Medium Owner	Small Owner
Size of farm	800 qasabas[a] (2 hectares)	300 qasabas (0.75 hectares)	100 qasabas (0.25 hectares)
Quality of qat	best	average	poor
Price/qasaba	1000 YR	500 YR	100 YR
Total earnings from harvest (every 3 years)	800,000 YR ($175,824)	150,000 YR ($32,967)	10,000 YR ($2,197.80)
Annual gross income	266,666 YR ($58,608)	50,000 YR ($10,989)	3,333 YR ($733)
Costs at 30%	79,999 YR ($17,582)	1,500 YR ($3,297)	999.99 YR ($220)
Annual profits	186,667 YR ($41,026) (233 YR/qasaba) ($51.20)	35,000 YR ($7,692) (116 YR/qasaba) ($28)	2,333 YR ($513) (23 YR/qasaba) ($5.13)
Realizable profits per hectare/year	93,200 YR ($20,484)	46,400 YR ($10,198)	9,200 YR ($2,022)

[a] 1 qasaba = 25 sq. meters (10 dirah al hadi)
400 qasabas = 1 hectare

gave us these figures as examples. They admitted that most farmers fall between the extremes portrayed here, and that most farmers have mixtures of qat quality. For example, there are families with 200 qasabas of high quality qat and 300 qasabas of medium grades, etc. Also, there are years when profits are higher or lower because of hail damage to competing areas, or to their own best plots. Additionally, it must be remembered that many of these farmers grow most of the qat chewed by themselves and their families and friends, removing considerable pressure from their budgets. In view of the living patterns in Yemen, this is an additional profit.

As another example of the profitability of qat let us look at some figures we collected in the region of Utmah, a region known as much for its coffee as for its qat. It is in a lush rainfall zone, good for both of these cash crops plants as well as for grains. Generally, in the Utmah region qat is grown in the easternmost exposed sides of the mountainsides while coffee is on the more shaded Western slopes. Coffee is generally grown farther down in the Wadis, which are wetter and more shaded. The Utmah area is divided into 5 or more or less equal sized divisions called *mukhlafs*, and the group of farmers we interviewed gave us the breakdown of crops in these as shown in Table VI.

TABLE VI

Mukhlaf	Qat	Coffee	Other (mostly grains)
Samah	1/3 (33.3%)	1/3 (33.3%)	1/3 (33.3%)
Himyar	1/10 (10.0%)	1/4 (25.0%)	13/20 (65.0%)
Beni Bahr	1/4 (25.0%)	1/8 (12.5%)	1/2 (50.0%)
Sumal	3/8 (37.5%)	1/8 (12.5%)	1/2 (50.0%)
Razih	1/16 (6.25%)	3/8 (37.5%)	9/16 (56.25%)

Thus, their overall estimate amounts to 22.4% in qat, 24.16% in coffee, and the other 53.24% of the land in food crops. The men of Utmah also provided us with estimates concerning various grades of qat in the area. They would not be more specific concerning holdings of individuals, but several agricultural experts who were advising in the region corroborated the general correctness of the figures given (see Table VII).

In this discussion of the profitability of qat, we have only demonstrated that it can and does yield rather incredible incomes to those farmers having decent sized fields of it, particularly when irrigation is available. Some figures produced by Revri which compare profits from qat to other crops which may be sold will assist us to better understand qat's position in the general agricultural picture.

Regarding Table VIII we should first note that taxes are not included in

TABLE VII

Utmah — Estimated income from Qat production

	Irrigated land		Rainfed land	
	Best Quality	*Good Quality*	*Average Quality*	*Poor Quality*
Price/*matrah*	2,000 YR ($ 400)	1,000 YR ($ 220)	500 YR ($ 110)	100 YR ($ 55)
Total earnings from harvest/hectare (every 2 years)	312,500 YR ($68,681)	156,250 YR ($34,340)	78,125 YR ($34,340)	15,625 YR ($3,434)
Costs estimated at 30%	93,750 YR ($20,604)	46,895 YR ($10,302)	23,437 YR ($ 5,151)	4,688 YR ($1,038)
Annual profits per hectare	109,375 YR ($24,038)	54,688 YR ($12,019)	27,344 YR ($ 6,010)	5,469 YR ($1,202)

matrah = 8 sq. meters (16 dirah)
56.25 matrah = 1 hectare

the expenses. The field tax for qat at the time of study was supposed to be 10%. This was assessed by inspectors who assessed the trees of each farmer who sold commercially. However, according to my informants the actual taxes probably never averaged more than 2.5 to 5% because market conditions could not be predicted and because often the tax collectors were local people, particularly in areas distant from the capital. In fact, such taxes were often evaded altogether. Collecting from the traders and merchants in the towns is also difficult, though this is a much more reliable means of securing tax revenue from qat.

It can be immediately appreciated that the tax revenues coming from a product accounting for 30% of the gross domestic product are immense, and constitute a major deterrent to efforts to bring about its abolition. However, even if taxes were factored into the table, the relative values would remain more or less the same, since the other crops are also taxed. Thus, Revri's major inference from this data is quite modest:

> Even if one insinuates two croppings per year for the annual crops the gross margin per hectare of qat in comparison with all other crops is at least tenfold (1983:84).

These estimates could prove wrong in detail, but they do accurately reflect relative differences. They enable us to better understand one of the frequent analogies one hears in Yemen: "Qat is our oil!" While the drug certainly is not comparable to oil in the prices it brings, or in its usefulness to industry,

TABLE VIII

Summary of variable costs and output of major crops Y.A.R. assuming 40% Hired Labor

Crop Variable Costs/Yemeni rials per hectare	Sorghum	Maize	Tomatoes	Vegetables	Fruits	Grapes	Coffee	Qat
Hired Labor	315	310	310	310	465	730	380	1380
Harvesting/Threshing	595	260	430	430	770	970	1190	1460
Drought/hire	350	350	350	350	220	120	350	420
Oxen feed	25	25	25	25	20	10	25	30
Seeds/Seedlings	40	60	70	90	140[a]	140[a]	90[b]	—
Fertilizer	—	—	150	150	—	—	—	—
Fungicide/Insecticide	40	40	60	40	40	310	40	470[c]
General Maintenance	30	30	30	30	120	120	120	120
Storage bags/packaging	45	35	1250	840	840	1250	60	60
Storage losses	470	165	—	—	—	—	80	60
Costs of irrigation	560	650	645	560	560	560	935	560
Total variable costs	2470	1925	3370	2825	3175	4210	3270	4400
Total return	8760	4800	14130	7235	11420	20560	16450	218400
Gross margin	6290	2875	10760	4440	8240	16350	13180	213900

[a] Depreciation of plantation in 20 years.
[b] Depreciation of plantation in 15 years.
[c] Plant protection by fine dust.

the little qat trees certainly provide a great number of people with improved incomes, and a substantial number of qat farmers are becoming very rich.

Additional evidence for these generalizations, as well as some other good reasons for qat's popularity with the farmer are given for the Khamr and Ibb regions by Richard Tutweiler, another good observer of the Yemeni agricultural scene:

> By far the most important cash crop during 1974—80 has been qat, which offers every relative advantage over other crops — at least to farmers on moderately watered mountain terraces. Some use values are provided in fodder and firewood, not to mention the aesthetic pleasure of shade. And the opportunity to interplant other trees and shrubs in the same grove is attractive. Qat is more drought-resistant (the plant goes dormant) than even some grain varieties. It is well-suited to domestic management because labor requirements are fairly low but some skill and familiarity with the trees themselves is important. Moreover, the system of marketing for qat is far more sophisticated and elaborate than for other crops (1981:164).

A final excellent example of how much economically better off the qat growing areas are than their grain growing counterparts is presented by Cohen *et al.* In a study comparing 25 representative villages from differing ecological zones in Hajja and Hodeida provinces, they found that in comparison with the subsistence agriculture and commercial villages, the four villages from the qat growing areas had the lowest migration rates, the highest wages for workers, and the most road building equipment owned by Local Development Associations (1980:180—210). As these authors summarize the situation with regard to the potentials for economic development:

> . . . It is clear that Hajja and Hodeidah governorates exhibit substantial subregional variation.
>
> Best off among these are the highland cash (*qat*) cropping areas which are characterized by substantial income and low emigration rates. So long as migration continues and qat prices remain high, they will progress toward their development goals at the fastest rate (*Ibid.*:210).

QAT VS. COFFEE AND OTHER CROPS

Has qat driven the famous Yemeni coffee from the terraces of Yemen? Among foreign planners and Yemeni officials one of the most persistent dogmas one hears is that (1) there has been a decline in Yemeni coffee production; (2) there has been a significant increase in qat production; (3) coffee and qat flourish under similar climatic conditions; (4) qat is so much more lucrative, and so much easier to care for that farmers have *en masse* uprooted their coffee trees and replaced them with qat trees; (5) this is harmful to the economy of the country because coffee brings in foreign exchanges and qat does not (e.g., Tarcici 1972, Yacoub and Akil, 1966; Econ. Report 1964, U.S. Embassy Taiz, Report #340a YAR World Bank, 1976). If true, such conditions would give strong economic support to those who wish to eradicate qat from Yemen. However, I will argue that there is little evidence to support these allegations, and though it is mixed, much of the data support the contrary thesis.

Another often heard argument is that qat is usurping other crops and thereby obstructing the Yemeni government's attempts to regain self-sufficiency in food production. This argument does not make much sense in light of the fact that qat still occupies less than 5% of the arable land in the country. Also Swagman has adduced data to show that grain traditionally was grown only for home consumption, as it is still (1985:76). Moreover, at the present time, imported wheat is considerably cheaper than local grains (Statistical Yearbook 1983). Grain production has been in decline for many years while importation of grain has been increasing (Swagman 1985:77). On the other hand, there have been steady increases in the production of cash crops other than qat. In the past decade the proportion of land producing vegetables has risen from 10,000 to 35,000 hectares. Grapes have risen from 7,000 hectares to 11,000 hectares and potatoes from 5,000 to 8,000 hectares (Statistical Yearbook 1983).

Even in places like Jabel Razih, where the amount of qat planted in the terraces has increased from 15% to 30% over a four year period (1977—1980). grain production was earlier declining on its own due to its low profitability and high labor expenses (Weir 1983:513). Weir's conclusion corroborates that of Steffen *et al.* 1978:

> I would argue further that qat is actually helping to sustain what grain production is still taking place. Many of those who still grow sorghum are able to afford high labor costs (which are a direct consequence of the high wages offered across the border in Saudi Arabia) precisely because they also grow qat. The revenues from qat are therefore helping finance grain production (Weir 1983:15).

Regarding the question of coffee and its decline, Weir also found no evidence that qat was replacing it in the Jabel Razih region. She noted that despite the temporarily high world prices for Yemeni coffee it still produces several times less profit than qat, but despite this, farmers have more than one reason to continue to produce it. One of these is the prudence of people who know from sad experience that the economy may change. They know that cash flow from Saudi Arabian migrants may cease and that they may well need the reliable income from the coffee. Also, coffee has great prestige value as a symbol of affluence and generosity. It is the favored gift to officials and strangers (1983:12—13).

This is essentially the same situation I encountered in the green and rich coffee and qat growing area of Utmah. I was assured by a large group of farmers that in spite of increases in qat production, no one in that region had *ever* replaced coffee with qat, and they gave good reasons for this. They showed me how the qat is generally found higher up and on the eastern slopes of the mountains and pointed out how these areas receive more sun and get less rain than do the coffee areas which are found more in the Western slopes and down towards the bottom of the wadis. Coffee needs more shade, as well as more water than does the hardy qat, which has been expanded into areas never planted before and onto some abandoned grain terraces.

A reason these farmers gave for retaining their coffee plantations was that in better areas of Utmah the yield is 2000 or more rials per matrah per year. This compares with the income from the best qat. These claims are partially substantiated in Table VII where it is shown that the percentages of Utmah land devoted to the two crops are estimated as being fairly equal. This same situation was described to me in Iryan which lies to the west of Yarim, and it coincides with data from Jabel Rayma in the mountains just west of Utmah as well (Swagman, personal communication).

In the village of Bani 'Awwam in the Hajja region Swanson found that coffee production had declined radically in some years, but coffee had not been replaced with qat. At the time of his study qat occupied only 5% of the land: "It is surprising that more qat is not being grown in Bani 'Awwam. While it is often said that coffee is being replaced by qat throughout most of Yemen, in Bani 'Awwam coffee is being replaced by subsistence farming." He guesses that perhaps this is because summer temperatures are too hot for qat (though they are well within the ranges we have mentioned), or perhaps the need for guarding it cannot be met under conditions of labor shortages. He thinks it may also be because men are absent in labor migration and it is men who handle cash crops (1981:17).

On the other hand, Gerholm claims that ". . . eastern Haraz is achieving a certain reputation for its qat, which gradually has replaced coffee, not only as the most profitable cash crop but also, literally on the terraces" (1977:54). He gives no data on the degree to which the decline in coffee production has occurred in Haraz, or on its direct replacement by qat, but he offers cogent reasons for the decline. During the early 1940s drought severely affected the trees in this famous coffee region, and this, coupled with low world prices for coffee over a long period, contributed to a heavy emigration of young men from the area. This exodus was further encouraged by the availability of high wages in oil producing Saudi Arabia. The consequent labor shortage has favored qat over coffee since costs for storage are much less, and less organized labor is necessary in proportion to the price secured. Gerholm notes also that while the volume of exported coffee from Haraz has remained nearly constant, the export income from it has declined (*ibid.*:53). Such factors, along with the development of roads, the growing import of motor cars, and the spreading popularity of qat chewing accompanying these changes, have led to the present supremacy of qat over coffee in Haraz.

Similar factors have been at work elsewhere, but in most areas the prudent Yemeni farmer has not replaced his coffee with qat. We inquired into this matter in many parts of the country during our study and were surprised to find that this common belief is largely unfounded. To be sure, I was shown some terraces where coffee had been eradicated and qat substituted, e.g., in Bani Yousef, down in Hujjariyya. However, here, as in other regions, coffee had never been very important historically, and the amount of land so replanted was miniscule. The people in Bani Youssef told me that 90% of the area recently planted with qat was too sunny and rocky for coffee, and too far from the necessary dependable water supply. Nothing had previously been grown there.

Yacoub and Akil in their study near Turba, which is close to Bani Youssef, made the ambiguous statement that Yemeni farmers "are moving away from planting coffee and replacing it with qat" (1971:31). This is generally true if it means that they are not planting new coffee trees and *are* planting new qat trees. However, we could find very little evidence of actual *replacement* of coffee with qat. However, an interesting insight into the motivations of growers is contained in the following statement by Yacoub and Akil:

> About half of the respondents in this study (48%) were found to be qat growers. When they were asked whether they would like to continue to plant qat all of them replied "Yes." However, one-fifth of them preferred to plant coffee instead if the government guaranteed to purchase all the quantity of coffee produced at a reasonable price. The reasons they gave us for refusing to replace qat with coffee, arranged in sequence of their importance included: "Qat is more adaptable to village soil and climate," "It is easier to grow and requires less care than coffee," and "Qat is much more profitable, and is needed for personal use" (1971:31).

A final bit of evidence which should be introduced here is provided by Revri. During our fieldwork he and I discussed this matter and since he was interested in looking at qat plantations over a wide territory (particularly the heavy qat growing regions of Hajja, Sanaa, Dhamar, Ibb, Mahwit, and Taiz), I asked him to keep a special lookout for the replacement of coffee by qat. His conclusion is as follows:

> Gradually in some areas, where irrigation facilities are available, it was observed that qat is replacing the less profitable practice of cereal cultivation. *Recent replacement of coffee with new plantations of qat could not be confirmed* (1983) (Emphasis added).

Thus, the evidence on this matter leads to the following generalizations: (1) The growing of qat has expanded significantly in many areas particularly during the past 20 years. (2) The production and export of Yemeni coffee has probably gradually declined during this century but have remained fairly constant at around 4000 to 5000 metric tons per year for the past 20 years. (3) There is no evidence that coffee trees have been uprooted and replaced by qat trees on any significant scale. It has, however, happened in isolated instances, and these have been blown out of proportion by planners and authorities. (4) The main reason it has not become general is because such replacement is not practical or necessary. The common statement that qat and coffee compete for the same ecological niche is not really true either. Actually, qat can be grown in areas suitable to coffee production, but since qat is more hardy, new plants generally are either placed on the less shaded and less watered areas where there were no crops before, or they displace unprofitable grain crops. Since the area needed by qat is so much smaller, the amount of such replaced grain is not significant, particularly when measured against the cash income from qat, which can be used to purchase food. Furthermore, it should be noted that if conditions should change, qat could be uprooted and immediately replaced with grain. Coffee, on the other hand, like qat, needs several years before it begins to be profitable. (5) While the production of qat has certainly increased in these coffee producing regions, it has had a share of the land in most of them for a very long time. Furthermore, some of the most famous qat growing areas, such as Wadi Dahr and Jabel Sabr, as well as other less famous qat growing areas, never had any coffee because they do not have the proper climatic conditions. In fact most of the recent expansion of qat plantations have been in areas, such as the Central Highlands, which are climatically unsuitable for coffee.

Thus, it is my conclusion that this whole issue is a bogus one. Yemeni coffee production has declined, but the role of qat in its decline is negligible. Given the limited areas in Yemen where coffee can be grown it is unlikely that, even with subsidies and help, coffee production can be increased much. Even if it could be increased Yemeni coffee has been only marginally competitive on a unpredictably fluctuating world market. There is little incentive to put in the long-term effort and investment necessary to make it productive under these circumstances. On the other hand, it is clear that most of the immediately profitable qat now growing in the coffee regions of Yemen cannot be replaced by coffee because the qat is growing for the most part in soils where coffee cannot.

It must be mentioned here that some foreign "experts" as well as some Yemeni officials, have proposed that qat be replaced by grapes, or some other relatively high profit cash crop. They propose that at first the government should support the price so that the incentive to produce qat would decrease. I have pointed out the impracticality of this in the case of coffee, but it does not take much thinking to conclude that for the same, and even more reasons, such a proposal makes little sense for grapes or other fruits. Not only are grapes less hardy than qat but they require far more care and the costs are much greater and the demand for them is less. For example, in Wadi Dahr we were informed that not only are grapes less resistant to drought, but they must be dusted with turab 15 times as opposed to two times for qat. In addition to this, each year many of the poles supporting the arbors must be replaced. When such factors are added to the lower price for the product and the fact that grapes have a much shorter season, are much more perishable, and cannot be consumed in large quantities, it is easy to see how difficult it would be to persuade the Yemeni farmer to switch from qat to grapes. This is particularly true in a country where wine can only be produced clandestinely because it is banned on religious grounds.

It is not necessary to carry such arguments further here. It should be plain why the long dreamed of profitable competitor which could supplant qat is elusive, and perhaps impossible to find.

MARKETING

The perishability of qat means that it must be gotten to market very quickly, and this has been much of the stimulus behind the expansion of the system of roads in North Yemen. Hundreds of small villages have built feeder roads with only hand tools in order to connect their areas with the main roads and highways, so that the local farmers and merchants could move their qat to the larger markets of cities and towns (Kopp, 1981).

The perishability factor has also contributed to the spread of the profits from qat among a relatively widespread segment of the population of the country. Unlike coffee, qat must remain in the trees until the last moment before marketing. It cannot be stored and witheld from the market by large speculators.

Gerholm makes a number of significant points relative to this in his discussion of why and how, since the recent civil war, coffee has been superseded by qat as the major crop in Haraz. Pointing out that a considerable amount of capital is needed by the coffee merchant because he must store the beans in the highlands until enough has been accumulated, and then organize transports of large quantities, etc., he goes on to say:

> In the history of Haraz, one often hears of great coffee merchants and even of a single merchant who for awhile was able to dominate the trade. Great qat merchants, however, are quite unknown. While the coffee trade seems to generate a structure with a few big merchants in control of the market, trade with qat apparently does not offer the same opportunities for a "big man" structure to develop. Borrowing the terms of another contrast between two crops (Ortiz, 1947), one could say that coffee is, in a sense, an aristocratic crop, qat a democratic one (1977:55)

The "small man" feature of qat marketing is something frequently noticed by most of us who worked in Yemen, and it applies to both the farmers and the traders. However, there are signs of change and Gerholm is again very germane when he states:

> The coming of the car may eventually lead to a certain change in this structure. It is now possible to reach the lucrative city markets where qat fetches much higher prices. Qat enters the long distance trade, and transportation costs rise far above those involved in local trade. This situation will favor the merchant with some capital to invest (1977:56).

Indeed this has already happened in some areas, particularly in situations where the distances between the qat fields and their markets are very great. In the northern reaches of Wadi Mawr in the Tihama the magnificent houses of two wealthy qat merchants were pointed out to us. These men were reputed to buy the produce of whole fields in Razih and Mahabisha, and to transport large amounts to Hodeida by means of a fleet of pickup trucks. The same is true in the south, where the qat from Sharab, Misra and Dhi Sufal is packed into large bales and trucked to the Tihama towns of Mokha, Zabid, Beit al Faqih, etc. These large traders, even if they account for a small fraction of the qat sold in the country, have certainly entered the "big man" stage of capitalistic enterprise.

In Razih, far to the north, Weir similarly notes the "small man" pattern:

> Although those who grow qat or trade it (who are often the same people) are among the wealthier members of the community, it is important to note that the expansion of the qat industry has not resulted in the accumulation of larger land holdings (as happened in the past in the coffee industry), nor has the qat trade become the monopoly of a few big men (as happened with coffee) (1983:8).

It must be noted that Weir is speaking of a region which is at the greatest possible distance from the larger markets. Like many other remote regions, merchants there experience great difficulties in anticipating the fluctuations in the distant market. If large loads were brought and shipped, there would be great risks of losing the entire investment if the market should be glutted. The farmers will not assume part of this risk and collect their money from larger traders before the qat is picked.

> The best strategy therefore for the trader aiming at an unpredictable market with a highly perishable product in which he has invested considerable capital is to buy and market it in relatively small quantities. This spreads the risk and makes him less vulnerable to a single gigantic loss (*Ibid*.:10—11).

In areas close to a large market, such as Wadi Dahr, Dulla, and Beni Hushaysh which are near Sanaa, or Jabel Sabr near Taiz, the matter of perishability is not really a problem. Farmers and traders in these areas have constant ready knowledge of the market, and as mentioned, this makes it possible for them to sell more qat in the winter season when there is greater scarcity. Weir notes that in the distant northern region of Razih, some traders buy as much as a pickup truckload of qat from the fields, even though they rarely speculate on much more than that. In Sharab, or Misra in the south, bigger truckloads of the drug are purchased by agents (*wakala*) because these areas are comparatively intermediate in distance from their markets in the Tihama cities of Hais, Zabid, Mansouria, Beit al-Fakih and Hodeida.

However, in the mountains and central highlands of Yemen the closer the qat growing area is to the market, the more likely it is that individual farmers and small traders with only a sack of 30 to 100 robtas can bring it in and sell it directly. They either pay a few rials for a seat in a pickup truck or they carry it on their own motorcycles. Since these petty traders can do this almost daily, in contrast with the larger speculators in distant regions, and since they neither have to sell to middlemen or to shopkeepers at a margin, nor must risk loss of freshness or loss due to market gluts, they often make as much profit as the owners of pickup trucks. These drivers not only must sometimes absorb losses, or just break even on the qat itself, but they must take into account costs of gasoline and truck maintenance as well.

In spite of these trends, however, the great majority of the qat is still grown by small landowners and taken to market by petty traders (*muqawatin*) or the farmers themselves. These individuals often find a place or a street of a town or city to sell directly. However, most of the small traders take their supplies to a wholesale commission agent (wakil) or to an established merchant (*tajir*) who rents a regular stall in the qat market, to whom they sell it at a small markup or stay to sell directly for a small profit. If the farmer sells to a wakil the latter gets 10% of the sale, and the farmer only gets his money only after the qat has been sold to a shop by the wakil. While such use of a middleman is sometimes most convenient, especially for those farmers coming in from long distances, most of those without larger amounts of qat prefer to sell directly to shops or to individuals. Their profit margins are greater and the loss of time is minimized.

An important fact to note, however, is that money can often also be made by a small qat farmer without leaving the community. A great deal of qat never passess through the hands of a middleman because it is sold or traded within the local communities where it is grown. This market exists because local conditions usually determine that not every farmer can grow his own qat, not all qat fields are producing at the same time, and there are usually members of officials, merchants, bankers, butchers, etc., in any community, who do not have fields. Thus, much qat is directly sold locally within qat growing communities. The prices are lower than they are in the larger market towns because there are no transportation or middlemen costs, but the grower is able to realize a little ready cash for his daily expenses.

If further evidence of the importance of qat in the economy of Yemen is needed, it is shown by the fact that in a study of the main market in Sanaa it was found that there were 95 qat shops out of a total of 527 shops in total. This constituted 18% of all the shops and accounted for 5.6% of all business in the market (Dostal *et al.* 1983:257).

As impressive as this figure is, by no means does it portray the actual amount of qat sold in Sanaa. At the time of this study, there were several major qat markets in other parts of the city as well, some of which had as many as 30 permanent stalls. Additionally, at these locations many farmers and petty traders simply arranged their qat in front of them on the street and began selling. The most extensive of these market areas were Bab al-Sabah, Bab al-Shu'ub, Bab al-Balagah, and al-Qa, the former Jewish quarter. Each of these markets had 20—30 permanent shops. Some of them, for example, Bab al-Shu'ub, also had as many as 50—60 street sellers on any given day, depending on the season. There were many other areas of the city where qat was sold and these shifted from time to time, or new ones developed according to ideas or whims of individual sellers. Other areas where there were more than 10 sellers at the time of the study were al-Mansouria, Bab al-Huria, al-Ta, al-Tabri etc. Thus, I estimate that at least 50% of the qat sold in Sanaa, was sold outside of the main market.

THE PLACE OF QAT IN FAMILY BUDGETS

It has often been alleged that the people of Yemen are squandering large percentages of their income on the qat habit and that this impoverishes them, contributes to the malnutrition of children, inhibiting saving and investment. This charge certainly makes sense when the high costs of qat (2 to 100 YR per robta during the time of the study) are balanced against monthly earnings of 500—2000 YR per month. In particular, one cannot help but wonder how poor people can chew regularly and still afford the necessities of life. One answer, of course, is that poor people buy cheap qat and do not chew every day, unless they live in the rural areas where they grow their own.

Though opinions abound, very little hard data is available on actual spending patterns in Yemen. A study on a random sample of 144 families in the old city part of Sanaa in 1972 reported that the average income was 816 YR/month per family and that 12% of family income was spent on qat and tobacco (C.P.O. Report 1973). Judging from the costs of these two items I estimate that about 10% of income was expended on qat for that sample.

In our study several years later we also attempted to gather information on this question. Though we were not able to make a random sample we used a variety of indirect as well as direct means of ascertaining both income levels and chewing habits. Figure 8 expresses the relationships between income level and qat chewing habits as they relate to expenditure on food apart from meat and qat. Meat was singled out for a separate comparison because, at the time, a kilo of meat and a robta of qat were comparable in price and it was felt that it might be interesting to compare these two “goods” in terms of trade-off choices by consumers. How does the very desirable protein for the family compete with the pleasurable euphoriant for the individual?

The first observation that strikes one in this set of comparisons is the amazingly high percentages of family income generally spent by Yemenis upon this recreational drug. Lower-income heavy chewers on our sample spend proportionately more money on it than they do on food; and even the more wealthy heavy chewers allocate a remarkable percent of their incomes to it. It is evident that even for the lighter users the sacrifice is considerable.

All of our chewers spend a considerably higher percent of their incomes on qat than was reported in the Sanaa study. In addition to the growing popularity of qat, this might be partially attributable to the fact that the authors of that study lumped non-users and users together. It may also be the result of their relying only on direct questions about income and expenditures. Since Yemenis are very secretive about such matters, our figures, which additionhally are based on a number of other economic factors, may be more reliable.

Figure 8 also shows that the higher the level of income, the more likely it is that the individual will spend more money on qat, but, of course, it is a lower proportion of his total income. In other words, the richer individual is

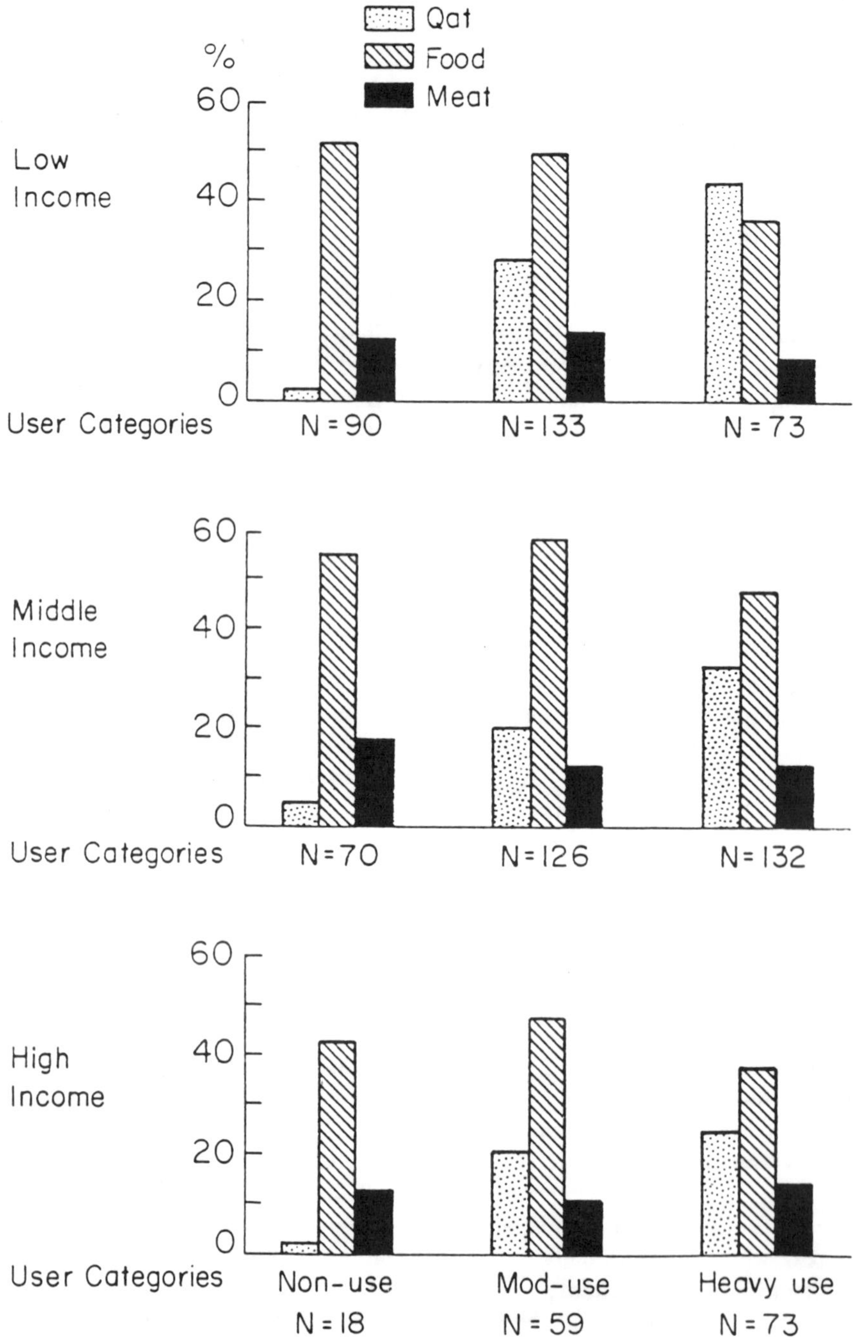

Fig. 8. Qat, food and meat expenditures expressed as % of total income.

likely to chew more, but can allocate money to other expenses and purposes, while the poor individual tends to sacrifice other amenities to participate in the qat experience.

As I said, at the time of the study the price of a kilogram of meat was about equivalent to that a bunch of fine qat. Since meat is highly desired as a principal daily food, indication of the trade-offs may be deduced by comparing the proportion of money which people said they allocated for meat versus the proportion they spent for qat. Figure 8 shows that as money spent for meat increased the percent spent for qat was reduced. As we would expect, this does not hold at the upper income level where the percentages spent for meat remained fairly constant. Correspondingly, regardless of income, there was a proportionate drop in reported expenditures for food as the heaviness of qat use increased, indicating a greater willingness to sacrifice as the habit grows stronger.

These data confirm our general observations that qat occupies an incredibly high place in the value hierarchy of the Yemenis, and provides some confirmation for those who claim that qat may have a higher priority than food for poor heavy users. If the data are at all representative of the country as a whole, as I believe they are, they further demonstrate the immense importance of qat to the Yemeni economy.

While these data do support the inference that expenditures on qat may well entail sacrifices of vital necessities for many families, this judgment should be tempered by the fact that our sample was primarily an "urban" one. Since perhaps only 10 to 15% of the country lives in these larger towns, and since qat is all grown in the rural areas, these figures are not quite as damaging as they may seem. In qat-growing regions the majority of the people have access to free, or at least, to cheap qat, and people in non-growing regions chew much less. Not only are they poor but they have less access to the supplies of the drug. The farmer's situation is also helped by the fact that he produces much of his own food, making his purchase of qat less of a tradeoff. Thus, while many of the poorest people in the larger cities of Sanaa, Hodeida, Taiz, and Ibb do undoubtedly spend more on qat than their meager budgets warrant, even by a liberal estimate this group makes up no more than 10% of the population in Yemen. At least 85% of the country is rural, and the middle and upper classes of the cities, even though they may choose to spend what we might think a high proportion of their incomes on a recreational drug, nevertheless cannot be said to be depriving their families of vital nourishment.

An example of how people cope under what at first appear to be impossible economic conditions may be seen in the case of a soldier we met in the town of Thula. His salary is 300 rials per month and he chews around 10 rials worth of qat per day. We were curious to understand how a man could live and support his family of four children on such wages. It turned out that he owned some land in a village nearby which, in most years, yields enough food for a meager livelihood. He even has a few qat trees which provide a little extra cash from time to time. As he told us, his 300 rial army salary per month certainly is not enough to buy food, but it is enough so that he does not have to use any of his farm income for his chewing pleasure.

Swagman provides another example. One of his informants in Kusma, who was director of schools in the district, admitted that his 2000 rial monthly salary would not cover his monthly expenditures for qat. Again, however, there were other sources of income. He received part of the profits from a family farm and further supplemented his earnings by settling disputes in the region, an activity which brought in considerable money in fees (1985:143).

When examined closely, the mystery of how people can chew qat on low incomes is not so mysterious. The judgment can be made that they would be better off accumulating savings or providing their families with a higher standard of living, but this is an outsider's opinion. Basic needs are usually met, and many apparently poor people are buying cars, radios and television sets. The rise of consumerism may well eventually diminish the demand for qat or lower its prices. However, until these economic forces gain momentum and alternative forms of recreation are developed, qat expenditures will probably remain an important part of the family budgets of Yemenis.

NOTES

1. This proportion has remained constant. In 1982 estimates by the International Bank for Reconstruction and Development were that the crop value for qat was about 800,000,000 dollars, or again almost a third of the Gross Domestic Product. "The estimated market value for all other crops in the country was no more than 15,000,000 dollars" (Varisco 1986:3)
2. More recent information from the Rida area (1983) indicates that at least some qat farmers of this region are now earning more than 37,000 dollars per hectare (data by Peter de Lange cited in D. Varisco, 1986:4). To some degree this reflects the inflation which has gone on in Yemen.

MARKETS AND TYPES OF QAT

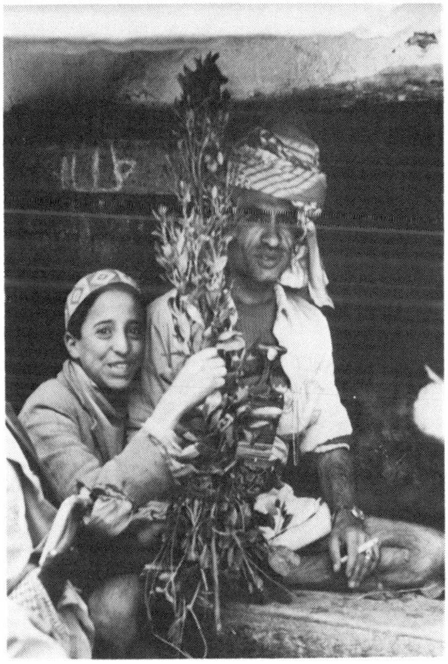

Qat from al-Wadi — Sanaa market

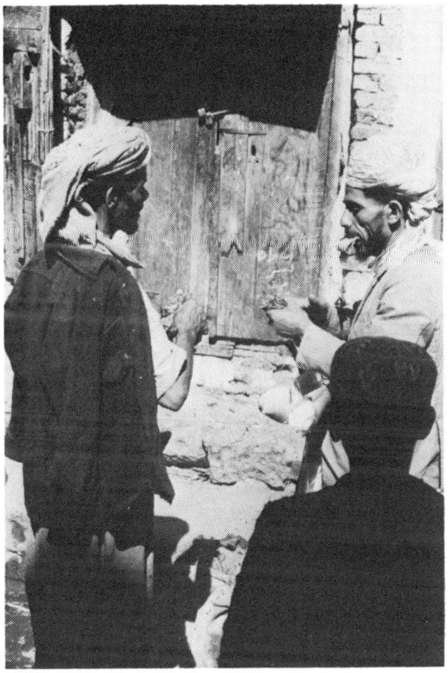

Paying for Sawti — Sanaa market

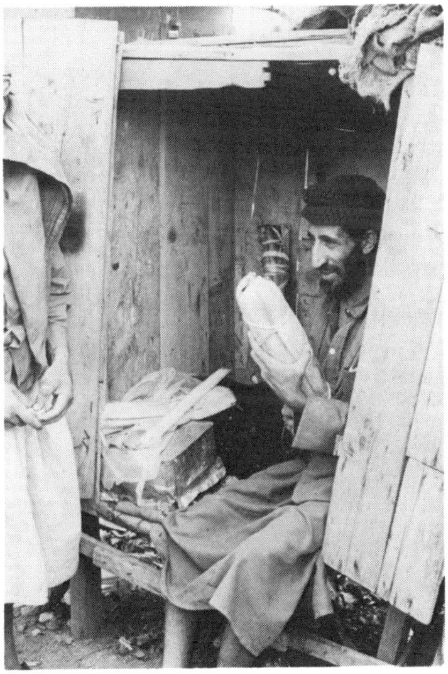

Qat seller in Sada market

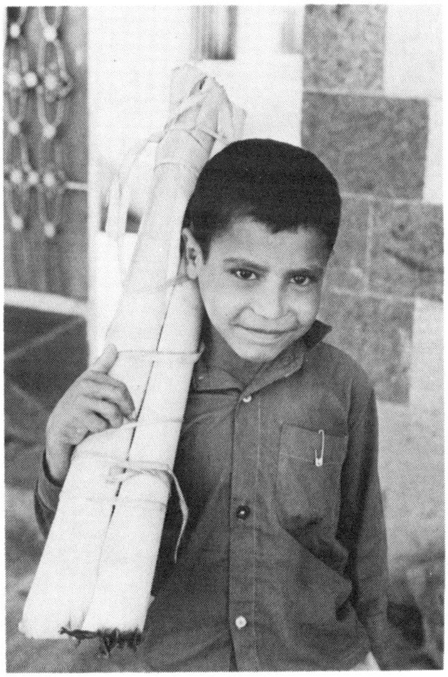

Two qarns of sawti for father and uncles — old city Sanaa

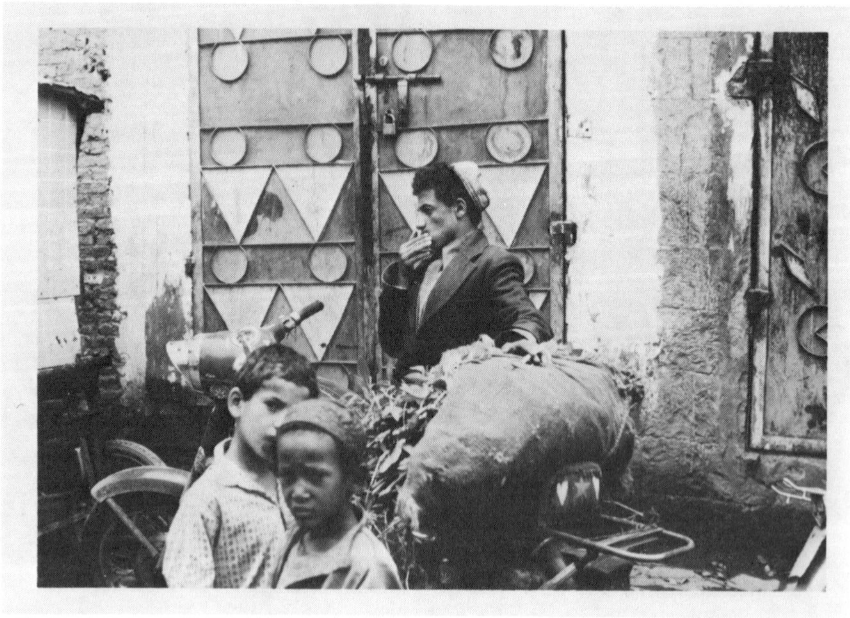

Small qat trader with motorcycle — Sanaa market

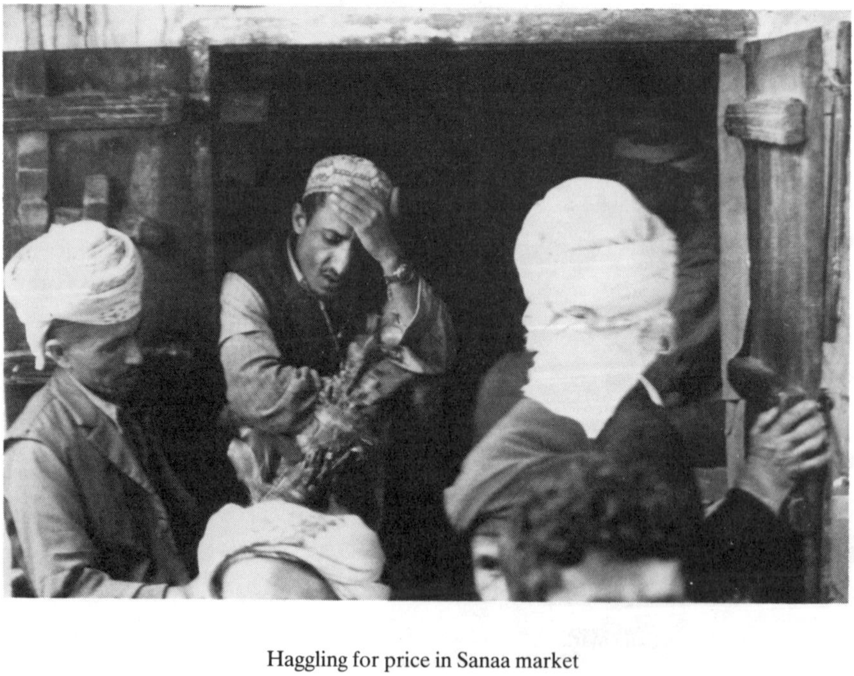

Haggling for price in Sanaa market

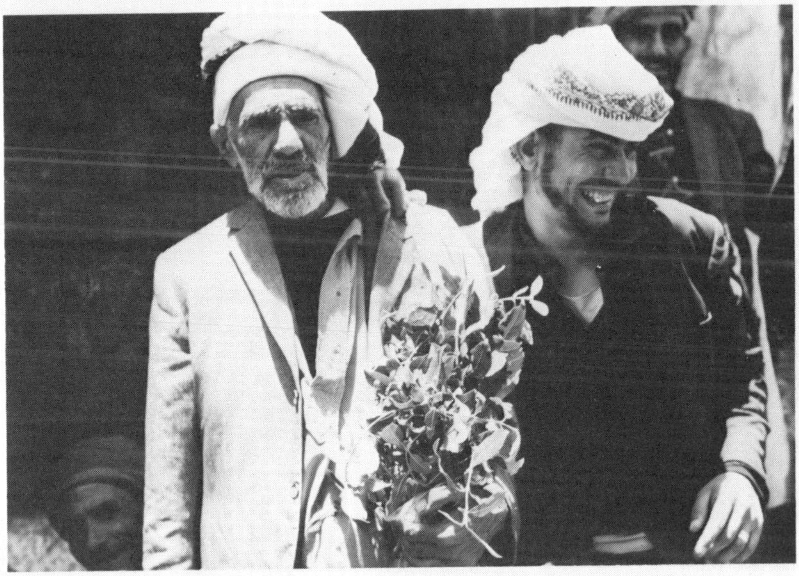

Satisfied buyers of Harazi qat — Sanaa market

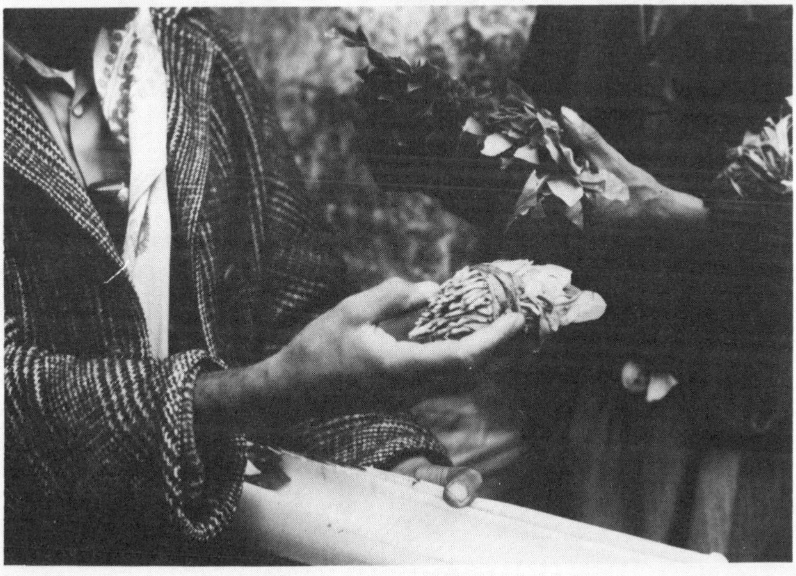

Selling Sawti from qarn — Sanaa market

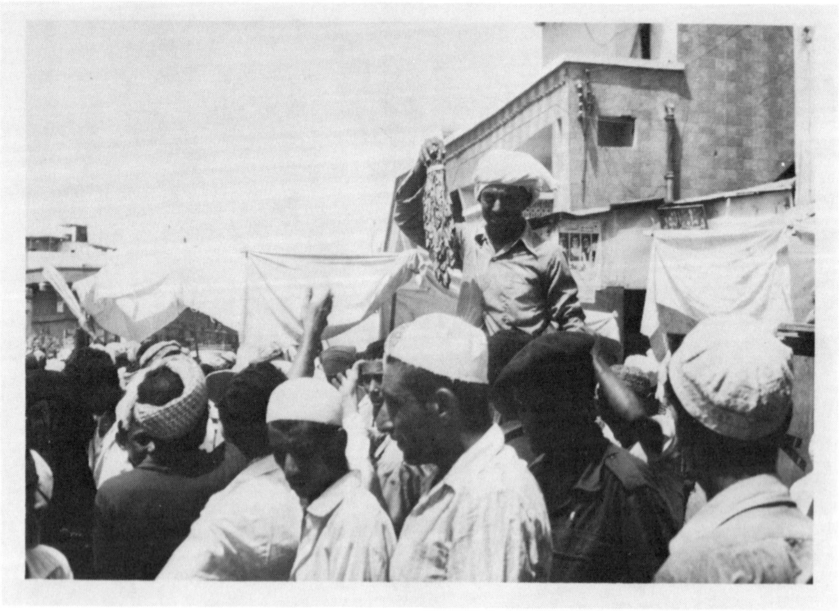

Vending harami qat in Hodeida

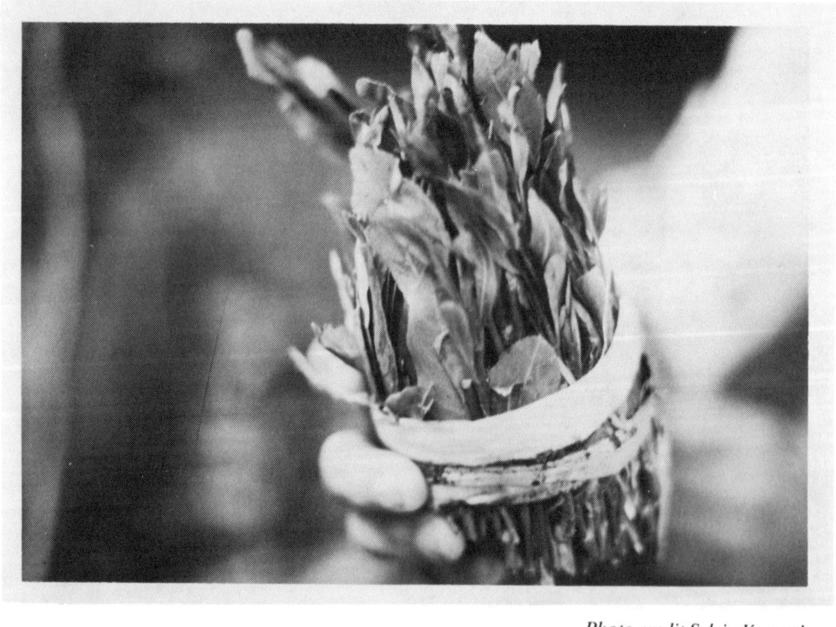

Photo credit Sylvia Kennedy

Ahmar (red) qat from Utmah in the Zabid market

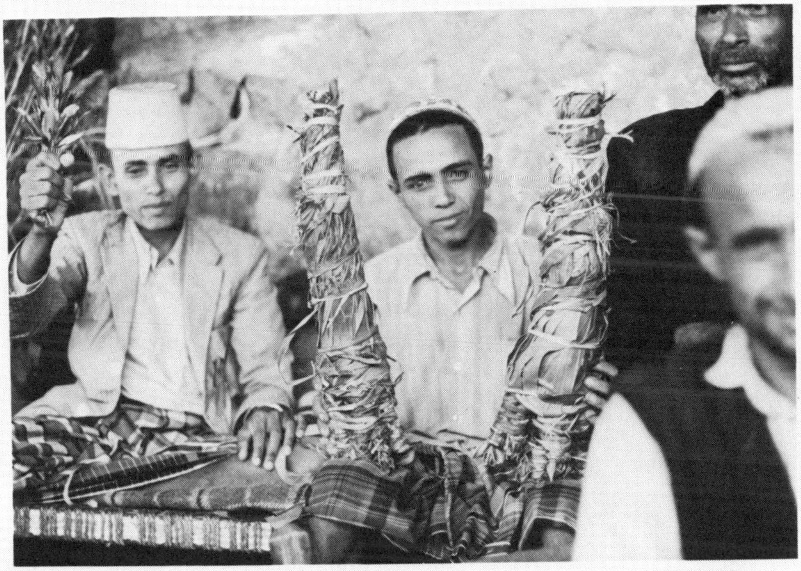

Qat from Dhi Sufal in the Zabid market

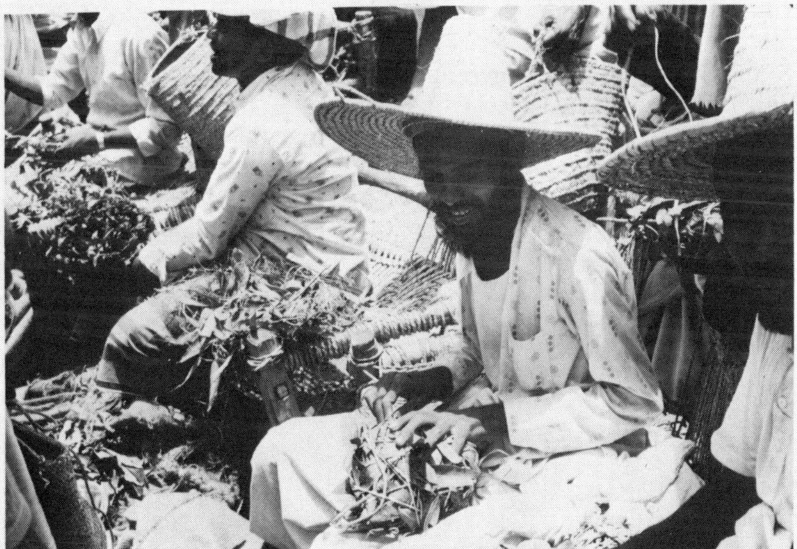

Raymi qat in the Bajil market

CHAPTER VII

THE BOTANY, CHEMISTRY AND PHARMACOLOGY OF QAT

Probably the most recurrent error in the literature on qat, aside from its mistransliteration as "khat," is the common designation of it as a "narcotic."[1] As the Latin root of this commonly misused word indicates, the term narcotic refers to a drowsiness-producing quality such as is typical of the opiates. But the most important experiential effect of qat is precisely the opposite. Like its close relatives the amphetamines, this substance stimulates mental alertness, wakefulness, and later, insomnia.

Though there has been some concern with its history, most of the past research on qat has been on its chemical constituents. The sociological, cultural, economic, medical and even the pharmacological aspects of the drug have been almost entirely neglected. However, in spite of the fact that work on the chemical properties of the drug began as early as 1887 and has continued sporadically to the present time, surprisingly little was known about the plant's constituents until very recently. The circumstances leading to this unusual situation derive not only from a prior lack of sophisticated techniques of analysis, but from the complexity of the alkaloids, the elusiveness of their qualities, and the fact that some of the active elements are lost within forty-eight hours after harvesting. Chewers have always maintained that the effects, as well as the taste of qat, are reduced greatly if the leaves are not fresh.

Despite this, before the present decade there were no reported chemical studies of freshly-picked leaves. If qat came exclusively from Yemen this would be understandable, since up until the 1980s they were no direct airline connections from that country to Europe, where the laboratories are. However, since the Catha edulis plant is common in East Africa, there has long been little reason for this neglect. Future studies will utilize freshly-picked qat, but most of the recent advances in analysis have been made with freeze-dried plant materials from Ethiopia and Kenya. Before discussing these experiments, however, the basic facts of its botany should be sketched.

BOTANY

In botanical terms qat (*Catha edulis Forssk.*), is classified as a dicotyledon of the celastraceae family. Within these classifications it belongs to the suborder celastrineae within the celastrales order. The celastraceae family contains about 40 genera and some 400 species, many of which are climbing trees and shrubs. These are widely distributed throughout the world and among them are a number of poisonous and medicinal plants known to the peoples of South Africa and other areas (Revri 1983:30—31).

Although Catha edulis, or qat is, by far the best known, the genus contains another member, *Catha spinosa*, which like Catha edulis, was also first reported by Forsskal in his *Flora Aegypto-Arabica* (1775). The existence of at least these two species has been corroborated in recent studies by Revri in Yemen (1983), refuting the frequent statements in the literature that the genus *Catha* is monotypic (e.g., U.N. Narcotics Lab report GE-79-10365, 1979:5, and Nordal 1980:51). Catha spinosa, however, is only observed in the wild state and at lower elevations (Revri 1983:35—30). Four different cultivars of Catha edulis are known, and the Yemenis recognize these by shades of color difference: *abyad* (white), *ahmar* (red), *aswad* (black), and *azraq* (blue).

On the basis of cytological studies made at the botanical laboratory at Hohenheim University in Germany, Revri has shown that Catha spinosa is probably the ancestor of Catha edulis. His basis for this rests on DNA analysis indicating that Catha spinosa is a diploid, and that it can be propagated from seeds, while Catha edulis is a triploid, whose seeds are sterile. This means that qat must be vegetatively propagated whereas this is not true of Catha spinosa (Revri, 1983: *op. cit.*).

Catha edulis is an evergreen tree with a straight and slender bole and white bark. The serrated leaves, ovate-lanceolate to elliptical in shape, are generally between 50—100 mm. long and 30—50 mm. wide. The plant has small petaled white flowers of yellowish or greenish tone. In Yemen the trees range from 2 to 10 meters in height, and some of them are claimed to be 100 years old. In the Ethiopian highlands and on Mt. Kenya, where rain is much more abundant, qat trees are often 10 meters tall, and some reach heights of more than 20 meters. In areas of Yemen where frost may occur on a succession of nights the aerial parts of plants may be killed, so that it never becomes more than a small shrub between three and five feet in height. In these areas, the tree is pruned back to ground level every few years.

By contrast with the Catha edulis tree, Catha spinosa, its probable ancestor, grows at lower altitudes and always remains a small shrub about 1 1/2 meters high. It has auxilliary spikes on the branches, smaller leaves and flowers, and is much larger and heavier, with more plentiful seeds. A main differentiating feature is the presence of the large thorns on the older branches (see Nordal 1980, Revri 1982) for much more technical botanical details. (See Figures 9 and 10.)

In addition to the ephemeral qualities of some of qat's active ingredients, there is another significant problem in securing definitive answers about its composition and effects. Due to differences of climate, soil, elevation, care, and the like, there are considerable regional variations in reported effects and in the proportions of alkaloids and other constituents of the plant. However, even if Yemen's qat produces some different effects than that of

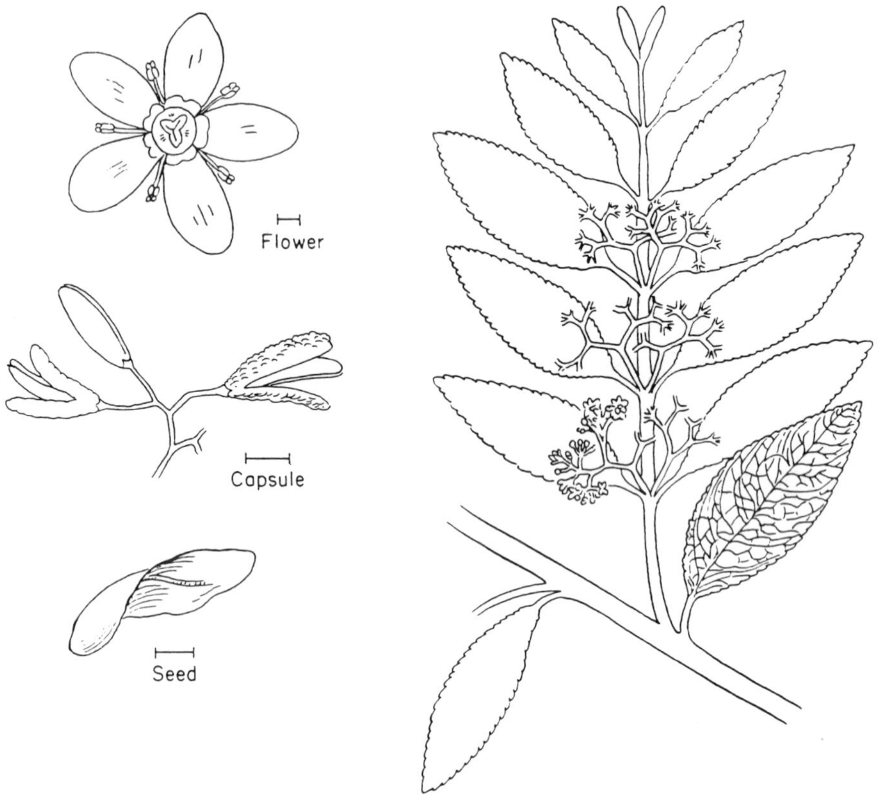

Fig. 9. *Catha edulis Forssk.* (from Revri, 1983).

Ethiopia and Kenya, it is still reasonable to assume an indentity of essential chemical properties with East African chat, marongi, etc. on the basis of the identity of botanical classification features in both areas.

Nevertheless, we must enter a caution here; it still needs to be established by laboratory tests that Catha edulis from these different areas is really the same, since some fairly consistent differences in behavioral effects are reported by chewers in East Africa and Yemen. For example, the isolated cases of extreme agitation, aggressive behavior, psychotic attacks and even death reported in publications from East Africa (e.g., Carothers 1945, Margetts 1967) are not paralleled by any reports or observations from Yemen. These cases are not supported by convincing evidence that the individuals were not mentally ill before chewing, but if they are accurate, such differences may well be due to differing amounts of the active ingredient in plants from the two areas. Some of them could also be the result of differences in the amounts and the parts of the plant ingested, or even to regional basic personality differences. In any case, such variations make it

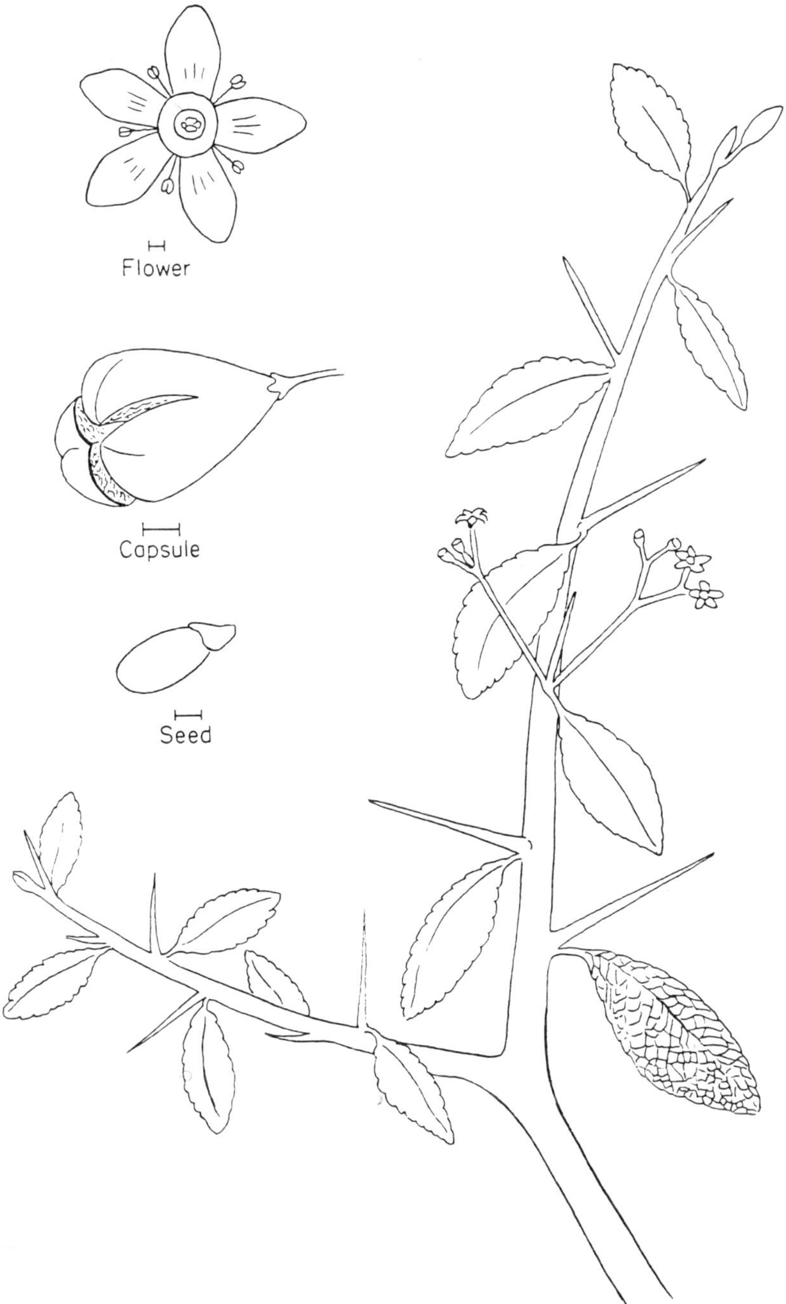

Fig. 10. *Catha spinosa Forssk*., plant, flower, capsule and seed (from Revri, 1983).

necessary to withold final judgment as to what may account for the different effects reported. Adequate samples from different areas must be analyzed in a comparable manner.

THE ACTIVE INGREDIENTS

Before the first scientific studies of this plant were made it was thought that, like, its sister plants, coffee, qat probably contained caffeine. In 1887, Fluckiger and Gerock laid that theory to rest, and none of the studies since that time have reported any trace of caffeine. These early investigators named the active alkaloid which they did isolate *katine*, a word which was later changed to *cathin* and Anglicized as cathine. This name is still retained by many investigators for the first verified active alkaloid of the plant: d-norpseudoephedrine (isolated in 1930).

Neither the work by Mosso in 1891, nor that by Beitter in 1900, did anything more to elucidate the alkaloid content of qat, though their studies clarified other features of the plant. Mosso, however, made a contribution by injecting a substance which he had isolated and called *celastrina* into a frog, producing motor and respiratory excitation and dilation of the eye pupil. This substance was apparently the same as cathine, later more fully analyzed by Wolfes. Beitter's thesis in 1901 attempted to ascertain chemical structures as well as the percentages of the alkaloid in qat samples from both Ethiopia and Aden, and though his formula has been questioned by later writers (Krikorian and Getahun, 1973: Wolfes, 1930), it was reasonably close to some of the recent ideas.

In 1912 and 1913, Stockman published results of experiments in which he claimed to have isolated three different alkaloid fractions. Besides cathine, he also named *cathanine* and *cathadine*. This work has been frequently and carelessly cited in the litertature without critical comment, which is unfortunate as much of it appears to have been rather poor, or even "inept" work (Alles *et al.* 1961).

As alluded to above, the next important step came almost 20 years after Stockman's analyses when Wolfes identified d-norpseudoephedrine (or (−) norpseudoephederine) as an active ingredient of qat in 1930 and referred to it as "cathin". This substance had been found in nature in certain *ephedra* plants in China by Smith in 1928. The biological effects of the ephedra are in many ways similar to qat, and several later workers have independently verified the existence of d-norpseudoephedrine in qat (e.g., Paris and Moyse, 1958; Alles *et al.* 1960; Winterfield and Bernsmann, 1960).

Some analyses have also been made of the urine of a group of four experimental subjects who chewed three bundles of qat each. D-Norpseudoephedrine was found unchanged in the urine, and the amount was equivalent to that in four control subjects who were given 30 mg. of synthetic d-norpseudoephedrine dissolved in water (Matai and Mugera 1975). Wolfes' work thus has led to the general use of the name cathine for d-norpseudoephedrine in the literature, and after 1930 it was widely accepted that cathine is the primary active ingredient in qat.

Nevertheless, even though d-norpseudoephedrine was the most clearly identified active ingredient in qat, even Stockman's early work had aroused a suspicion that there are probably other phenylakylamine derivatives in the plant which are more volatile. It did not seem to investigators (e.g., Von Brucke 1941) that d-norpseudophedrine in such small amounts could account for the reported effects of qat, nor could the chewers' conviction that fresh qat is more powerful and desirable be easily explained.

In 1958 Paris and Moyse showed that a tincture prepared from the qat plant, but with d-norpseudophedrine removed, had almost as powerful effects as whole plant material. More evidence supporting the suspicion of other more volatile active ingredients came from the work by Friebel and Brilla (1963) in which they obtained an alkaloid oxalate present only in fresh plants. The locomotor effects of this on mice were found to be greater than that of d-norpseudoephedrine, and these authors suggested that this other cathine-like substance is a labile d-norpseudoephedrine precursor which changes into d-norpseudoephedrine on drying. However, on the basis of their data they could not formulate a structure for it.

In 1968, Elkiez *et al.*, working independently, found cathine in qat but additionally isolated an alkaloid they called *cathenine.* Again the differences between the extractions from green and dry leaves of each alkaloid supported the hypothesis of a precursor. Elkiez *et al.*, also claimed to have isolated three other alkaloids — *cathedine*, as well as *ephedrine* and *eduline.* However, in the judgement of Krikorian and Getahun some of this work is of doubtful validity (1973:395).

Cais *et al.*, carried the search further in 1964 when they isolated a substance they called *cathedine D* and determined a partial structure for it. They saw a possible relationship of this to other complex alkaloids such as *eronine* and *maytoline* which came from the same plant family but whose structures were still undetermined.

In the last few years, the whole matter relating to the alkaloids in qat has been greatly illuminated. At least four different laboratories have done important work to elucidate its properties, but only since 1970 have experiments been done which help to clarify the behavioral effects of the newly isolated alkaloids. This work was all made possible by the recent determination of the structures of eronine and maytoline, since these served as keys to many related structures of substances in a number of celastraceous plants (Szendrei 1980:7—8).

Several research groups have participated in the new chemical work on qat. A group in Israel has worked with Yemeni-type qat brought to Israel by the Jews migrating from Yemen after 1948. They isolated and determined complete structures not only for cathadine D, but also cathadines A, B, and

C. Of these, cathidine D appears to them the most interesting (Cais, Ginsburg, Mandelbaum and Smith, 1975). The University of Nottingham group led by Professor Crombie, and another team at the United Nations Narcotics Laboratory under the direction of Dr. Olaf Braenden, have recently pushed the investigation even farther. Working entirely independently of each other these two groups were researching questions similar to those being investigated in Israel. By the late 1970s all three laboratories were sharing information.

Further refinements of analysis have now been made which indicate that one of the new compounds, *cathinone*[2], is much more important than d-norpseudoephedrine (cathine), in producing effects, and this would help to explain some of the problematical effects of qat. Cathinone has been shown to be identical with alpha-aminopropiophenone (United Nations Narcotic Laboratory Report No. 8, 1978 and Schorno, X. and E. Steinegger, 1978, Szendrei, 1980:16). The results of these findings are best stated in Schorno and Steinegger's own words:

> Whereas no prediction can yet be made concerning the possible physiological activity of the high molecular weight polyester alkaloids of khat, it would seem likely that the phenylakylamine derivatives are mostly (or entirely) responsible for the stimulant-like activity of the plant. The main component of the phenylakylamine fractions was found to be (−) — cathinone (alpha-aminopropiophenone). Cathine in varying amounts was also present in all the plant samples examined (1978:2).

They then went on to synthesize this substance to produce isomers and the "dimer" of cathinone, which they suspect may be formed in the human body as one of the metabolites of cathinone (*Ibid.,* 4 and 6).

U.N. Report No. 9 by Schorno and Steinegger further states:

> Comparison with other CNS-active phenylalkylamines (e.g., amphetamine, phenmatrazien, ephedrine, norpseudophedrine) shows that, of the optical antipodes, than an S configuration at the asymmetric center bearing the amino groups is always the more active (Brilla, 1962). It is also clear from Brilla that the CNS-stimulation properties of cathinone are appreciably different from those of (+) — norpseudoephedrine. Further, pharmacological research now is needed to determine whether (−) — amino-propiophenone is really more active than (+) — oxamino-propiophenone with regard to CNS stimulation (1978:3).

Szendrei has summarized the implications of this work as follows:

> Based on its structure, relationship to cathine, and the high instability in the presence of oxygen as well as under alkaline conditions, cathinone may be considered as the long sought labile cathine precursor in Khat. However, it is not yet clear if it is, or under what conditions it could be connected to cathine in the plant.
>
> It may also be suspected that if cathinone is the main CNS stimulant principle in Khat, its CNS stimulant actively should be similar to but probably stronger than that of norpseudoephedrine (Szendrei 1981:17).

Later studies of qat from Kenya (Guamtain and Matai 1982 and Schorno *et al.* 1982) have shown that (−) cathinone is mainly present in young qat leaves, and that it rapidly transforms into (+) norpseudoephederine in adult and particularly wilted leaves, and more slowly transforms in young leaves (cited in Kalix and Braenden, 1985:153—154).

With regard to chemical research on the "active" constituents of qat, then, it is clear that significant advances have been made in the past few years. Important strides are being taken which are leading to new chemical understandings. With the isolation of cathinone in two forms (l-cathinone and dl-cathinone) as the most significant active ingredients in qat yet found, pharmacological work has also lept forward. Some recent results in this area, summarized in reports of 1979 conference, convey the quality of the work going on.

Tests with rats by Knoll and Yanagita demonstrated that cathinone is very similar to d-amphetamine in its ability to increase locomotor activity, oxygen consumption and other central nervous system functions. The two drugs are also similar in increasing blood pressure and heart rates of rats and rhesus monkeys. Yanagita also found that the self-stimulation pattern in monkeys was of the "spree" type, like cocaine. That is, the monkeys would keep stimulating themselves to exhaustion up to 24 hours, and then repeat this after a rest period (1979:327).

Schuster and Johanson reported that l-cathinone and dl-cathinone were about half as powerful as d-amphetamine in reinforcing the food schedules in rhesus monkeys. However, in an interesting test with substitutions of various substances in cocaine-habituated monkeys, they found that while each of four drugs — cocaine, d-amphetamine, dl-cathinone and l-cathinone — maintained responding levels significantly above those of a saline solution, both cathinones were significantly more effective in this than either cocaine or d-amphetamine (1979:324—5).

The following concise summary of their findings helps to explain the hunger and sleep depressing qualities which have been frequently noted for qat in humans:

> (1). In summary, dl-cathinone shares with d-amphetamine the ability to (1) disrupt food-reinforced, lever-pressing in monkeys; (2) serves as a positive reinforcer in drug self-administered experiments; (3) produces a decrement of milk intake in rats; and (4) produces tolerance to its anorexic effect. In addition, there is a cross-tolerance between cathinone and amphetamine (1979:325).

Another set of experiments performed by Rosecrans, Campbell, Dewer and Harris at the University of Virginia showed that l-cathinone had little effect on norepinephrine turnover in the brains of rats, while it had an effect much like that of d-amphetamine on dopamine turnover. Also, in a stimulus discrimination experiment: ". . . l-amphetamine-trained rats responded as if they were given d-amphetamine when various doses of dl-cathinone were administered."

However, experiments with an antagonist, haloperidol, showed that ". . .

while dl-cathinone and d-amphetamine were indistinguishable behaviorally, their mechanisms of action appeared quite different" (Rosecrans *et al.* 1979:329).

The conclusion of Rosecrans *et al.* clearly expresses the importance of these findings:

The studies presented by Schuster (this symposium) clearly indicated that dl-cathinone is self-administered at lower doses than d-amphetamine in disrupting the operant behavior of primates. One hypothesis generated in this laboratory over the last couple of years suggests that behavioral disruption produced by drugs such as d-amphetamine and morphine is related to agonist effect on DA [dopamine] neurons. Taking this into consideration, the data presented here concerning dl-cathinone would predict that this drug would be less able to disrupt behavior than d-amphetamine as was demonstrated. Thus, dl-cathinone appears less disruptive of behavior, which might explain why this drug was more potent than d-amphetamine in our discrimination study and in self-administration research. From this, one might also predict that individuals using this drug would be less disrupted and better able to function under its effects. In addition, this drug might produce fewer long-term, d-amphetamine-like problems because of its apparent lack of a DA agonist action. However, this is not to say that cathinone could not produce psychological problems following chronic administration (1979:329).

In an extensive and parallel set of experiments on rats, mice, and rabbits, Kalix and his associates in Geneva have shown that (−) cathinone produces hypermobility effects that are the same in quality but weaker (about 50% less) than those produced by (+) amphetamine, that cathinone is about eight times more powerful than (+) norpseudoephedrine in producing these effects, that both (−) cathinone and (+) amphetamine act similarly in the same receptor releasing site in the brain (control dopaminergic synapses, peripheral noradrenaline storage sites, and the caudate nucleus, nucleus accumbers septi), that the same agents block the brain synapse effects of cathinone as block those of (+) amphetamine and that ". . . the sympathomimetic side effects seen during khat consumption are probably due to release of neurotransmitter at cardiovascular sites" (1983c:143). (See also Kalix 1980, 1981, 1982; Valterio and Kalix 1982; Kalix 1983, a, b and c).

It is clear that the new studies of qat's active ingredients, particularly the isolation of cathinone, and the initial pharmacological work on it, are carrying our knowledge rapidly forward. The search for other yet unisolated active ingredients in the plant still goes on, especially since the presence of such ingredients was suggested by the side effects of experiments on the "decomposition" of cathinone. Work on this is still in progress (Szendrei 1980:17—29). Indeed new discoveries seem imminent which are quite exciting. Szendrei expressses this in the following excerpt:

In addition, one more phenylalkylamine derivative (its trivial name cinnamoylethylamine) not found before in nature was described after derivatization and gas chromatography-mass spectrometry (GC-MS) analysis from a Kenyan khat sample. The compound could not, however, be isolated and characterized definitely and its existence remained questionable until further confirmation. Studies now in progress indicate that the structure proposal was probably correct. In this case compound (5) may become and interesting new contribution to khat chemistry for it has most probably similar CNS stimulant properties as cathinone and it might also serve as a useful chemotaxonomic marker for certain khat types (Szendrei 1983:97).

Thus, though it may well be that cathinone accounts for most of the psychoactivity of qat, norpseudoephedrine combined with other phenylalkylamine-type components may contribute in some as yet undetermined way to the overall effects. Certainly, further pharmacological studies on cathinone and the cathedulins are needed to verify and amplify these findings (Szendrei 1983:102) but it is clear that we now are in a much better position to understand the effects of qat on behavior than ever before. It is also possible that the newly-discovered drugs may prove useful to medicine as well[3].

I have taken some pains to review the technical literature which deals with the ingredients of qat which primarily affect the central nervous system. Clearly the alkaloids cathinone and norpseudoephedrine are of most psychopharmacological interest, but there are other ingredients of the plant which also have important implications for health. For example, as early as Beitter's work in 1901 a considerable quantity of tannins were identified in qat, and it was suspected that these adversely affect the gastric system. Since then, the presence of tannins (mainly flavenoids) has been confirmed a number of times (Paris and Moyse, 1958: Alles *et al.*, 1961; Sissy and Abdalla, 1966; Elkiey *et al.*, 1968; Revri, 1983). The Alles group found a range of between 5.58 percent and 7.4 percent tannins in different types of qat (1961), and Sissy and Abdalla in 1966 reported 14.52 percent. Revri's more recent work using representative samples from five widely dispersed qat areas of Yemen fell within the range of previous studies, i.e., between 6 and 11% (Revri 1983:48). Thus, we can say at the present time that the tannin content is generally high, probably varying between 5 and 15%. Recently Gellert *et al.* have continued this work, identifying two new flavenoids, but the meaning of this is not yet clear (1981).

Another important health-related finding regarding chemical constituents of qat is the significant percentage of Vitamin C which it contains. This was reported in two different investigations. Mustard found 1.36 percent of this vitamin in the leaves and twigs, and 3.24 percent in the leaves only, while the National Nutrition Survey of Ethiopia found 1.61 percent in an undifferentiated sample. Mustard's findings led her to one of the few optimistic statements in the literature on the possible health effects of the drug: "Depending of course on the quantity consumed, the ancient custom of qat chewing in Arabia may be inadvertently supplying the people of that country with some of their daily requirement of ascorbic acid" (1952:34). This is another matter which certainly should be followed up, particularly in view of the problem of adequate nutrition in Yemen, the large amounts of leaves ingested and the adverse press which the drug has received. The National Nutrition Survey of Ethiopia also found fairly large amounts of Beta-

Carotene in qat samples (0.0018 g/100 g plant material). Additionally it should be mentioned that 17 amino acids were isolated from fresh qat leaves, though the quantities of these are probably insignificant to nutrition (Winterfeld and Bernsmann, 1960).

Raman Revri has also shown that the variatons in the tannin content and the d-norpseudoephedrine content of qat are due primarily to environmental differences rather than to the genotype, i.e., to differences between cultivars (*Ibid.*:48). This is important in terms of preferences and costs for qat from different regions. For example, a high percentage of tannins accounts primarily for several of the negative side-effects of qat, particularly gastro-intestinal problems, while a high percentage of d-norpseudoephedrine, such as is found in older and wilted leaves, and perhaps in certain varieties of the plant, seems to produce the confused states experienced by chewers of larger amounts of "poor" quality leaves (Kalix and Braenden, 1985:161).

Revri also analyzed the relationship between the important soil nutrients in the qat plant. His complex analysis cannot be reproduced here but some of the main results are as follows. First, the percentage of nitrogen in the soil has statistically significant positive effects on the percentage of d-norpseudo-

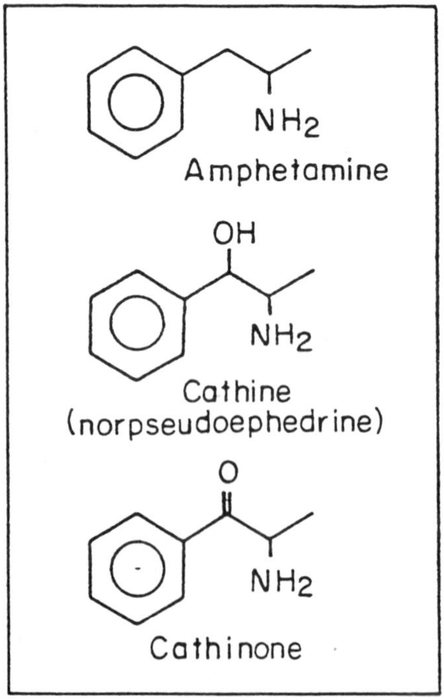

Fig. 11. Chemical structures (from Revri, 1983).

ephedrine in the plant. Various relationships between the interactions between the calcium, sodium, potassium and phosphorus which are also found in qat are proposed to account for this effect of nitrogen (*Ibid*.:49—58).

The amount of tannins in qat leaves were shown to be affected by the amounts of calcium in the leaves and soil and by altitude. The higher the percentage of calcium the lower the tannin content, and the higher the altitude at which it is grown, the lower the tannin content (*Ibid*.:59—60). Revri points out that: "This observation is further confirmed by preferences among qat chewers for tender shoots produced in the central highlands and higher altitudes of the Serat Mountains. Qat leaves low in tannin content are less astringent than those rich in tannin" (*Ibid*.:60).

While this does afford one important explanatory dimension to differences in qat quality and preference it should be cautioned that it is only part of a more complex story. While it is true that many of the better qualities of qat come from the high plains, e.g., the "champagne" qats of Dula and Wadi Dahr, some others nearly as fine come from such lower elevations as Jabel Sabr in the south, and from near Hajja (e.g., shami qat) in the North. At the same time some cheap "strong" types such as sawti come from higher elevations. Perhaps variations in tannin content as well as in proportions of cathinone to norpseudoepdrine can be partially explained by high or low percentages of calcium in the soil, but the matter may be much more complex and more work needs to be done. It does seem generally true that Yemeni qat from lower altitudes is cheaper and has more adverse side-effects than does that from higher elevations.

The search for qat's constituents as well as investigations of variations in the effects of the drug has proved to be more difficult than anyone had suspected. However, studies of the chemistry and pharmacology of the plant are moving forward rapidly. We may soon know as much about the obscure constituents of this plant and about the conditions contributing to different effects, as we now know about the more famous consciousness-altering plants such as coca, opium, cannabis, and the various hallucinogenic mushrooms.

NOTES

1. For example, this error even appears in the article by Hess in the *Encyclopedia of Islam* 1976.
2. There appears to be differences between the chemical nomenclature of the U.S. and Europe. Whereas in U.S. publications the most important substances in qat are labelled d-norpseudoephedrine, l-cathinone and dl-cathinone, in the European publications they are labeled (+) norpseudoephedrine, (−) cathinone and (+) cathinone. There are other inconsistencies, such as some authorities simply using the shorthand terms norpseudoephedrine or cathinone, etc.
3. By far the best and most complete review of the chemistry and pharmacology of qat is Kalix and Braenden, 1985. However, it is only authoritative when dealing with strictly technical matters and the results of laboratory testing. For example, with regard to effects

of chewing, they perpetuate several of the unfounded exaggerations that are found in the medical literature, e.g., that habitual use of the drug is "compulsive", that malnutrition is directly attributable to it, that it results in impaired sexual function and impotence, that periodontal disease results, etc. (pp. 150—151). These assertions are all based on a literature which is itself suspect, since it relies primarily on heresay and unscientific opinion. However, anyone interested in the biochemistry and pharmacology of qat can discount these sections and should certainly consult this article for a most thorough and expert review of recent laboratory studies.

CHAPTER VIII

QAT AND THE QUESTION OF ADDICTION

Qat is pleasant
There is nothing worse than it!

— Yemeni proverb

Earlier I remarked that among the other problems they perceived in Yemen, outsiders have been nearly unanimous in asserting that the Yemenis are massively "addicted to qat," and that they often find the cause of the country's social and economic problems in the qat habit (e.g., in addition to those quoted in Chapter I, we may cite Bury 1915, Rihani 1936, Helfritz 1936, Farrago 1938, and Shaffer 1952). Surprisingly, some ordinarily more responsible sources have echoed these opinions, without checking the documentation. For example, the FAO/UNICEF report in 1971 from the People's Democratic Republic of Yemen states without qualification that: "Qat, unlike coffee, has an overwhelming power on its consumer. It is extremely difficult for a qat chewer or addict to give it up as long as it remains within his reach" (1971:1).

A search of the literature revealed that these statements reflect no grounding in research, but rather are founded on prejudice and on the obvious fact, apparent to any visitor to Yemen, that qat is found everywhere in the country, and that it provides a major focus of interest to a high proportion of Yemenis. Such unsupported indictments nevertheless have continued to accumulate, and the question as to whether the heavy investment of time, money and activity on qat implies mass drug addiction in any precise sense is still unanswered.

The data presented in Chapter VI regarding the high proportion of income spent on qat are some evidence in favor of a hypothesis of widespread qat dependence, but the purpose of this chapter is to ask whether the concept of "addiction" applies in the Yemeni context. Does the Yemeni case have something to offer concerning such concepts as "drug dependence" in situations of widespread substance use? This turns out to a complex issue, and to require the exploration of a number of interrelated topics.

CONCEPTS OF ADDICTION

At the more extreme end of the scale of conceptions of addiction is the model based upon the opiates. This is the theory that some substances produce biologically-based "cravings" which create strong motivations and consequent behavior to satisfy them. The notion is that "true addiction" is signaled by the experience of physical “withdrawl symptoms” when the drug is withheld from the habitual user. A concomitant idea is “tolerance,” the notion that as the body becomes accustomed, a continuously increasing need is felt for more of a substance, with consequent driven “seeking” to procure the needed “fixes.” This then leads to continually greater neglect of ordinary behaviors in favor of drug experience and further drug seeking.

In 1956 a group of WHO experts (Eddy *et al.*) attempted to replace the term “addiction” with that of “drug dependence.” They divided the general concept into “physical dependence” and “psychic dependence”, specifying a set of subtypes corresponding to characteristics, effects and use patterns of several “prototypical” drugs. The categories of drug dependence they produced were: (1) morphine type; (2) barbituate-alcohol type; (3) cocaine type; (4) cannabis type; (5) amphetamine type; (6) khat type; (7) hallucinogen type.

Whatever the merits of the other categories in the WHO list, the logic of including “khat (sic) type” as separate and comparable to the others in the series was very weak. Evidence to back up this judgment will be presented later, but here it should be noted that the effects described for the “khat type” are essentially equivalent to those of the “amphetamine type,” though of lesser intensity. According to the authors, both amphetamine dependence and qat dependence fall under “psychic dependence”; they do not produce “physical dependence.” These two types are distinguished primarily on the basis of the development of a considerable degree of tolerance in the case of amphetamines, and the absence of tolerance in the case of qat.

The concept of “psychic dependence,” is less well-defined than is “physical dependence.”

> ‘Psychic dependence’ of a substance generally refers to most of the same qualities as does ‘physical dependence,’ but to be less powerful in its grip on the user because it does not produced physiological withdrawal symptoms or inevitable tolerance (Eddy *et al.* 1965:723).

The following judgment was made about qat, apparently on the basis of traveler’s reports:

> . . .the pleasurable effects afforded by khat are a strong inducement for many to procure by any means the necessary supplies at least once a day or to repeat or prolong the periods of chewing, often at the expense of vital needs such as food. Such behavior is a manifestation of psychic dependence (Eddy *et al.* 1965).

This is an unsupported statement, and according to our experience, it is extreme, but before addressing it the question should be asked: What are the Yemenis’ own conceptions of degrees of dependence produced by the drug? It is true that a general cultural concept of dependence on qat does exist. In Yemeni usage, the word *mula’i* signifies one who is “tied to” qat; that is, dependent upon it, but rarely is one so designated regarded negatively. Another term *mut’wala*, used more in the Taiz region, also refers to dependence, but has a less strong implication. It more closely approximates our concept of "habituated". The term *mudman*, on the other hand, literally means "addicted," but it is generally reserved for either opium or alcohol dependence, and is rarely used in connection with qat.

A common pattern we observed in many villages, particularly in qat-producing areas, is that there are a few individuals who are known to chew excess amounts of qat. These people chew huge quantities and are found to be chewing morning, noon and night. These make up a small subcategory of users above and beyond the "heavy use" category of this study. They are regarded as deviants and, somewhat as we regard alcoholics, are not held entirely responsible for their behavior. To these individuals, the term mudman was often applied, and it seems, accurately so.

Despite their use of the above terms, the unanimous report of the many Yemenis we encountered who had gone abroad to study, or for labor migration, was that they were able to cease chewing without any difficulty whatever. They claimed to be able to forget about qat altogether until they returned to Yemen. Mancioli and Parrinello who remained in Yemen over an 11-year period similarly noted this phenomenon:

> We should also mention the ease with which habitual users are able to temporarily abstain under specific circumstances (no smoker would be able to do the same with cigarettes). . . . The same case of quitting, at least temporarily, was observed in our private practice as the result of medical prescription (1967:162).

A number of migrants who presently go regularly to Saudi Arabia even said that one reason they emigrate is to *escape* for a time the social pressure to chew qat. Of course, the main reason for migration is to earn more money, but even if they earn the same salary in Yemen, the high prices of the drug, coupled with unavoidable pressures to chew, discourage saving. Pressures to conform are so strong that many university graduates who returned from Europe with new found disdain for the qat habits of their parents, nevertheless have found themselves chewing again within a few weeks. They reported feeling ostracized and cut off from the society of their fellows if they do not participate.

Despite much testimony that no physiological withdrawal symptoms occur, however, the issue is complex. Very heavy chewers produced many descriptions of experiences which appear to qualify as true withdrawl symptoms, even if they are relatively weak. Many of these heavy users described attempts to stop chewing qat more than once during their lives, and they gave three main reasons for having begun again.

First, they felt a profound lassitude, a lack of energy and general sluggishness. For several days they experienced difficulties in initiating their normal activities. They also experienced a slight trembling which could last up to several days. A third experience they reported was the occurrence of extremely unpleasant dreams for several nights after abstaining. For example, they often had rather paranoid dreams of being attacked, strangled or followed.

Some heavy chewers reported only one or two of these symptoms, while a few said they had experienced all three. All of them voluntarily attributed the onset of these negative experiences to the cessation of qat chewing. Yemenis who are not extremely heavy daily users did not report these symptoms; in fact, on direct questioning they denied experiencing them. However, they were aware that very heavy users report them.

One question in the sociomedical survey was intended to probe this issue. Respondents were asked whether they had stopped using qat at some point, and if so, whether the immediate results were good or bad. "Good" was defined as feeling physically better, "bad" was defined as having "symptoms" such as lassitude, weakness, nightmares or trembling. Figure 12 tabulates the results of this inquiry.

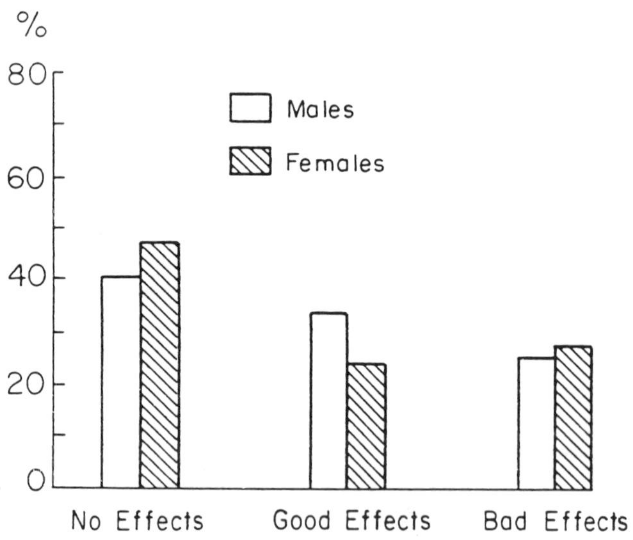

Fig. 12. Immediate effects of stopping on chewers.

These data certainly are not decisive, but they support the common belief among Yemenis that stopping is generally not problematical. However, more than 25% of the users did report "bad effects". More of those reporting these effects were among the heavy users, but differences did not reach a statistically significant level.

Thus, though the literature on the clinical effects of qat claims that it produces only "psychic" dependence and no physical dependence, I would assert that the nightmares and trembling which many very heavy users report after ceasing to chew cannot be explained away entirely as "rebound phenomena" (cf. Halbach 1972:27). The mildly depressive feelings with lack of energy and experienced powerlessness are probably partially due to psychological conditioning, supporting a notion of psychic dependence; but the general malaise, trembling and bad dreams appear to be purely physiological responses to drug deprivation. These data support the hypothesis that a mild form of physiological dependence does result from extremely heavy use. However, as long as the percentage of people using qat at this very high level remains small, true physiological dependence will continue to be relatively unimportant in the overall Yemeni picture.

TOLERANCE

Just as with the question of dependence, the self-limiting nature of the use patterns creates problems in dealing with the concept of tolerance to qat. The amounts normally chewed are relatively standard and fall within fairly narrow limits. At a typical session most individuals chew one robta of the long branch-type or the equivalent amount of leaves of other types. The larger robtas are the 18 to 30 inch bunches from the Wadi Dahr near Sanaa, or those from Hadnan on the mountain of Jabel Sabr near Taiz. Two or even three small sawti bundles of leaves, or two bundles from Haraz or other areas may be chewed to gain an effect equivalent to that from one large marbita from Wadi Dahr. By "small", I mean bundles from six inches long and four or five inches thick, such as the sawti or hajaji from the Sanaa market, or the small sacks of loose leaves (mandil), sold in Taiz by the female traders of Jabel Sabr. In attempts to estimate more precisely the amounts used it was found that chewers averaged about 100 grams of picked leaves during a session. However, some users chewed more than 200 grams, and some as few as 50 grams.

Despite such variations, the customs of use automatically create a general limit on the amounts of active ingredients which can be ingested. Ingestion is by absorption of the active ingredients in the juice through the mucous membranes of the mouth as the fresh leaves are chewed, and by swallowing. During the chewing period, a gradually enlarging cud or bolus of leaves is retained in the cheek. Even the distendable cheek of the average Yemeni, unbelievably stretched by long term use, can hold only a few ounces of chewed leaves, and as mentioned, the normal-sized robta or mandil is well calibrated for the customary three-to-four hour chewing period. When the time of the session has elapsed, most chewers have gauged their supply so that they are just finishing or have just finished their qat. Some may stay on a bit longer, quickly finishing what they have left — perhaps even refreshing what remains in their cheeks with a few fresh leaves donated by a neighbor who has brought an excess amount. After lingering for perhaps another half-hour, the remaining few guests inconspicuously expectorate their chewed leaves into the small brass receptacles and silently depart. The customary length of the session, which in turn roughly follows the cycle of drug effects, is another condition placing limits on the amount chewed.

An mentioned earlier, a number of exceptions to the general afternoon-session pattern exist. Merchants, taxi drivers, stone-cutters and other laborers often empty their first cheekloads after several hours and reload them at least once. This enables them to maintain the feeling of energetic well-being which qat provides. All these individuals consider qat as necessary to their productive activities, and even though they chew more than the average Yemeni, they too are limited by the sheer impossibility of chewing large amounts of leaves. They find it difficult to chew more than twice as much as the ordinary chewer.

THE LATENCY EFFECT

Many foreigners who chew qat for the first time claim to feel no psycho-physiological effects at all. They concur with the traveler Niebuhr, who, in the mid-18th century reported that: ". . . its insipid taste gives no indication of extraordinary virtues, the only effect we felt from the use of this drug was the hindrance and the interruption of our sleep" (1792, orig. 1774).

This raises another important issue, the question of the degree to which a cumulative buildup of the active ingredients in the body is a part of the qat experience, i.e., whether there is "tolerance" to the drug. One explanation for the often-reported lack of experience on first chewing could be what has been called a "latency" characteristic, and El-Mahi has proposed that qat has precisely this quality:

> From the historical down to the contemporary (period) khat has been known to have a definite threshold, i.e., a latent period varying in time from two to six weeks before its action become clearly and subjectively manifest in the taker. . . . Khat chewing practised for the first time would not produce any effect at the outset; the effects appear after a period of latency during which there is evidently an imperceptible building up of the "reaction" (El-Mahi 1962:13—14).

At least two questions are involved here. One reason for the often-reported lack of perceived reaction on first chewing could be the proposed latency or cumulative effect, but another might be that a period of learning is necessary in order to identify effects, to respond to them and finally to enjoy them (Becker 1963:46—58, Weil 1972:83—85). The evidence suggests that both of these factors are operating.

As Becker and Weil have so well described for marihuana, for many drugs some period of experimentation is required to learn to distinguish experiential changes, as well as to understand the range of feelings which are possible to experience. As is the case with marijuana and other drugs, some novice chewers of qat report no initial effects, but this is by no means always true. Many people, myself included, report a heightening of mood within the first hour, while others report that they do not feel any changes of mood of behavior.

Subjective unawareness of their own behavior changes seems particularly noticeable in some normally talkative and intense individuals. One typically verbose and active professor, visiting the research site in Yemen, for the entire duration of his first chewing session kept vehemently claiming that he was experiencing no effects at all. But those of us who knew him agreed that his normally mildly "manic" traits became much more pronounced during the afternoon. Ordinarily he is much more responsive to feedback, but on this occasion, as one Yemeni intellectual aptly remarked, "It was like talking to a radio." It was also noticeable that the volume on the "radio" was turned up.

These considerations of learning do not rule out the possibility that cumulative effects may also be important. Indeed, we have some evidence which is confirmatory of the "latency" hypothesis. Figure 13 is taken from our EKG monitoring of the changes in heart rate of a subsample of 55

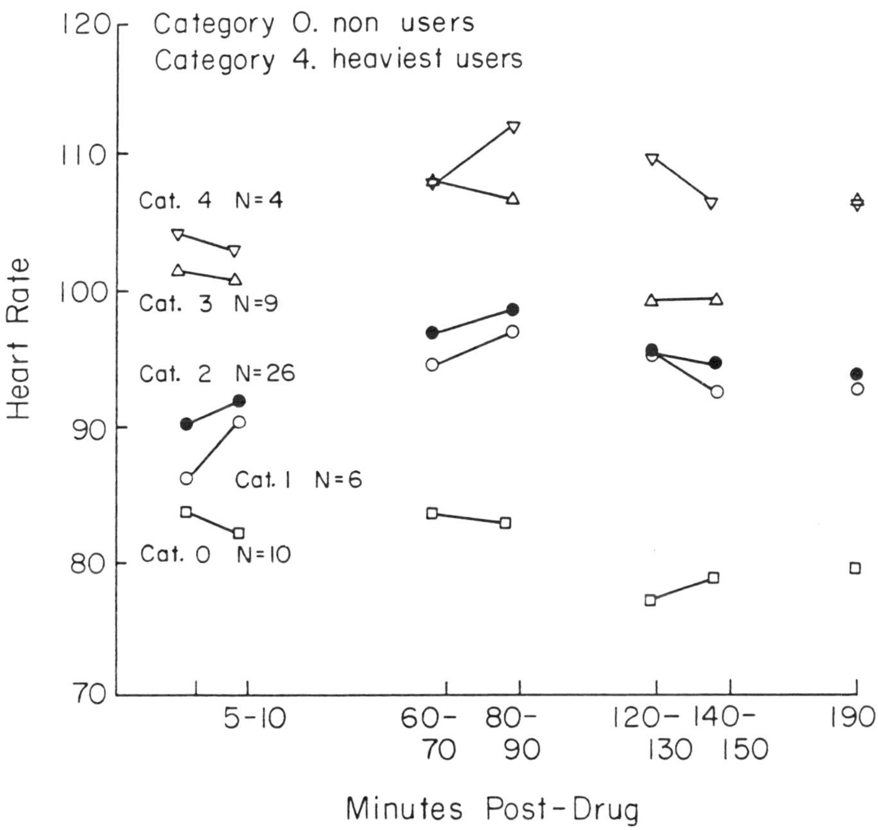

Fig. 13.

subjects who chewed qat under experimental conditions in our field station in Sanaa.

These categories of individuals were at first classified from 0—4 on a scale of heaviness of chewing.[1] It is most interesting that the pattern at the beginning of the session is exactly what we would expect if a latency effect were being produced. The non-chewers of the control group were recorded at about 83 beats per minute at the beginning while the heaviest chewers are over 100 bpm, and the others ranged between these in appropriate order. Each group held its relative position throughout the pattern of rise and decline during the three-hour chewing period. This provides provisional evidence that each group of chewers began the session with a different and category-consistent level of the active ingredients in their systems, which was proportionately augmented by chewing.

From all of this it is clear that the "tolerance" question is more complex than might have been supposed. In many publications it is stated bluntly that no tolerance factor exists for qat (e.g., Halbach 1972). However, it is clear that the amount of active ingredients of the drug which may be ingested by an individual user is automatically limited by the customary means of use, and we could find no evidence in the literature for these statements that there is no tolerance build-up. Some recent pharmacological research, in fact, supports my own cautious hypothesis: ". . . from this study we can infer that tolerance develops to pharmacological effects of khat, even if some caution is needed" (Nencini *et al.* 1983:151).

The evidence from this study on the "latency" question leads towards a hypothesis of what might be called "stabilized" or "controllable" tolerance. That is, each individual appears to attempt to achieve a level of the active ingredients which "feel right" to him. This is achieved, or maintained, through a self-regulated pattern of intake. Qat chewers seem to make partially unconscious choices regarding the optimum levels of the psychoactive substance for the sensation they want to achieve. Cultural use patterns, regulated somewhat by natural limitations upon amounts of active ingredients which can be ingested, enable Yemeni users to gauge and anticipate the effects upon their systems fairly accurately. Each person learns to produce his own individually comfortable kayf, in terms of its intensity and duration.

This assessment is also supported by the fact that chewers can easily classify themselves as to how much and how often they chew, and their neighbors also are well aware of their customary patterns of consumption. Without hesitation informants said that they chew once a week, three times, or seven, and they chew a preferred amount each time. They consciously make decisions based upon a number of factors in addition to the desired state: income as it relates to cost, immediate economic needs, future plans, allocation of time, etc. The vast majority are able to control their intake according to rational criteria, and this supports the hypothesis that people try, and generally succeed, to hold steady the levels of active ingredients they judge to be optimum. They are not led down an inevitable path of increasing dosage to a state of hopeless "addiction."

We may even propose that these levels of active ingredients which accumulate in the body, and the accompanying feeling states, may be geared to particular types of qat. I have pointed out that in Yemen the qats from many areas are regarded as distinctive in their effects. In Sanaa, for example, expensive types such as those from "the Wadi" or from Dula are held to produce a better kayf, and to produce many disagreeable side effects, than for the cheaper sawti or hajaji from farther north. In Hodeida, the shami is much superior to the harami; the jeddi and hadnani are among those with good reputations in Taiz, while sharabi, maqtari and jashani are among those reputed to be "strong" and of poor quality.

There is also a common belief that "the qat is best in its own country." This aphorism means that the best effects are achieved with the qat one is used to, and which is taken in familiar surroundings. However, in keeping with our hypothesis of "controllable tolerance," we found that after only a very short period of experimentation, strangers in an area are soon able to select the types and amounts of local qat which suit their individual preferences and pocketbooks.

AVAILABILITY

A variable which may confound studies of addiction is that of availability or access. In most countries laws against various substances, and variable degrees of success in enforcing them, may make for a large unknown factor, and costs certainly are another aspect of the equation. The situation in Yemen is very interesting because qat is legal, and it is harvestable over a period of several months. In addition, the staggered planting practices, differences in microclimate, irrigation in some areas and the construction of new roads all have worked to create a situation in which qat is virtually always available in most parts of the country. Contributing to this availability is the fact that in almost any qat market one can find a cheap kind of qat as well as an expensive one, with a complete range of prices in the larger markets.

For the majority of Yemenis, therefore, the availability factors is nearly a constant. Qat is readily available most of the time to most people at a price which they regard as within their income capabilities. This is particularly true in Sanaa, Taiz and Hodeida, even though as has been shown, at lower levels of income the choice to chew regularly may mean a sacrifice of some amenities of life. Access to the drug is not completely uniform, however, and differential availability does sometimes play a role. In the rural areas where qat has long been grown there are considerable numbers of people who may chew two or three times in a single day, and a few who do this several times each week. People from the northern part of the country claim that inhabitants of Hujjariyya, particularly the inhabitants of of Jabel Sabr, spend most of their time lying around chewing.

Our observations in this region did not completely bear out this stereotype of general excess, but they did give it some support, adding evidence that availability is a factor relating to frequency of use. For example, we observed that at weddings and other special occasions, people of Jabel Sabr, like those in some other qat-growing areas, chewed two or three times daily during the harvesting seasons. We were also shown individuals in these areas who chew several times a day throughout the year, but this degree of heavy use is much more common during the rainy season when qat is abundant and the price is low.

It must be emphasized, however, that such a high level of qat consumption is not a universal pattern anywhere in Yemen. Even where qat is most plentiful the majority of people do not chew anywhere near the maximum which would be possible, and there are always some non-chewers and light chewers in addition to the heavy users.

Adding to the evidence from qat growing regions the importance of availability is the fact that in a survey of nearly 300 qat merchants in and around the three cities of Hodeida, Taiz and Sanaa, approximately 96 percent were heavy chewers, with most of them chewing more than one robta daily. Thus, the proposition is supported that if a person has a high degree of access to qat, either by growing it or selling it, there is a strong tendency towards habitual heavy use.

We have said that though there are seasonal fluctuations in amount and therefore price, a majority of Yemenis have access to a more or less continuous supply of qat. Moreover, there are few attitudinal or cultural restraints against using the drug. Nevertheless, the generally high cost does work to induce restraint. At the time of our study the prices averaged from two to eight rials per robta for the inexpensive types, and from 12 to 50, or sometimes even 100 rials per robta for the more expensive types. These prices more than doubled over the next few years (Revri 1983:82—83). Even if people stick to the cheaper varieties, qat certainly constitutes an important proportion of the budget of most families. This is reflected in Figure 8 in Chapter VI.

The question of addiction to qat has been discussed in somewhat general terms, but it is useful now to take different perspectives on the dependence question, and to ask whether there is anything which this analysis might suggest concerning general theories of drug abuse. Theories of addiction are for the most part predicated on the assumption that people ingest psychoactive substances or engage in other similar "compulsive" behaviors because they feel threatened, anxious, in pain and/or inadequate in some sense. The actions of the substances permit them to temporarily forget these feelings, by providing them with an "escape from reality." The escape experience then tends to become so highly rewarding as to be "craved" and repeated (e.g., Kielholz 1973:8—9).

It has struck me as curious that while authorities and investigators have nearly unanimously placed most explanatory weight on the notion that drug addicts are motivated primarily to escape their problems through blotting out the pain of "reality," the users themselves often speak of "kicks" and emphasize the pleasurable side of drug taking. When reduced to their essence, most explanations turn out to be some variation of the simple pleasure/pain theory. It may seem obvious that both pain and pleasure are involved, in varying proportions; that different drugs vary in their actions of either deadening pain or enhancing pleasure. However, explanations seldom attempt to sort out and assess these differing effects.

The assumption that the major motivation for drug use and abuse is escape from the realities of a harsh environment or from facing the consequences of an inadequate self-image arise with monotonous regularity in the literature, and most authors writing about qat in Yemen also routinely fall back on to some form of this argument. The impression conveyed is that Yemen is a country of qat addicts, and that the explanation for this behavior is that it is a response to the universally miserable conditions existing in the country. For example, although Mancioli and Parrinello are not dogmatic at all, they employ the same stereotype:

> Undoubtedly the desire for qat is conditioned by environmental factors: the monotony, the harshness of life, the general low cultural level which inhibits various interests, etc., are elements which are present in Yemen and foster the spread of the use of qat (1967:161).

Stanton Peele has sharpened and elaborated this commonly held general set of causal assumptions by describing what he calls the "analgesic effect":

> The definitive characteristic of every sort of addiction is that an addict takes something that relieves pain of whatever kind. This 'analgesic experience' goes far towards explaining the realities of addiction to a number of very different substances (1978:61).

> Addiction is an extension of ordinary behavior — a psychological habit, dependence or compulsion. Just how pathological or addictive that behavior is depends in part on a person's life. When an involvement eliminates choices in all areas of life, the addiction has been formed (1978:67).

The analgesic theory clearly puts priority on pain avoidance, and though relief from distress may be said to be in some sense pleasant, this emphasis on pain makes the pleasurable side of the drug experience secondary and actually removes it from a causal status.

This analgesic concept does, of course, account for much drug dependence that we see. It obviously works fairly well in the context of the urban scenes of large American and European cities where substances such as morphine, heroin and other opiates are used on a large scale. It also works, to a limited degree in Yemen. However, the pain reduction concept seems much too rigid and simple for a general theory of all drug habituation. For example, it does not take account of individuals like legendary Oriental potentates and many others whose pain and malaise are not demonstrated.

These people may take opium for pleasure. But the weakness of such attempts to stretch this a narrow theory to cover *all* forms of habitual substance use can more clearly be seen in Peele's strained attempt to apply it to the stimulants. Referring to recent research by Paul Nesbit, he says:

> How can we analyze addiction to cigarettes and other stimulants in terms of experience when that experience is not analgesic? The answer is that cigarettes free smokers from feelings of stress and discomfort just as heroin does, in a different way, for heroin addicts.
>
> The person who becomes addicted to cigarettes (and other stimulants) apparently finds the rise in his heart beat, blood pressure, cardiac output and blood sugar level reassuring. This may be because the smoker becomes attuned to his internal arousal and is able to ignore the outside stimuli that normally makes him tense.
>
> Coffee addiction has a similar cycle. For the habitual coffee drinker, caffeine serves as a periodic energizer throughout the day. As the drug wears off, the person has not changed his inherent capacity to deal with the demands which his day demands of him, and the only way for him to regain his edge is to drink more coffee. In a culture where drugs are not only legal but generally accepted, a person who values activity can become addicted to nicotine or caffeine and use them without fear of interruption (*Ibid.*:66).

Though it is hard to see why increased heart rates etc. are automatically reassuring, Peele's argument is attractive in some ways. However, it does not probe deeply enough. The blanket use of the analgesic model inhibits a more penetrating inquiry. It fails to distinguish the stresses coming from the environment from those stemming from the poor self-image of the individual in dealing with the environment, or from the "conditioned" response of lack of energy, etc., i.e., the rebound phenomena, which may accompany cessation of a stimulant. Even more important, it assumes without proof that the negative desires to avoid rebound effects are more important than any desires to achieve positive feelings.

How far does this "analgesic hypothesis" actually take us in accounting for widespread qat use in Yemen? Recent pharmacological studies have indicated that cathinone has some analgesic action on mice (Abdullahi *et al.* 1983), that qat raises beta-endorphin (Nencini *et al.* 1983), and that it reduces fatigue (Elmi 1983).

Some of our data also bear on this general problem, since in our interview schedule we asked a number of questions which relate to motivations for chewing. These had been previously derived from participant observation in many qat sessions where we had probed people's attitudes. For example, the sociomedical interview contained the general question: "Are there any situations, apart from normal social ones, when it is beneficial to chew qat?" Among a number of items which informants had spontaneously listed prior to the sociomedical survey were five which referred specifically to pain relief in a broad sense (colds, fevers, headaches, body aches and sadness). Thus, in the interview informants were specifically queried as to whether qat produced these benefits and when they had last experienced each benefit. The answers enable us to propose that, if chewers tend to use qat to relieve pain, this will be reflected in the heaviness of their chewing. The hypothesis may be stated more specifically as : *Heavy chewers will tend to report more pain-relieving benefits than will light chewers.*

Before examining the breakdown by heaviness of chewing, it seems significant to note that 72% of the chewers in our sample see qat as providing some kind of relief from pain. This gives support to the assertion that some analglesic effect is being experienced by users and is part of the answer to the question of why many people chew qat. On the other hand, it seems quite remarkable that in a country where qat is so available, where there are widespread beliefs about it as an antidote to sickness, and where everyone has considerable experience with it, as many as 28% of the regular users reported no pain relieving benefits at all. This is even more remarkable when we break down the group reporting "no benefits" and find that 30% of them are heavy users and 17% of them are moderate users. That is, nearly half of them are those whom we would expect to be believers in its efficacy. Now let us look at a finer breakdown.

Figure 14 shows that more heavy users are among those reporting more pain-relieving benefits, and that significantly more of those reporting "no benefits" are among the light users. Thus, these data do provide some provisional support for the hypothesis of analgesic effects. However, this effect must be very weak, and it could be argued that Figure 14 shows also that the heavier the use, the more one is likely to *believe* there is some pain relief in it. Perhaps the more one chews, the more he tries to justify the high expenditures of time and money involved. However, at present, it seems reasonable to assume that both placebo and analgesic effects may be contributing to this finding.

Such questions cannot be completely resolved with data from this study but we can still look at the analgesic question from other perspectives. One of these is to conjecture that poorer people are likely to suffer more general distress and exposure to sickness than are wealthier people. If indeed qat is a drug which facilitates significant alleviation of pain and distress, or is perceived to do so, poor people would be more likely to use it for that purpose than would wealthier people. The reasoning here is that the poor are more likely to chew for the alleviation of distress than are the rich, who may also sometimes chew for that reason but who will not be subject to as much distress, and would therefore be more likely to cite other reasons. We can frame this hypothesis as follows: *Chewers who are poor will tend to report more pain-relieving benefits than will wealthier chewers.* When our data are applied to this hypothesis, Figure 15 results:

It shows that, contrary to the hypothesis, the more wealthy the chewer, the more he or she is likely to report pain-relieving benefits. This may be interpreted to indicate that the Yemenis in the sample do not chew more if they are poor, i.e., they do not chew for the purpose of alleviating the generally stressful conditions of poverty. However, caution is indicated here

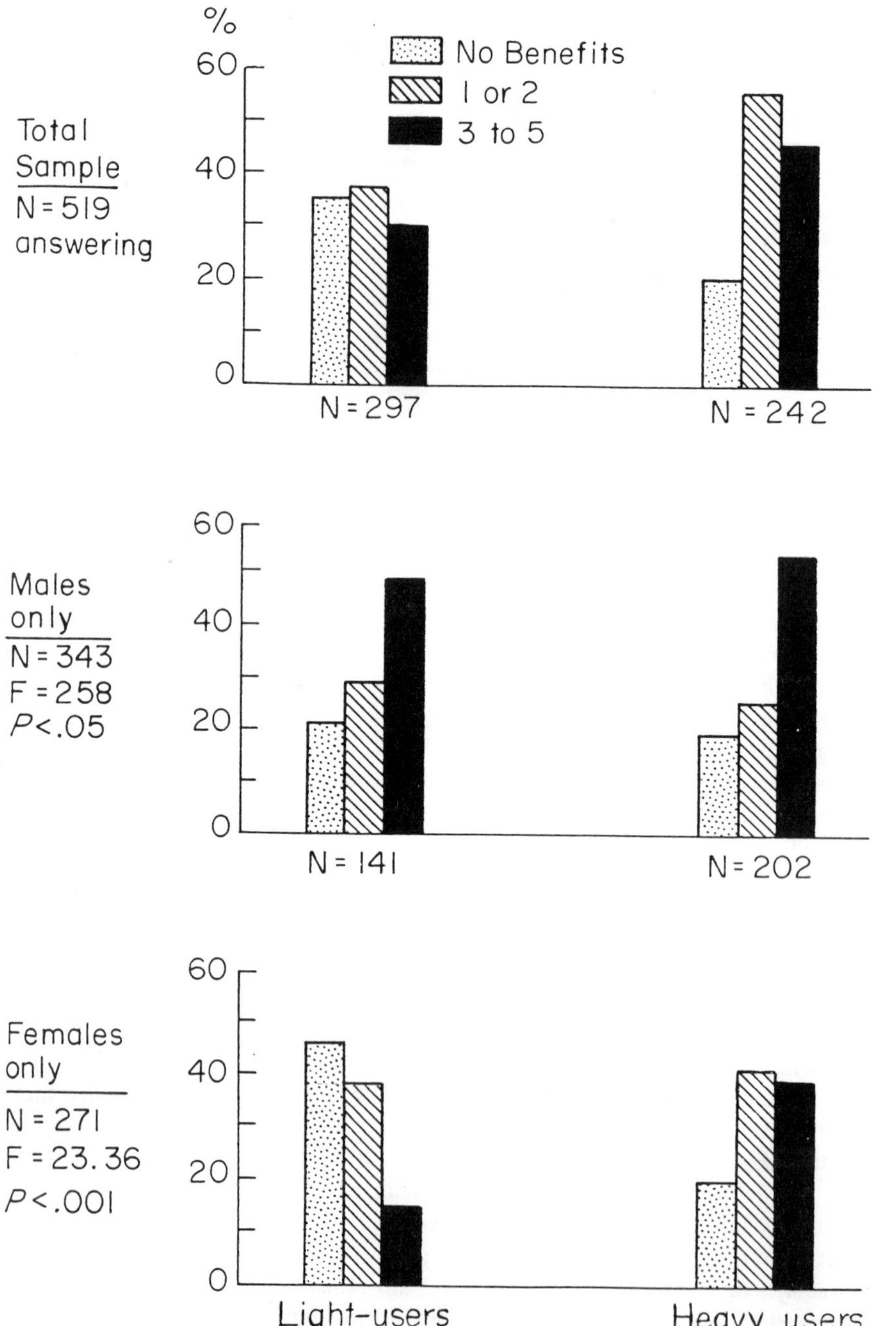

Fig. 14. Number of pain-relieving benefits by user category.

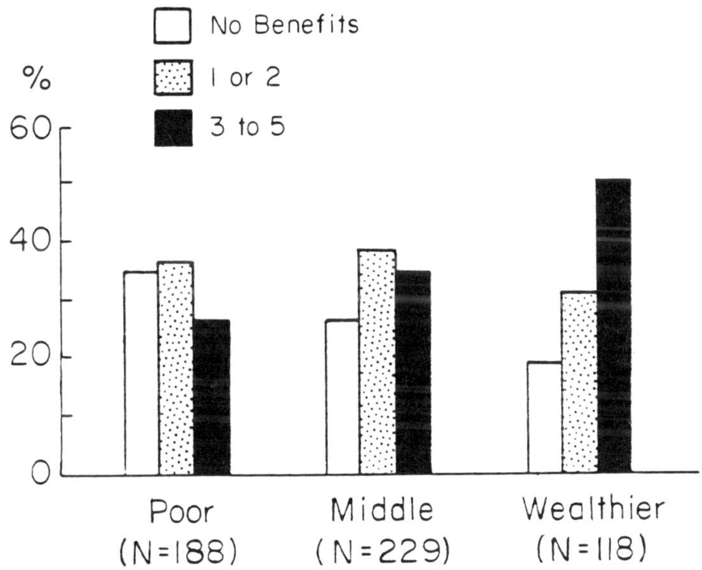

*males: F=26.05, p.< .001, females: F=0.035, n.s.

Fig. 15. Number of reported benefits by income category.

as well. It could be argued that wealthier people's experience with the drug is more meaningful since they can afford enough of the drug to provide the analgesic effect. This goes along with the observations that the greater the *access*, the greater the propensity to chew more. Contrary to the above interpretation it is our consistent observation that the *amounts* of qat ingested do not vary much between rich and poor. However, it seems possible that the cheaper qat chewed by the poor produces less analgesic effects along with the greater number of negative side effects, and that this could partially account for the differences. This opens up a question which should be pursued in future research.

A third method of partially testing the analgesic hypothesis with our data is to examine the propositon: *Chewers who are more ill will tend to report more pain-relieving benefits than chewers who are less ill.* This is based on the assumption that ill people will be likely to experience more distress than well people, and will, therefore, tend to be found more in the ranks of the heavier chewers. Our sample was classified into (1) those who are well or only suffering from minor complaints; (2) moderately ill people who can still function fairly well; and (3) severely ill people. Looking at these classes in terms of the frequency of pain-relieving benefits reported, the situation depicted in Figure 16 emerges.

These results are somewhat ambiguous with regard to an analgesic

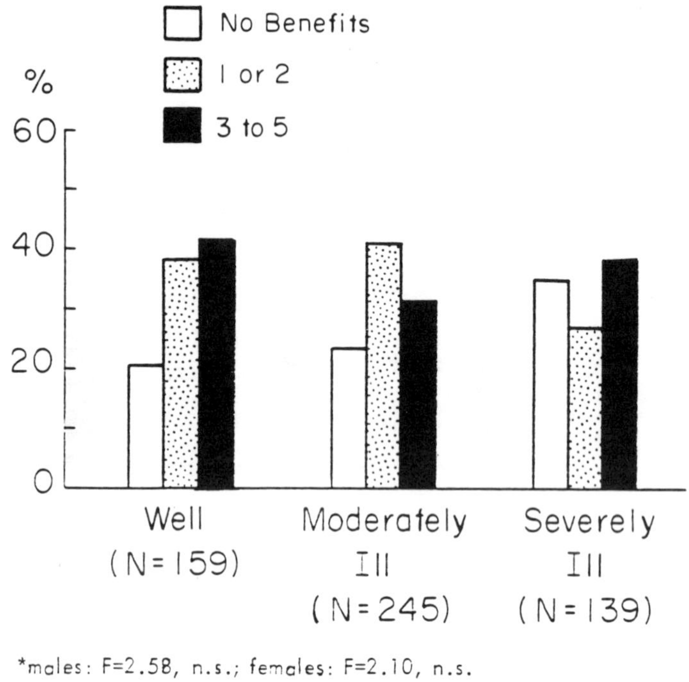

Fig. 16. Number of reported benefits by degree of illness.

explanation. There are few differences between the illness categories, but those that do not exist are in the opposite direction. That is, well people actually tend to report more pain relieving benefits than do sicker people. In fact, 87% of those classified as "well" report at least some pain-relieving benefits, while only 65% of the "severely ill" report them. This may reflect the fact that severely and chronically ill people do not find the mild analgesic properties of qat much of a relief, while "well" people do find relief in it for transient aches and pains. These figures could thus be interpreted to support an analgesic hypothesis. However, since the "well" category contains a disproportionate number of "wealthy" people, this may further confound the results.

In a final effort to approach the question of analgesic motivation for chewing qat, the physician member of our team (Teague, M. D.) classified all of the illnesses diagnosed by the doctors in our study as to their pain-producing potential. Each was classified on a 3 point scale: 1 = no pain potential; 2 = some pain potential; 3 = high pain potential. Figure 17 shows how this scale relates to chewers' perceptions of pain relief.

The results of this breakdown are much like those which emerged with the general overall illness categories. The distributions are again mixed, and again a contrary result emerges; the lower the pain potential, the more

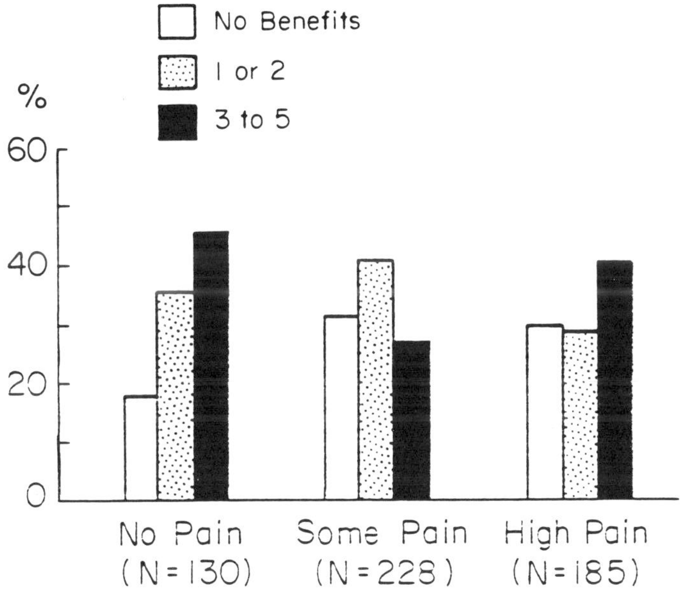

*males: F=0.68, n.s.; females: F=0.77, n.s.

Fig. 17. Number of reported benefits by pain rating.

likelihood there is of perceiving pain-relieving benefits from qat chewing. These data along with those in Figures 15 and 16 are fairly conclusive evidence against a simple analgesic hypothesis. Qat seems to provide some relief for minor distresses, but it may be concluded that attempts to escape harsh reality, although they may be important in particular cases, are motivations operating within a complex constellation of causes, and are not major factors accounting for the massive chewing of qat which characterizes North Yemen. Of course, motivations for drug use are rarely simple, and this indeed, is one of the reasons why the oversimplified "analgesic hypothesis" was challenged.

Let us now turn to the question of positive motivations or reward characteristics of qat. While again admitting that no definitive answers can be given, some of the data can be applied to the problem with the hope of moving a step forward.

In addition to our early informal interview questions about the possible relief from pain which the drug might afford, we also asked about the feelings of the "kayf" or state of pleasure, which chewers experience. As indicated in a previous chapter the pleasurable feelings upon which considerable consensus emerged were (1) increases in the flow of ideas, (2) alertness, (3) ability to concentrate, (4) contentment, (5) confidence, and (6) friendliness.

In our more formal interview respondents were then routinely asked to choose as many of these six as they thought applicable to their own kayf experiences. It may be inferred that the numbers of such experiences listed by chewers should be some measure of the pleasurable effects of qat chewing.

Following reasoning similar to that used with the problem of pain relief, the hypothesis proposed is that: *Heavy chewers will tend to report more pleasurable experience effects than will light chewers.*

In Figure 18 we observe a definite trend: heavier chewers do tend to report more positive effects than do light chewers. It may be inferred from

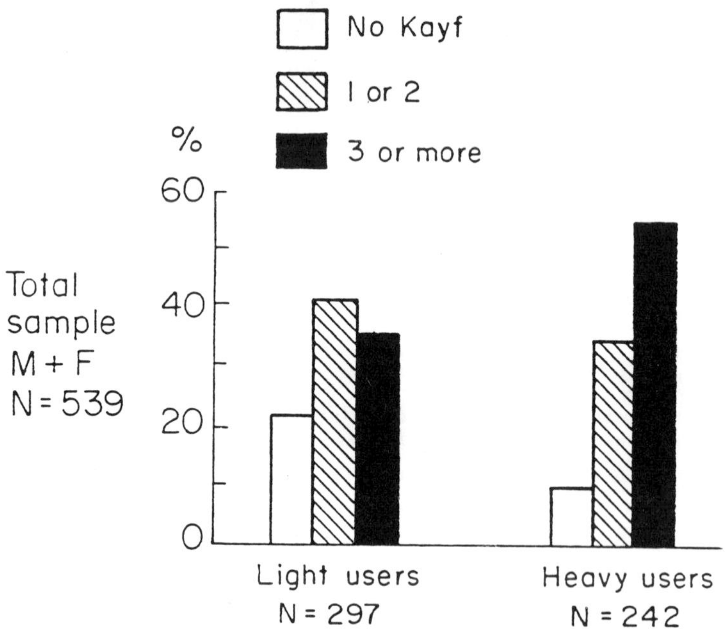

Fig. 18. Number of positive kayf effects by user category.

this that greater pleasure is generally associated with heavier use. The finding that 9% of the heavy chewers and 21% of the light users (14% of all users) report no pleasurable kayf effects is a bit enigmatic, but perhaps is explained by the fact that a number of those classified as light users chew less than a robta, and only once or twice a week. It is also true that the norms and pressures on people are so great that a number of individuals who either derive no pleasure from chewing qat, or have attitudes against it, still feel it necessary to chew.

The foregoing data and discussion have neither convincingly disproved the analgesic hypothesis nor have they strongly supported an alternative "pleasure-seeking" hypothesis. The evidence is mixed. There certainly are minor analgesic benefits from qat use, but these do not seem adequate to explain the widespread and intensive use of this drug in Yemen. Thus, though it must be admitted that there is considerable usefulness in the analgesic hypothesis, in order to push our understanding of drug use farther it would seem necessary to distinguish carefully between drugs, and to introduce other ideas. It seems clear that we must not only consider the question of drug effects on alleviation of pain and the production of pleasure and their interrelationships, but we must also look more carefully at the particular *kinds* of pleasure and the *kinds* of pain or discomfort involved.

For example, we spoke of the necessity of distinguishing between "conditioned" drug-related discomfort responses, and the discomforts and pains which impinge more directly from the environment. It also seems necessary to break down the *kinds* of dependence or addiction according to the *kinds* of rewards involved. To begin this type of analysis we may distinguish at least the following motivations are potentially related to the "choice of drug."

First there are those drugs which specifically relieve corporeal pain or discomfort without affecting consciousness directly; asprin, codeine, etc., come to mind here. Second, are those drugs which may not only deaden pain, but are primarily used for their consciousness-altering properties. Some of these have a pain-reducing capacity as well, but with them the motivations of the user generally are to either "escape from reality" and/or to enter "another reality," This experience holds the promise of being very pleasurable and may be sought for its pleasure alone, or since its alteration of consciousness also removes the perception of pain, discomfort and/or failure, it may also be sought, at least in part, for these indirect analgesic properties. Of course, the powerful effects of these drugs may combine a number of these motivations, a feature giving them tremendous appeal. Not only are pain and the feeling of inadequacy in the face of an intractable environment made to disappear, but a world of drowsy womblike numbness, or one of interesting fantasy images and activities is made available. Pain removal and pleasure-producing characteristics are combined in a powerful dose of positive reinforcement. In this class we would place morphine, heroin, the psychedelics, etc.

A third type of drug does nothing directly to block pain, nor does it, in itself, produce any alterations of perception, escapes from "reality," or journeys to the hidden layers of personality. Instead, the main effects of such drugs are to elevate mood, and to speed up cognitive processes. Rather than facilitating an escape from consciousness and from "ordinary reality," they facilitate awareness of, and perceptions of *connectedness with* that reality. They can induce a sustained focus of attention and high concentration, along with increased sense of capability and control of the environment. In controlled dosages these substances heighten both mood and cognitive process to produce an outward, active orientation of external reality. They facilitate extroversion, sociability and communication, rather than introversion, passivity and self-preoccupation.

In other words, their relationships to pleasure and pain are of a different order than is the case with the other two classess of drugs I have outlined. A period of cessation of the *awareness* of pain, discomfort and inadequacy is certainly facilitated, but it is accomplished not by a numbing or an alteration of consciousness, but by an intense focus upon the "real" ideas and activities valued by the culture. Sometimes these substances do indeed transfer attention away from some "real" problems, but more often they stimulate intensive efforts to solve these. Such effects are facilitated by feelings of enhanced self-worth and a heightened sense of ability to master the situation, while at the same time transferring energy and attention away from one's own person. A sense of mastery and control is certainly rewarding, but it is a different *kind* of reward from the childlike pleasure or nirvana produced by the direct stimulation of pleasure and fantasy. It is a reward directly relevant to socially validating self-reinforcement and outward socially-valued goals, rather than to narcissistic indulgence.

In the case of institutionalized stimulant drugs like qat, the basic theory of pain and pleasure surely must be utilized, but kinds of pleasure must be distinguished as well as kinds of pain. We must devise ways of assessing the relative weight of these and even think of reversing their usual explanatory order in some cases. Chewing qat is a pleasurable experience and contributes to one kind of "pleasurable reality," and anything which gives intense pleasure temporarily assists the user to transcend his surroundings. For example, the near total absorption achieved in active sports, rituals, etc., have the accompanying, rewarding "side effects," of reducing levels of anxiety. They assist in the forgetting of pain by allowing escape from mundane reality for the moment.

What is proposed is really only a case for a more complex theory. In the case of stimulants we need to shift away from a simple negative focus upon the "analgesic" reduction of pain with the reinforcement this offers, an explanation which might be appropriate with other drugs. Instead a theory in which the pleasures of enhanced mastery of reality are given a proper role in the complex equation should be developed.

As is probably evident by now, personal experience with qat along with our more objective study is what led to my thinking on these matters. It seems evident that Yemen has evolved a cultural institution around the qualities of the third type of drug outlined, and that these qualities have shaped major features of Yemeni culture and experience. I now want to conclude the discussion with some further reflections on the problem of "massive addiction" and institutionalized drug use in Yemen. It seems evident that this important feature of Yemeni society cannot be explained by reference only to the drug effects themselves. A more comprehensive view must be added.

I propose that a social institution has been created which provides rewards to people over and beyond those which may be associated with drug use *per se*. At the qat session, people are entertained and may express themselves in a relatively uninhibited and spontaneous manner. It is a place, where as at no other time, each person has license to be himself or herself. The person who is ordinarily ignored can command attention, and anyone may argue without being held fully to account. The shy are encouraged by others, as well as by the stimulus of the drug, to come forward socially. At the same time, the session is a place where there is a general expectation that mundane concerns may be transcended, and this is encouraged. The senses are heightened, attention is fully aroused and focused; the essence of this experience is the feeling of mastery, of being fully alive, fully social, and therefore "meaningful" in an existential sense. Since this state is rarely attainable for most people much of the time in any society, it is not surprising that Yemenis look foward to it. The qat session is an institution which temporarily produces that "sociability" in Simmel's connotation, or "communitas" in Victor Turner's terms, which is so valued by human beings everywhere. Thus, it is not, as "addiction" concepts would have it, simply the drug effects upon which people are "dependent," though these effects certainly do have positive reinforcing value. Clearly, these feelings are a predictable physiological symbol of the sought for, valued state. They identify its presence. However, what users are "addicted" to is the *qat session* itself as a sustained *set* of pleasurable experiences, a many-faceted reward system. It is this ever newly created micro-world of personal meaning which has become associated with its most tangible feature, the mood-enhancing qat leaves.

Of course, the actual situation is not quite to simple as this. Certainly, group interaction *in itself* can produce such euphoric feelings and temporarily raise feelings of self-worth. Qat and other stimulants can also surely generate some of these effects in isolation. What I am arguing is that when the natural excitement of group interaction is joined with the mood-enhancing effects of the drug, a synergistic effect is produced which is many times more powerful and rewarding than either in isolation. As has been pointed out for other substances, both setting and psychological set are important to an overall drug experience (Weil 1972:29—30), but these set-and-setting effects vary in their roles with different drugs. With psychedelics a supportive environment may help to induce a "good trip," but with a stimulant like qat environmental features of sociability act powerfully to reinforce the mood-elevating and cognition-enhancing drug effects.

When viewed in this way the concept of "withdrawal pain" and "withdrawal symptoms" also can be seen in a broader way. It is not simply the pains of physical withdrawal from the drug which pull the Yemeni qat user back again and again, but even more powerful negative effects of "social withdrawal symptoms," i.e., experiences of deprivation of the joys of companionship and comraderie which the qat session almost unfailingly provides.

Concepts of social reward and its synergistic power help us to understand the widespread, regular use of qat, but they still do not seem sufficient. There is more to the issue than millions of individuals, each simply satisfying his or her own needs for physical and social stimulation.

In Yemeni culture it is universally accepted that it is "proper" and even quasi-obligatory to go to qat sessions. The social pressure is to go rather than not to go, and those who do not participate are seen as somewhat deprived, though they are not ostracized. Many people reported that they go to qat sessions because they *should* go. We have talked to numerous people who do not particularly like qat and who rarely or never chew enough to achieve a kayf. Some think qat is far too expensive for their budgets, yet they feel constrained to chew at least once or twice a week. Regardless of preference, however, it is certain that if a person does not chew he or she will miss out on most of the interesting behavior and communication which the society has to offer. Such individuals are seen by peers as people who are "out of it," and only strong personalities can stand against such pressure to conform. Most people feel it necessary to be where the social action is — in the qat session.

The point should not be belabored, but it bears emphasis as a part of any overall attempt to account for why the majority of Yemenis use the drug qat to the extent they do. A concept of "cultural drug dependence" or "drug-facilitated sociability dependence" needs to be added to the equation containing physiological and psychological effects of the drug. Qat may well originally have become institutionalized largely on the basis of the qualities of drug effects and interaction rewards we have outlined, but once institutionalized, the social norms themselves began to exercise their powers as important forces in the motivational configuration. The cultural behavior patterns relating to use are fine examples of the qualities of "exteriority" and "constraint" in Durkheim's terms; they are invested with the character of true social norms. It is necessary to add the social and cultural components to the psychopharmacological theories of drug dependence to achieve an adequate understanding of the widespread, institutionalized use of qat, and this is probably true of several other drugs as well.

Given the manifold cultural, social, psychological and physiological functions of qat and the institution which has grown up around it, it is understandable why, under the stimulus of recent culture change, the importance of it has increased, and the use of it has continued to spread. A significant proportion of the new money coming into the country from migrant remittences and development projects is channeled into the growing, trading and consumption of qat. Though she overstates the case, I believe Weir is essentially correct in stressing these economic factors behind "recent efflorescence" of qat use (1985:168). Varisco also makes a valid point for at least some Yemenis when he argues that "the meaning of chewing is that it gives the chewer a meaning, a sense of his or her own identity in rapidly changing world over which he or she has little or no control. . . . The modern Yemeni has a need to identify himself in a positive way. Chewing qat is distinctively Yemeni and shared with no other Arab Culture" (1986:3).

It is important, however, to maintain a balanced perspective in order to understand this many sided phenomenon. As we have seen, the motivations for chewing qat are complex. They derive from numerous mutually reinforcing sources, which vary for individuals. When the psychophysiological importance of the drug is underplayed, as it is by these authors, as much distortion is produced as when cultural, sociological and economic factors are not accounted for.

CHAPTER IX

QAT AND HEALTH

What effects may qat have upon the health of individuals? Certainly, the possibility of health effects is one of the more important questions which can be raised about the use of any ingested substance, and in this instance many health problems of Yemen have been laid at the door of qat. On the other hand, it has been asserted by many, particularly Yemenis, that to associate health problems with qat-use is absurd. On more than one occasion in qat sessions, young intellectuals upbraided me for bothering to study such a trivial subject as qat and its uses. "You should be spending your time and money studying our serious economic problems, rather than our recreation," one young man told me during a qat session in Taiz. However, such opinions were not frequent since many Yemenis are aware of the criticisms that have been leveled against their precious plant. Many wonder what its long-term effects might be. Our team usually received strong support and cooperation, and a strong curiosity was frequently expressed about what adverse health effects there might possibly be. In this chapter some more health related findings of the study are presented. It will be seen that drawing clear-cut conclusions on these matters is very difficult.

GENERAL HEALTH CONDITIONS IN YEMEN

Reliable health statistics from the Yemen Arab Republic are not available, but the general health picture in the country is dismal. There is a lack of adequate sewage systems, and the negative effects of this are naturally to be found primarily in the growing cities. However, the capital, Sanaa, which has traditionally depended upon packs of roving half-wild dogs to clean the garbage from the streets at night, is protected somewhat from the effects of poor sanitation by its high elevation (2,250 meters) and its low humidity. The port city of Hodeida, on the contrary, must cope with heat and high humidity, both of which exacerbate the problems of pollution which prevail there. Since there are no rivers, lakes, or reservoirs in Yemen, surface water is scarce, and is mostly obtained from wells and cisterns. The water sources of the country are often contaminated with schistosoma and other parasites (Arfaa 1972, Kuntz *et al.* 1953). The country is 100% Muslim and ritual washing in contaminated mosque pools promotes further spread of water-borne diseases. Poor nutrition, deriving from deficiences of protein and of fresh vegetables containing vitamins, in combination with high frequencies of endemic parasites, severely affects the health of the Yemenis. These conditions are mostly unchecked due to the general lack of adequate health facilities and the low level of medical knowledge and education among the people (Bornstein 1974).

The meager health data which are available reflect under-reporting since no surveillance system or vital registry exist, and no adequate health surveys have ever been undertaken. The Government of North Yemen reported in 1975 that the five most prevalent diseases were gastroenteritis (17,909 cases), malaria (8,119), amoebiasis (6,789), bilharzia (3,932) and typhoid (3,705) (Nyrop *et al.* 1977:182). Some estimated disease incidence rates from WHO for 1975 were: tuberculosis 25/1000, dysentery and intestinial parasites 850/1000, and malaria 20/1000. Thus, though statistics are inadequate, there is ample information to support Nyrop *et al.*'s statement that:

> The efficiency of most Yemenis is impaired because of both parasitic and enteric disease and diseases caused by vitamin deficiencies. Night blindness from lack of Vitamin A, scurvy from lack of Vitamin C, and rickets from lack of Vitamin D are common. Niacin, riboflavin, and iron deficiencies are the norm. Because of the widespread malnutrition and the constant barrage of enteric ailments to which they are subjected, Yemenis are very susceptible to death from prosaic illness (1977:182).

Our findings regarding the possible relationships between qat-use and health must be considered in the context of the appalling picture of Yemeni health in general. The purpose in this chapter is to provide information which may assist in assessing the extent to which qat-use may play a role in that overall picture.

As stated earlier, the Yemenis are nearly unanimous in the opinion that qat is *not* an important threat to their health. On the contrary, as we have seen, the majority of them feel that qat is beneficial for minor ailments such as headaches, colds, minor body pains, arthritis, fevers and depressions. A few of the more educated people even claim that the plant is preventative of diabetes and hypertension.

Not all Yemenis regard qat as without danger to health, however. Most of the 22 doctors that we interviewed felt that excessive use may lead to transient gastric difficulties. Nonetheless, these doctors were generally in agreement with the majority of the general population in their opinions that negative effects of qat use are largely economic rather than health related. Most of those Yemenis believing that qat is harmful to health come from the small minority who have traveled or been educated abroad, where they have come in contact with Western notions of drug "abuse."

THE MEDICAL CASE AGAINST QAT

It is primarily foreigners who have proclaimed the harmful health effects of qat, though some Yemeni intellectuals are of the same opinion. Most of the condemnations have been the anecdotal impressions of non-medical people, but some medical writers, most of whom have never spent any appreciable time among qat chewing people, have also dwelt upon negative physical effects. These authors have been so adamant and so "authoritative" that questions arise as to why the Yemenis, Ethiopians and other East Africans have continued to chew it for centuries, and why the patterns of use still continue to spread. Why have not rulers of Kenya, Somalia, Ethiopia, and Yemen stamped it out before now, or at least made it illegal?

Halbach, the most noted and cited medical authority on qat, asserts unequivocally that certain ailments are "common" among qat chewers: gastric problems such as stomatitis, esophagitis, gastritis, constipation, malnutrition, and cirrhosis of the liver. He claims that anorexia, sexual problems and anemia also definitely result from chewing the drug. Basing his conclusions largely upon anecdotal evidence, this authority generalizes that qat-use produces "a vicious circle — Khat-destitution-hunger-anorexia-malnutrition-digestive troubles-anorexia, etc." (1972:25—26, 1980:319).

In 1977, physicians Luqman and Danowski wrote an article essentially repeating Halbach's list of harmful effects of qat, but adding "occasional schizophrenia," "confused speech," and "spermatorrhea" (247—248). Again, no research to support this conclusion was cited. Mancioli and Parrinello, were physicians who stayed in Yemen for some 10 years, and they also indict qat for its effects on health. However, their actual evidence on the matter is somewhat mixed.

Prevalences of any of the allegedly qat-related health problems among chewers and non-chewers are rarely mentioned in this literature, and most figures presented are sheer guessing or are inadequately documented. Yet readers of these medical writers cannot easily escape the conclusion that many diseases are unequivocally caused by qat-use. If one considers the more than 500 years during which large groups of people of this area have used this drug on a regular basis, it is very strange that such a mild stimulant could be so rewarding that millions of people would ignore the terrible medical consequences which are alleged. This apparent paradox was one of the questions which led us to make a study of qat-use in Yemen. In addition to some of the other questions already taken up in this book we wished to address some of these medical questions in a more systematic way then had been done before.

ASSESSING HEALTH

The basic methodology of this study has been outlined in Chapter I. Here we need only present some of the more specific methods for dealing specifically with issues of health.

In order to handle the question of overall health status for users and non-users of qat, a classification scheme was developed based upon the relative potential of the various conditions for inducing functional incapacity, disability, and death. Under the scheme, the subjects were each classified as severely ill, moderately ill or well, based on the aggregate of their disease conditions. To avoid neglecting possible effects of qat-use in inducing illnesses of lesser import, tallies were also made for each participant of the number of conditions in each level of severity. Both the assigned severity classifications and the number of conditions in each severity category were then tested with chi square tests for association with qat-use.

A total of ninety-five different diagnoses were made in the research population and many individuals were diagnosed as having two or more illnesses. However, for many of the diagnoses which the literature links with qat-use, too few cases were diagnosed even to allow valid chi-square tests to be made. This in itself raises doubts regarding the prevalence of the problems alleged to be associated with qat-use. Particularly for diseases with generally moderate to high incidence, if qat is substantially increasing the relative risk, the prevalence should increase as well, and be reflected in our data. Despite the limitations of using general physical examinations as a diagnostic modality, it is remarkable that this should not have occurred.

Figure 19 indicates that for males there is a suggestion that qat-use is associated with modest increases in the prevalence of severe illness. On the other hand, there is a strong association between poor health and use among women. This association can be seen even more clearly in Figure 20 which selects "qat-related" diseases and problems, i.e., those which have been particularly cited as resulting from qat-use.

Figure 20 shows that for males, there is no association of severity of allegedly "qat-related" illness with qat-use in general, or with the degree of qat-use. On the other hand, Yemeni women's health is generally worse than men's, and our data indicate that they are more affected by the use of qat, whether they are light or heavy users. What can account for this?

It can be proposed that because men get preference in quality and amounts of food (Bornstein 1972:33), the nutrition of women may suffer in comparison to that of men, and this potentiates the effects of qat. It is also true that the female role puts women at greater disease risk by exposing them to contaminated water sources. They are the ones who carry water daily from the cisterns and wells, who wash the clothes and dishes, etc., in addition to cleansing themselves for prayer. How this might affect women's susceptibility to "qat-related" illnesses must remain conjectural at this point, and no definitive evidence to support this hypothesis is yet available.

Results in this chapter will focus primarily on what have been termed "qat-related" disease categories, and on organ system based groupings of health problems. The tables include only those diseases and medical conditions which occurred in sufficient numbers in the sample to warrant statistical tests. Individual diseases were also grouped by the general organ systems within which they induce pathology. The groupings by system serve to moderate the problems of diagnostic misclassifications which may occur in

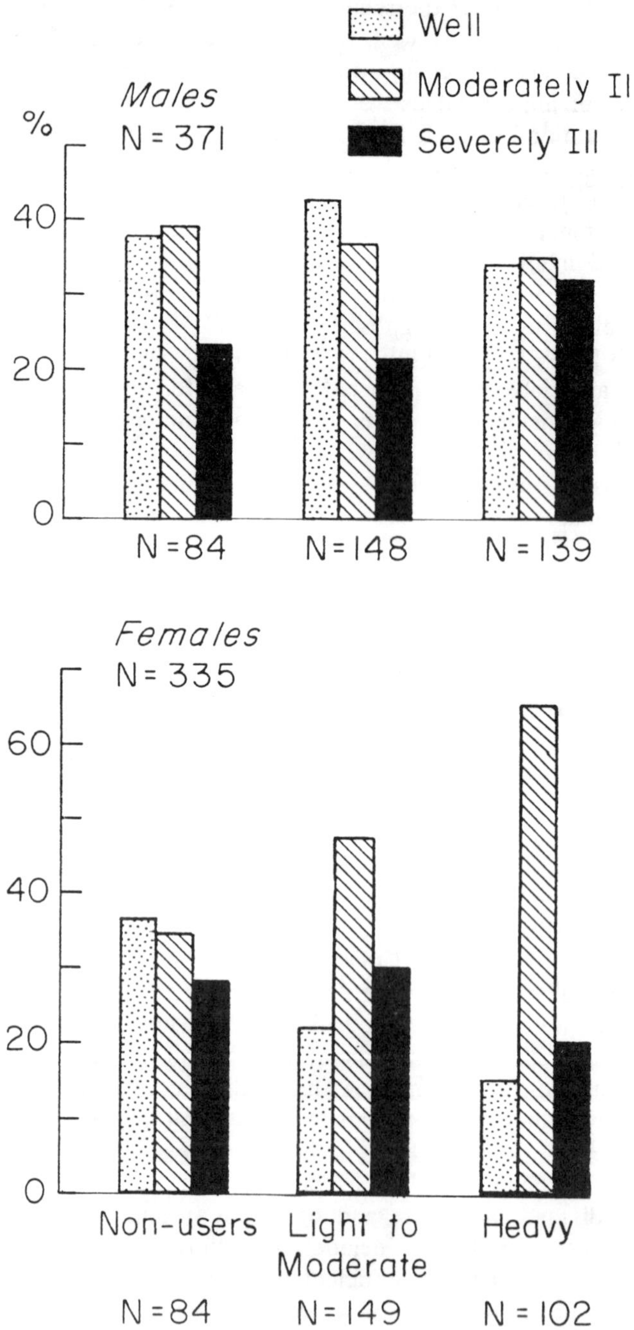

Fig. 19. Final diagnosis scale by use categories.

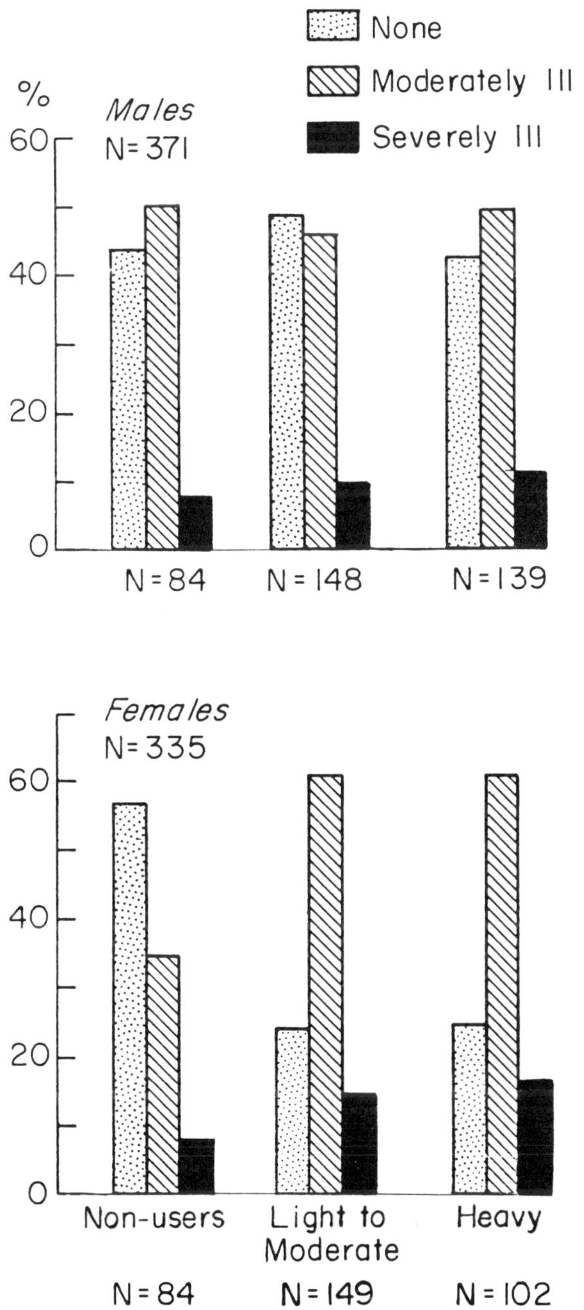

Fig. 20. "Qat-related" illnesses.

single physical examinations. Thus, if increasing levels of qat use are associated with increasing prevalences of pathological conditions in an organ system, this would tend to support a proposition that the particular body system, as a system, may be vulnerable to qat effects.

The tables also reflect the two types of data: diseases and problems detected during the physical examination, and diseases and problems which through the medical history by which the physician judged the patient to have suffered, the ailments in the past. These types of data are designated "dx" (diagnoses) and "hx" (histories) respectively. Since the histories (hx) refer to the entire cumulative life-span of the patient, they are more likely to have occurred in any given case than the diagnoses (dx), which were identified at the time of examination. History items thus seem likely to be less accurate because they depend upon memory and self-report. Some ailments may have been omitted from the histories, and misclassification is somewhat more likely to occur.

Our measures of economic status did not show any strong associations with disease. This obviated the necessity of controlling for them in this part of the analysis. It also confirms our observations that differences in wealth in Yemen are not reflected in vastly different styles of life. For example, diet, sanitation, and probability of exposure to infectious diseases do not vary significantly by class, and thus Yemenis have been fairly uniformly subject to disease regardless of their economic levels.

The order of reported findings here is as follows: On the basis of existing literature (1) hypothesized qat-related problems are classified by organ systems; (2) within each organ system statistically associated findings, including those exhibiting a dose-response gradient are tabulated by individual diagnoses, individual histories, and by organ system groups as wholes; (3) in diseases with strong crude associations, effects of age and area factors are controlled for by Mantel-Haenszel odds ratio estimates.

GASTROINTESTINAL PROBLEMS

Of all the ills which have been attributed to the use of qat, those associated with the gastrointestinal system are most frequently mentioned by foreigners and by the Yemenis themselves. Medical writers on Yemen agree that gastritis and constipation are the most frequent problems of the gastrointestinal system, and they implicate the irritant effects of the tannins in the leaves as a main cause of these problems (Halbach 1972:25, Luqman and Danowski 1977:248, Mancioli and Parrinello 1967:144—146).[1] Qat has at least two modes of producing gastrointestinal effects. The first is the direct physical effect of the material ingested, with the tannins being the most important ingredient, and second, secretory, muscular and absorption activity are probably effected via the active alkaloids: cathinone, cathine, and the cathedulins.

Anorexia and hemorrhoids are two related gastrointestinal problems which have been attributed to qat (Luqman and Danowski 1977:248). However, Mancioli and Parrinello believe that "... gastric and duodenal ulcers are exceptionally uncommon" and that this may be a positive effect of qat use (1967:147).

Such allegations make it reasonable to propose that the following gastric conditions identified by our doctors should be positively related to levels of qat-use: acute gastritis, chronic gastritis, hemorrhoids, colitis, and avitominosis. Ulcers, on the other hand, should be negatively associated with levels of use. Table IX depicts those findings where sufficient numbers of cases were diagnosed that statistical tests could be made.

Six specific gastrointestinal ailments appeared as diagnoses in members of our sample (chronic gastritis, hemorrhoids, colitis, ulcers, esophagitis, avitaminosis), but none of these were found in high enough frequencies to warrant statistical tests. Gastrointestinal history items which occurred infrequently were ulcers, and diarrhea. Those specific diagnoses and specific histories with sufficient numbers are listed on Table IX. They show that the only strongly associated individual diagnosis was acute gastritis in females. In males a weak trend in the predicted direction was found. In the gastrointestinal histories a reversal is evident; here males were significantly affected, whereas females were not. In all these cases evidence supports some qat involvement. When we group the entire series of gastrointestinal history items as a body system we get the results arrayed in Table X.

The data in Table X indicate that the prevalence of gastrointestinal system conditions in the sample generally are very high, and that they increase with the level of qat-use. Among females both the G.I. diagnosis groupings and the G.I. history groupings are strongly associated with increasing use. Among males the prevalence of the G.I. history group is strongly associated with increasing use, and though the G.I. diagnosis group is weakly associated, it shows a dose-response gradient in that direction. These data thus tend to support the hypothesis that qat-use is contributory to gastrointestinal problems in Yemen. However, this confirmation is not true for all gastrointestinal conditions; many specific conditions were present only in very low numbers, or were not correlated with use as expected.

The overall rates for stomach ulcers for the diagnoses were males — 2.4%, females 2.7%. For the histories they were: males 1.9% and females 2.2%. Though the numbers were too small to make statistical tests meaningful, it can be noted that the comparative percentages between non-chewers and both levels of chewing were virtually identical. Thus, the hypothesis of a negative correlation between ulcers and use was not given even provisional support.

TABLE IX

Gastrointestinal problems (specific disease categories)

Condition	Males N = 371				Females N = 336			
	Non	Lt	Heavy	Sig	Non	Lt	Heavy	Sig
Dx Acute gastritis	10.7%	11.5%	17.3%	$\chi^2 = 2.116$ $p = 0.251$ n.s.	1.2%	22.1%	22.3%	$\chi^2 = 19.784$ $p = 0.0001$
Hx gastritis	22.6	25.9	42.0	$\chi^2 = 12.39$ $p = 0.002$	42.2	62.8	57.8	$\chi^2 = 9.40$ $p = 0.009$
Hx constipation	34.5	54.7	64.0	$\chi^2 = 18.45$ $p = 0.001$	53.7	65.8	64.6	n.s.
Hx anorexia	14.3	25.7	50.5	$\chi^2 = 11.6406$ $p = 0.0030$	42.2	39.6	53.5	n.s.

TABLE X

Gastrointestinal groups (*Dx* and *Hs*)

Condition	Males Non	Males Lt	Males Heavy	Males Sig	Females Non	Females Lt	Females Heavy	Females Sig
GI Dx group	22.6%	19.6%	28.8%	n.s.	21.4%	46.3%	46.6%	$\chi^2 = 19.784$ $p = 0.001$
GI Hx group	52.4	66.9	80.6	$\chi^2 = 19.76$ $p = 0.0001$	73.8	91.9	91.3	$\chi^2 = 18.03$ $p = 0.0001$

PARASITES

The literature on the medical effects of qat does not postulate any relationships between parasites and qat-use. However, since qat is ingested orally and since our doctors diagnosed parasites with considerable frequency, it is of interest to see whether such an association might exist. Those parasites which logically could have a more direct relationship to qat-use have been classified as Parasite Diagnostic Group I. Diagnostic Group I includes Ascaris lumbriocoides, Giardia lamblia, Entamaeba histolytica, Hymenolepis nana, Entamaeba coli, Enterobius vermicularis, and Chilomastic mesneli. These might conceivably be connected with qat-use since they usually enter the body orally, through food and drink. Because qat is an orally ingested drug, it might act as a vehicle, or as an agent facilitating colonization by some of these parasites. Of this group only three appeared with sufficient frequency that a statistical test was possible, and none of them exhibited a strong association with use in either the male or female sample. When treated as a group the percentages shown in Table XI were found.

TABLE XI

Parasites

Condition	Males Non	Males Lt	Males Heavy	Males Sig	Females Non	Females Lt	Females Heavy	Females Sig
Dx Group I parasites	19.0%	13.5%	20.0%	n.s.	15.5%	28.9%	23.3%	n.s.

URINARY TRACT PROBLEMS

The attribution of urinary tract problems to qat use has been put forward by a number of writers (e.g., Halbach, 1972:25, Luqman and Danowski,

1977:248, Mancioli and Parrinello, 1967:147). The specific diagnoses in this category uncovered by our physical examinations were: acute cystitis, chronic cystitis, urethritis, renal colic, kidney stones, and prostate problems in males. Not one of these diagnoses was found in sufficient numbers for statistical analysis, nor were there any apparent associations with use levels. When the urinary system is taken as a whole, however, we get the figures in Table XII, which for women are at least suggestive.

TABLE XII

Urinary system

	Males				Females			
Condition	Non	Lt	Heavy	Sig	Non	Lt	Heavy	Sig
Urinary Dx group	15.5%	21.6%	17.3%	n.s.	8.3%	19.5%	21.4%	$\chi^2 = 6.40486$ $p = 0.0407$
Urinary Hx group	32.1	35.1	36.0	n.s.	25.0	33.6	37.9	n.s.

These data indicate that in both diagnoses and histories there is a slightly greater prevalence of urinary problems among qat users, particularly among female chewers. There is thus some evidence to contradict the hypothesis of no association. We have so far been unable to account for the observation that increasing use in females is associated with a relatively higher prevalence of urinary disease than it is in male users. Again we must fall back on the surmise that perhaps females generally have poorer diets and are more vulnerable to poor sanitary conditions than are males, and that qat-use tips the balance in favor of poor health.

ORAL CAVITY PROBLEMS

In informal conversations foreign physicians and Western trained Yemeni doctors often mention the negative effects of qat chewing on the oral cavity. The literature on qat tends to support this view. For example stomatitis is mentioned as frequent by both Halbach (1972:25) and Luqman and Danowski (1977:248). The latter authors most clearly state the common opinion: "Stomatitis is common among those who begin to use khat, then persists with chronic use, producing local irritation and secondary infections." Periodontal disease is also said to have a high rate among male qat users (Halbach 1972:25), while dental cavities are claimed to be rare (Luqman and Danowski: 248).

In line with this latter finding is some research by a German dentist, E. Schafer. After examining the teeth of 140 people of various ages from the small Yemeni village of Al-Djaddaijah, he stated that 90% of the villagers were regular qat users and that use has a cleansing effect on the teeth which is beneficial (cited in Makki 1975:1). On the other hand Ina Makki, a dental surgeon working in Yemen in 1969—71, claimed that qat chewing is carcinogenic. In her unpublished thesis she reported 74 cases of mouth and tongue tumors in a clinical series of 5757 patients in the coastal city of Hodeida. She found that the majority of these patients were men over 40, who had chewed qat *or* used *shama* (finely ground tobacco placed between gums and cheek for stimulant effects) for 20 or more years. Furthermore, the tendency for the carcinomas to be in the areas of the mouth where qat is used was to her highly suggestive of a causal role for the drug. However, she used no control groups, and no formal sampling techniques or statistical methodologies were employed. Most questionable, in view of the known carcinogenic potential of tobacco, is the fact that she could not distinguish the possible effects of shama from that of qat. Nevertheless, her contention that the use of qat and shama are implicated in mouth cancer in Yemen certainly should be given serious consideration in future studies.

We had no dental specialists among the team of examining physicians, but it is interesting that our medical examinations, which included careful attention to the mouth, found very few cases of severe oral disease and no cases of cancer. In our sample there were five different diagnoses of oral cavity problems (discolored and rotting teeth, missing teeth, gingivitis, glossitis, and stomatitis). Two of these, "discolored and rotting teeth" and, "missing teeth" occurred with enough frequency to warrant statistical tests, but neither of them showed any association with use. Nor did the oral cavity dx group as a whole show any association. It is particularly interesting that stomatitis was so rare in this sample, since it is so widely assumed to result from qat chewing. Oral cavity problems constitute another case in which the literaure-derived hypothesis concerning the negative effects of qat-use is not supported by our data.

LIVER PROBLEMS

The liver has been suspected to be particularly vulnerable to negative effects of qat use. For instance, both Halbach and Luqman and Danowski think that cirrhosis may be a result of heavy use (1972:25; 1977; 248). Mancioli and Parrinello do not speak of cirrhosis, but citing radiological evidence from a series of more than 20,000 of their patients, claim other hepatic malfunctions are related to qat-use.

> In essence, the cholecystographic examinations show alterations considered favorable to the development of cholelithiasis itself." . . . and ". . . in Yemen a small hepatic insufficiency is clinically detectable in not less than 50% of the population . . . (1967:147).

Our examinations revealed only three dx categories of liver problems in the Yemeni males of our sample (cholecystitis, hepatic insuffiency, and hepatitis), and only two diagnoses in females (cholecystitis and hepatitis). The prevalences are quite low and the few positives which turned up are in the heavy user category. This is true for both males and females, weakly supporting the proposition that specific liver problems are related to qat-use. However, as Table XIII shows, the individual history "jaundice", and liver history problems as a group were strongly associated with qat-use in women. Again we note the curious male-female differential.

TABLE XIII

Liver histories (*Hx*)

	Males				Females			
Condition	Non	Lt	Heavy	Sig	Non	Lt	Heavy	Sig
Hx jaundice	13.1%	13.5%	15.8%	n.s.	8.4%	23.3%	16.8%	$\chi^2 = 8.11515$ p = 0.0173
Liver Hx group	13.1	13.5	15.8	n.s.	9.5	22.8	16.5	$\chi^2 = 6.613$ p = 0.0356

As a related set of problems, it has long been thought by both physicians and educated Yemenis that diabetis is rare in Yemen and many have felt this is related to the widespread use of qat. A group of Egyptian scientists working in Sanaa have now given support, if not yet complete confirmation, to this belief. In their first study they selected 15 male non-qat consuming diabetics at the Kuwait Hospital in Sanaa, and collected samples of blood from each of them following an overnight fast. Then each subject drank a 250 ml. glucose solution, and blood samples were taken each half hour up to 2 1/2 hours. The blood was then analyzed for glucose concentration. The same patients were then kept on a diabetic diet with no drugs for one week, after which the experiment was repeated with 250 ml doses of the same amount of glucose mixed with an extract from 50 grams of qat.

The results showed that the qat extract significantly lowered the rise in the blood sugar count in all patients. For example, in the first experiment the mean gluclose immediately after fasting was 205.9 mg. After one hour it was up to 320.5 mg, and by 2 1/2 hours had dropped to 270.3 mg. In the experiment where qat extract was mixed with glucose, after being kept on a proper diet for a week, the count started at 181.3 mg., then went up only to 237.8 mg. after an hour, dropping again to 201.9 mg. at the end of 2 1/2 hours. The differences at each 1/2 hour were significant at the 0.001 level of significance, showing a dramatic effect of the qat in keeping blood sugar low (Ramadan *et al.* 1978).

Encouraged by this finding, the group then went on to do another experiment with groups of qat users differing in degree of use. This was done on 80 male volunteer blood donors at the Kuwait Hospital, who were divided into four groups: non-users, and those who reported using qat costing 10, 20 and 30 or more Yemeni rials per day. Blood from each of the subjects was frozen and sent via air to Ein Shams University in Cairo for testing.

The results of this experiment showed that non-users and light ("mild") users were about the same (fasting blood sugar at 85.3 and 83.5 respectively). However, in the moderate (20 rials) and heavy (30+ rials) groups fasting blood sugar was lowered significantly (76.14 and 72.2), i.e., to the point of mild hypoglycemia (Ramadan *et al.* 1979). These findings lend provisional empirical support to widely held beliefs that the widespread use of qat may contribute significantly to the low incidence of diabetis in Yemen.

There is, of course, the further implication from these findings that heavy use may result in hypoglycemic conditions. It may be proposed, however, that the heavy meals of starch and fat taken before chewing may mitigate these potential effects by helping monitor adequate blood sugar levels. There were also significant increases in lipids, decreases in triglycerides and high increases in potassium (see Ramadan *et al.* 1979 for details).

This research is certainly preliminary, and it needs adequate replication as well as expansion. It should be noted that the authors do not attribute the blood sugar lowering and other effects to the alkaloids, but instead implicate the tannins and minerals in qat (Ramadan *et al.* 1979, 1980).

CARDIOVASCULAR PROBLEMS

With regard to relations between cardiosvascular problems and qat use the existing opinions tend to be contradictory. For example, Halbach reports that:

> Migraine, cerebral hemorrhage, myocardial insufficiency and infarct, and pulmonary edema have been described after the intake of khat, particularly in older and predisposed individuals" (1972:25).

and

> The assumption that hypertension in *young persons* without other apparent etiology is due to the *chronic intake* of khat is supported by the observation that spontaneous remission occurs after consumption ceases" (1972:25).

However, most writers, as well as the 22 Yemeni doctors interviewed in our study uniformly believe that cardiosvascular problems are rare in Yemen, and that this may be related to the common use of qat. Luqman and Danowski point out that hypertension is "not observed" among chewers (1976:248), while Mancioli and Parrinello state that: "cases of angina or disorders of the peripheral circulation have never been detected" (1967:144).

On the other hand, short term effects in the cardiovascular system do occur. It has been reported by many writers that qat ingestion produces transient conditions of tachycardia and raises blood pressure (e.g., Luqman and Danowski 1976:248, Mancioli and Parrinello 1967:144). In the present study we monitored EKG changes over three hours of chewing in a subsample of 60 men. The average heart rate increased a total of about 10 beats per minute during the first 90—100 minutes of a session, and then gradually tapered off to its previous level over another 90—100 minutes, even though some qat was still being chewed during this latter period (see Figure 13, Chapter 8). Whether such regular increases in EKG and other such effects conduce to strain on the system, or possibly have beneficial or no effects over the long term, remains a question.

In line then with the hypothesis that cardiovascular problems would not be associated with increasing use, we found that only one, cardiopathy, among our diagnoses (which included heart trouble, hypertension, caridopathy), and only one (heart trouble) of three histories (heart trouble, stroke, hypertension) occurred with sufficient frequency that statistical tests could be applied. Neither of these was associated with qat use in either males or females. Furthermore, though there were slight positive gradients among males of the dx group, and among females in the history group, neither of the cardiovascular disease groupings was significantly associated with use. In view of the prevailing opinions about qat and cardiovascular problems, these negative results are interesting enough to present in Table XIV.

TABLE XIV

Cardiovascular (groups)

Condition	Males				Females			
	Non	Lt	Heavy	Sig	Non	Lt	Heavy	Sig
Cardio-vascular Dx group	4.8%	6.8%	11.5%	n.s.	15.5%	15.4%	10.7%	n.s.
Cardio-vascular Hx group	10.7	13.5	11.5	n.s.	9.5	14.1	15.5	n.s.

These findings do not strongly support the frequently heard opinion that qat use may be protective against cardiovascular difficulties, but they are not inconsistent with it. They do, however, undermine implications of the drug in the causes of cardiovascular problems.

RESPIRATORY PROBLEMS

The literature is silent on the question of whether there should be any relationship between qat use and respiratory disease. However, since people tend to smoke much more heavily during qat sessions than at other times, it seems logical to look at the respiratory data. Our doctors diagnosed five respiratory dx ailiments in our sample: (bronchitis, bronchial pneumonia, chronic bronchial asthma, respiratory vescularis, emphysema). Of these, only bronchitis was found to the frequent enough to allow a statistical test. As Table XV shows, it proved to be in the direction of positive association but was of only moderate strength. However, as seen in Table XVI, when all of the respiratory ailments are grouped together increasing levels of qat use appear to be strongly associated with increasing prevalence of respiratory problems.

TABLE XV

Respiratory problems (*Dx*)

	Males				Females			
Condition	Non	Lt	Heavy	Sig	Non	Lt	Heavy	Sig
Dx bronchitis	8.3%	6.1%	13.7%	$\chi^2 = 4.9855$ p = 0.082 n.s.	4.8%	10.7%	14.6%	$\chi^2 = 4.793$ p = 0.0911 n.s.

TABLE XVI

Respiratory problems (*Dx*)

	Males				Females			
Condition	Non	Lt	Heavy	Sig	Non	Lt	Heavy	Sig
Respiratory Dx group	20.2%	11.5%	23.0%	$\chi^2 = 6.9946$ p = 0.0307	15.5%	17.4%	23.3%	n.s.

Since females usually do not smoke, this clear association in males may well be simply an indication of the heavy smoking which takes place during the qat session, rather than any direct result of the drug. However, further research is needed to clarify the relative roles of smoking and qat use in respiratory disease susceptibility.

EMOTIONAL PROBLEMS

The doctors in the study were instructed to look for clear cut mental symptoms and for psychosomatic complaints. Nothing unequivocally emerged from the diagnoses, but as indicated in Table XVII, the histories yielded some results of interest.

Since insomnia is one of the most frequently reported effects of qat chewing, it is not surprising to find that sleep problems are correlated with the heaviness of use in both males and females. Also, in view of the common belief in Yemen that qat is analgesic for headaches, the figures here could mean either that the more headaches one has the more he or she chews, or that heavier chewing produces more headaches. It is likely that both of these factors work together to produce this strong association.

"Emotional instability" in Table XVII is a general category in which the physicians recorded any difficulties of a psychological nature which they

TABLE XVII

Emotional problems (*Hx*)

Condition	Males Non	Males Lt	Males Heavy	Sig	Females Non	Females Lt	Females Heavy	Sig
Hx insomnia	15.5%	22.3%	33.3%	$\chi^2 = 9.78$ p = 0.0075	30.8%	33.1%	46.5%	$\chi^2 = 6.065$ p = 0.0484
Hx headaches	16.7	28.4	46.0	$\chi^2 = 33.42$ p = 0.0000	45.1	58.1	57.6	n.s.
Hx emotional instab.	11.9	20.5	31.	$\chi^2 = 4.86$ p = 0.0030	24.7	55.9	44.0	n.s.
Hx frequent illnesses	13.3	17.7	24.8	$\chi^2 = 4.86$ p = 0.0479 (n.s.)	24.7	27.3	31.6	n.s.
Emotional Hx group	29.8	45.9	61.9	$\chi^2 = 22.14$ p = 0.000	72.6	83.9	74.8	n.s.

could detect from the medical histories and examinations of the respondents. Here they put any bizarre behavior, such as psychotic or hysterical reactions, hypochondriasis, etc. It is interesting to note the generally very high percentages of women which are reported to be afflicted by such disorders, and that percentages of men so classified is also very high. The fact that the male psychosomatic problems are strongly associated with increasing qat use while those of females are not, e.g., in the cases of "headaches", and "frequent illness" are interesting findings. They may mean that males tend more to believe in the efficacy of qat for alleviation of these problems, perhaps because of their more regular and consistent exposure to the drug. Again, it could mean that because of heavier use, men are more prone to generalized tensions and anxieties.

In all three of these categories much larger numbers of women generally are afflicted than are men, supporting the common opinion of doctors in Yemen that a large percentage of women there suffer from psychosomatic and hysterical disorders. Table XVII also shows that when these disorders are grouped, the support for the opinion is very strong.

Such problems are generally frequent in the female sample (72% to 84%), and the number of factors playing a possible role in the causation of such problems which could influence diagnosis is large. Attitude and belief of the diagnosing physicians could also play a role in inflating the numbers of such problems among women. It is interesting however, that our two female doctors diagnosed about equal proportions of such problems as did the nine male physicians. At any rate, for a number of reasons, any contributory role of qat to such conditions might well be obscured. Males in the sample not only show substantial increases in the group of psychosomatic variables with increasing qat intake, but they show this on each individual dx as well. The general prevalence found among men is lower and we would expect less bias among physicians toward them. Because of its anorectic and insomniac effects, as well as its effects on sexual performance, these results are in the expected direction.

AGE AND AREA OF RESIDENCE

To assess some of the implications of the fact that age are residence were independently associated with disease, these factors were controlled in a separate analysis using Mantel-Haenszel odds ratios as seen in Table XVIII. This procedure is limited to pairs of variables, so the two levels of use were collapsed into one category and compared with non-users. The resulting odds ratios represent the relative prevalence of the diseases in question among qat users as compared to non-users.[2]

This analysis clearly emphasizes our previous conclusions regarding the associations of qat use with problems of the gastrointestinal tract for both men and women. The Mantel-Haenszel odds ratios compared with the crude odds ratios in these cases also reveal that, with the exception of the female G.I. History group and G.I., diagnosis group, controlling for the effects of age and residence does not eliminate the effects of qat use. For example, for the gastritis history item the crude odds ratio shows that males who chew show a 1.74 times higher relative prevalence of such problems than those who do not chew. When age and area of residence are controlled by the Mantel-Haenszel method, the relative increase drops to 1.39.

The clearest findings in this table are those for the acute gastritis diagnosis among women. The crude odds ratio indicates that women using qat have a

TABLE XVIII

By use controlling for age & residence

Condition	Chi Square Value	p Value	Crude Odds Ratio	Mantel-Haenszel Odds Ratio
		Males		
Gastritis Hx	1.738	0.0543	1.738	1.39
Constipation Hx	2.756	0.0001	2.756	2.28
Anorexia Hx	2.697	0.0025	2.697	2.64
GI Hx group	1.747	0.0519	1.747	1.49
Emotional Hx	5.257	0.0145	2.389	2.64
Headaches Hx	2.928	0.0005	2.928	2.56
Insomnia Hx	1.853	0.0593	1.853	1.84
Emotional Hx group	1.705	0.0533	2.5	2.29
		Females		
Acute Gastritis Dx	19.783	0.0000	23.714	6.89
GI Dx group	18.401	0.0000	3.039	1.08
GI Hx group	8.879	0.0029	2.128	1.11
Jaundice Hx	6.332	0.0119	2.811	3.58
Liver Hx group	5.612	0.0178	2.537	2.94
Urinary Dx group	5.446	10.90	2.79	1.29
Insomnia Hx	1.2154	n.s.	1.41	1.06

nearly 24 to 1 chance of having a diagnosis of acute gastritis. When age and areas are controlled it still remains a dramatic 7 to 1. Table XVIII should be inspected in like manner for each case, but overall it is clear that these particular associations of qat use with various problems stand up. However, most of the associations certainly are not strong.

The situation with regard to gastrointestinal and urinary problems among females deserves some comment. The crude ratios (approximately 3 to 1 for the gastrointestinal dx group, 2 to 1 for the gastrointestinal dx groups, and 3 to 1 for the urinary dx group) are each reduced to a negligible level when the odds are corrected for age and residence. This simply implies that area and age are more likely to account for the differential distribution of these diseases than is qat use.

CONCLUSION

The data we have presented here indicate that the argument that qat is responsible for the health problems of Yemen is exaggerated, but it also shows that they are not without foundation. In order to put the accusations to the most rigorous test possible with our data, we selected for special examination here the diseases and body systems which according to the literature are most likely to be affected by this substance. We then compared nonusers, moderate users, and heavy users with respect to both final diagnoses and histories in each cateogry. We also compared the user categories with diseases grouped by these organ systems allegedly most affected by the drug.

These comparisons confirmed the adverse effects of qat in rare conditions, and few of these are very severe or enduring. Prevalence of effects on the gastrointestinal system was associated with increasing qat use levels in both males and females, as was insomnia. However, many of these associations were relatively weak, and more importantly these diseases are those which can be lived with and which can be fairly easily be alleviated by various means. Since gastrointestinal problems are so generally prevalent in Yemen, and because it is obvious to people that there are many causes of them other than qat, they do not see why they should stop chewing on their account. The same reasoning applies to insomnia which is associated with use in both sexes, and to the psychosomatic problems which are strongly associated among males.

The most serious negative health findings of this study are those pointing to associations of liver and urinary problems with qat use among women and the extremely strong association of use with acute gastritis among them. These differential effects can only be reported here, since a fully satisfactory explanation for them has not been forthcoming. As was suggested earlier, the hypothesis could be put forward that the more adverse effects on women are due to inferior diet and the more difficult female life conditions, which, coupled with the effects of the qat, might render them more vulnerable to these problems. Why this should occur is still obscure, and future research should address the issue.

In the meantime, it must be evident that while the medical case against qat use is weaker than the literature would lead us to believe, the drug clearly cannot be discounted as a health threat. The heavy use of qat seems definitely to add another risk factor, albeit a mild one, to the heavy burdens of illness-producing factors with menace the Yemeni people. Nevertheless, the evidence presented here makes the majority view of the Yemeni people plausible on the whole, particularly since most of the people are moderate or light users. That is: the adverse effects of qat on the family economics of poor people can more accurately be named as negative effects of the drug than can the health problems which have been alleged by foreign experts.

NOTES

1. "The digestive system is seriously affected by the prolonged use of qat. Tannins and the essential oils exercise an irritating action on the mucous membrances, thus facilitating the incidence of gastritis, insufficient secretions and stypisis . . . there develops over the longer range, serious gastritis of the hypertrophic type, with atony, ectasy and ptsosis of the stomach which, as previously mentioned, further inhibit nutritional conditions" (1973:146).
2. It must be re-emphasized that diagnosis outcomes here represent the product of the probability of contracting a disease and the probability of surviving to examination once ill. The "history" variables represent the cumulative chain product of probability of contracting a particular disease, recovering from it, and surviving to examination. Confidence intervals for those odds ratios were also computed, but their generalizability to the general population of Yemen, or other populations depends on the randomness of this sample. As this is not certain they are not presented; situations where the 95% confidence interval exceeded 1.0 are indicated by an asterisk.

CHAPTER X

CONCLUSION

Knowledge about qat and its uses is still rare and is found largely in superficial newspaper articles or obscure technical publications. Therefore, it has been necessary to describe the customs of use, economics and chemical constituents in more detail than would be necessary in a study of a more well-known drug. It has been shown that the effects of the institutionalized use of this stimulant ramify in countless ways throughout Yemeni society, influencing the scheduling and content of social activities, the structure of economic life, architectural styles and even the perception of reality. I believe that it has been demonstrated that qat deserves much greater attention than existing histories and studies of Yemeni life have accorded it. If the argument for this has been convincing enough to bring about needed corrections and a recognition in future works of the true significance of this substance, one of my main tasks will have been accomplished.

Additionally, through presentation of a rounded and accurate picture of this still relatively obscure stimulant plant, I have tried to dispell some of the prejudices toward it, and to challenge some of the accepted but unconfirmed beliefs and dogmas about it as well. For example, it has long been accepted on the basis of slim inferential evidence that the use of qat originated in Ethiopia and diffused to Yemen in the 15th or 16th centuries. My assessment indicates that use of the drug may well have begun in Yemen at least as early as the 12th century and diffused to Ethiopia at that early period. There are at least enough data for this to stimulate a more thorough search of the early sources by specialist scholars.

On the economic side, I have pointed out that qat is not only presently the most important cash crop in North Yemen, it is the most important crop of any kind. This fact is known to many, but nowhere is it officially admitted, and its significant implications for the society have not been studied. I hope that the finger I have pointed toward this may result in detailed field research by economists. One of the obvious implications of this is that facile talk about banning qat or replacing it with other crops is totally unrealistic at this time. Not only was total rejection of al-Aini's anti-qat campaign indicative of this (see Chapter 1), but the opinions of the individualistic Yemeni farmers are clear. They will continue to plant it as long as there is a market for it. As one typical farmer from Wadi Dahr phrased his feelings after the abortive anti-qat campaign: "People need qat . . . If anyone, even the Prime Minister tries to take even one tree of mine, I will kill him. I am willing to die under one tree!" (Obermeyer, 1973:17).

I have also challenged the prevailing dogma which holds that the use of qat was restricted to the noble class of Yemen up until the recent civil war. It is true that use of the drug has spread since then to areas where it was never used in the past, and that the total amounts used have increased greatly in recent years. However, much evidence points to heavy and widespread use among the populace in many areas of the country for at least 200 to 300 years, and perhaps longer. The myth that widespread use is a new phenomenon serves the purposes of those bent on using the drug as a scapegoat for Yemen's economic problems, but it does not stand up to close scrutiny. The historical depth of this culturally entrenched institution helps us to understand the continued spread of chewing under the stimulus of new capital, and alert us to the extreme difficulties which will be encountered by any programs of eradication.

Another set of beliefs challenged by this study is the commonly heard allegation that the decline of coffee production in Yemen, with the consequent reduction in the trade balance of the country, is due to the replacement of coffee trees with qat trees. The Yemeni people are said to be sacrificing their long range national interests to short term individual economic advantages and the satisfaction of their drug habits. It has been shown here that this is largely a bogus issue, which despite the lack of evidence in its favor has been repeated endlessly by the foes of qat, whether government officials or foreign experts.

Instead, the data point to an opposite conclusion; the growing of qat has not replaced coffee, rather, being a hardier plant, qat has been planted in areas where coffee cannot grow. The net effect has been that the personal income from qat growing has not only replaced the income lost from a dying coffee industry, but has provided supplementary support for a much larger number of farmers than were ever able to profit from coffee farming. In addition to this, income is also provided for a vast number of traders, merchants, guards, etc. In some areas, the production of qat has even, in a sense, "subsidized" the continuing growth of grain where it is now unprofitable.

Of course, we do not want to take an oversimplified view of this, since abilities to profit from qat growing and trading are clearly related to the fact that hard currency has been coming into the country through remittances from migrants, and through many foreign aid programs. To the consternation of some officials much of the increased money which has been made available has been channeled into qat use and this in turn makes it more profitable to grow and trade. If these experts truly grasped the importance of the qat institution in Yemen they might not be so surprised that added resources resulted in its expansion, rather than in "investment" in the Western sense, or in increased savings. With the discovery of oil reserves in the Eastern desert we may expect a continuation of this expansion.

It is true that since the cessation of qat exports in 1972 the plant brings in no foreign exchange. However, this appears unrelated to the decline in coffee production. Clear and viable alternatives, as well as better arguments than these must be brought forward before the Yemeni farmer can be induced to uproot his qat crop.

It has also been shown that oversimplified notions of drug addiction or other one dimensional theories of motivation such as prestige emulation (Weir 1985) or group identity needs (Varisco 1986) cannot adequately account for the popularity, persistence and spread of qat chewing in Yemen. I have argued that stimulant drug effects are indeed important in the motivational picture, but that they take on their importance only in the context of the institutionalized qat sessions. Prestige emulation and nationalistic identity feelings are often important aspects of complex motivations which also include the powerful rewards of communitas and general ego enhancement, along with pressures towards conformity. All of these motivations to chew are reinforced by the lack of alternative institutions, as the Yemenis frequently explain to the visitor. However, when all socio-psychological explanations have been given, it is important to remember that the chemical effects of this drug still remain one of the most important reasons that the people of Yemen chew qat.

Certain of the allegations about the negative effects of qat have been partially confirmed by this study. For example, our data point to some negative health effects which may result from heavy and prolonged use. There is a clear link between use of the drug and temporary gastrointestinal problems, as Yemeni doctors have claimed, and there are other probable negative effects on the urinary and hepatic systems of qat using women. Yet overall, most of the severe problems predicted by Western medical authorities were not encountered.

This does not mean that further studies of a more intensive nature will not uncover other, perhaps more subtle health hazards associated with qat chewing. Our study is only a beginning in what should be long-term well-financed research on these questions. However, the data do indicate that the use of qat in Yemen should not be equated with patterns of "drug abuse" in America or other countries. It suggests that the Yemenis have "domesticated" the use of the qat plant over a period of hundreds of years. Their customs of use make it difficult to "abuse" the drug. Eating a fatty meal before chewing, the gradual ingestion of the juice from a limited amount of leaves over a 4 to 6 hour period in a restful setting, and the drinking of water as it is being used, all make for a situation where the usually mild psychophysiological effects can be controlled and bent to the furtherance of social purposes. Used in this manner, qat has neither the runaway potentials of alcohol, nor the carcinogenic effects of tobacco, though it combines many of the desired features of both of these drugs.

On the other hand, there is no denying that some poor people, particularly in the cities of Yemen, sacrifice money on qat that could probably be better spent on food. However, the percentages of people so affected is presently small, and there are no data showing that these people are more malnourished than their counterparts who do not chew qat. This suggests a study to be carried out in the future.

It is often said that the time spent chewing qat in Yemen is a major contributor to the economic backwardness of the country. It is alleged that if that time were utilized for labor and useful economic pursuits a major step towards development could be made. This is a much oversimplified argument. It assumes the existence of a complex industrial infrastructure where rigid eight hour work days could be utilized. In an agricultural country at Yemen's stage of development there are simply not enough "Western" type occupations to absorb the daily scheduled work of the majority of the people.

The argument also assumes that nothing of value is accomplished in qat sessions. It assumes that they are simply recreational "parties" in a Euroamerican sense. I have pointed out that in addition to the obvious entertainment functions which they often do provide, these sessions are also the arenas of communication, where serious exchanges of ideas and information take place. The stimulant properties of the drug have the potentiality of enhancing these functions, and do so more often than not. It should be mentioned that while in most of the Arab world, as in southern Europe and other places as well, most people are taking a siesta during the part of the afternoon in which the Yemenis are intensely interacting in their qat sessions. Serious comparative time-use studies must be made in many parts of the world before accusations that the Yemenis are "wasting" their time can be considered to have any substance.

It is probably evident by now that I am not among those who call for an immediate abolition of qat growing and use in Yemen. A balanced assessment of the harmful effects versus those which may be considered beneficial in some sense does not yield clearcut answers, but there is certainly little support for the extreme condemnations cited at the beginning of this book. For example, though there is clearly a potential for abuse of this substance, such potential is relatively low in comparison with other drugs such as alcohol, tobacco, and the "hard drugs" which cause such serious problems in Euroamerican societies. Both the customs of use and the amounts of active ingredients available in the plant material make abuse difficult. This does not mean that there is no danger. As Iman Yahya's poem states, and as we know from the occasional abuse of caffeine in our own society, there are certainly always some people who can find ways to abuse any substance.

However, a far greater danger of abuse is now possible and perhaps imminent. Because the major active ingredient cathinone finally has been isolated from the qat leaves, the stimulant properties and lesser side effects of this pure substance create the conditions for a future course similar to that of the history of cocaine. Of course, it would be ludicrous to condemn chemical and psychopharmacological research on cocaine or on cathinone, even though the dangerous consequences of the pure substance cocaine have undoubtedly far outweighed its beneficial uses. The possible useful properties of cathinone and other ingredients of qat could very well have as yet undreamed of benefits for medicine. Nevertheless, the more immediate potentialities for dangerous abuse of cathinone in the modern drug oriented world are infinitely greater than any such possibilities for abuse of the natural qat plant in Yemen. This study, in addition to the Yemeni and Ethiopian experiences of hundreds of years of controlled use, lends weight to that conclusion.

Also, given the agricultural and economic conditions in Yemen, the lack of viable alternatives, etc., the economic arguments against the drug are not convincing. Indeed, the evidence can be more effectively interpreted as showing that the "qat system" with its rapid and widespread distribution mechanisms, still largely in the hands of thousands of small capitalists (farmers, traders, transporters and merchants), is providing a much more equitable redistribution of the wealth generated by remittances, foreign aid and traditional sources of income than could be brought about in any other way at this time.

The usual bleak picture of qat is not supported by this study, but I have made no claim that it is entirely harmless, or that the Yemenis universally support it. In many places I have pointed our contrary opinions and ambivalences about it. Further evidence of this comes from answers to two of the questions in our sociomedical survey. Towards the end of it we asked the following:

"If you stopped using qat forever, do you believe your life would be better or worse?" "If you could prevent your children from chewing qat would you do so?" The answers to these questions are summarized in Figures 21 and 22.

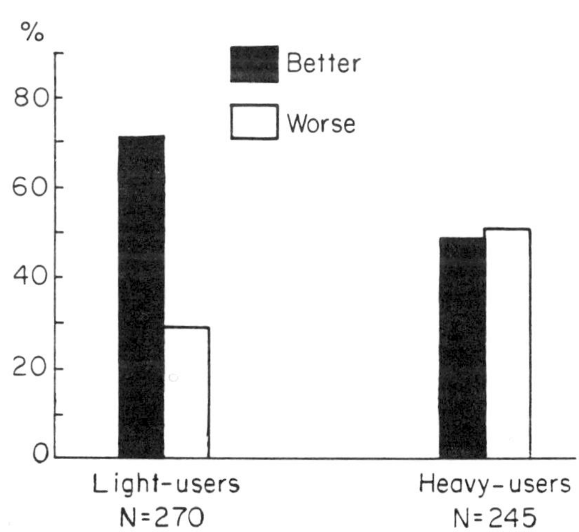

Fig. 21. If stopped chewing forever, life would be.

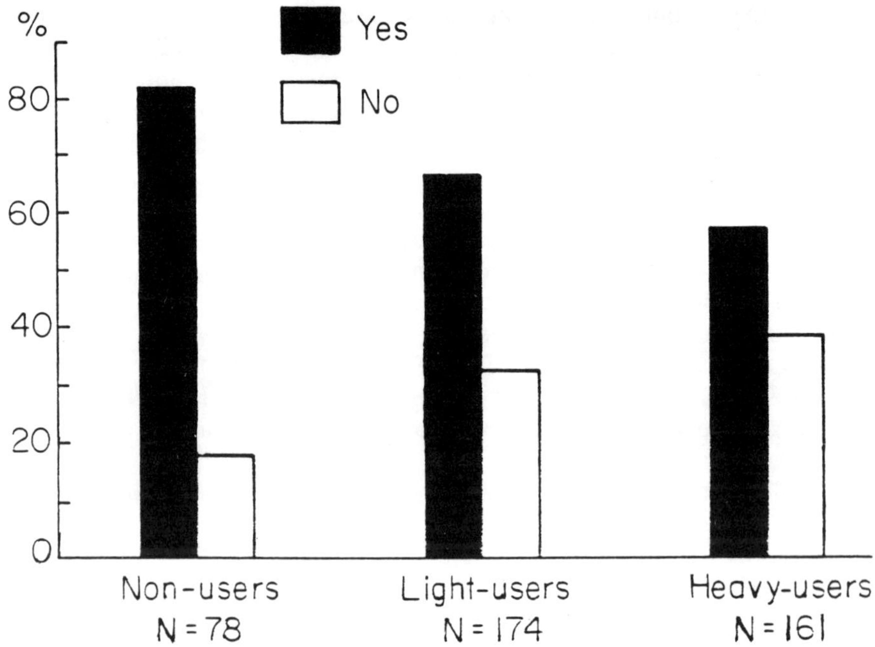

Fig. 22. I do not want my children to chew qat.

Figure 21 shows that nearly three-fourths of the light users and nearly half of the heavy users said they believed that their lives would improve if they could quit chewing. Figure 22 indicates that nearly two-thirds of the users with children would prefer their children not to chew. Taken together these figures contradict the expressions of overt support for the qat institution that one usually hears in casual conversations or while chewing qat. They reflect ambivalence, but they should not be overinterpreted. Observations of actual behavior and hundreds of conversations about qat use indicate that the answers probably do not indicate deeply held convictions.

Nevertheless, these answers perhaps reveal that many Yemenis are questioning the need for such heavy outlays of scarce cash for qat. The increasingly frequent newspaper articles against the drug, coupled with the growing desires for the many consumer goods now flooding the country, are undoubtedly deepening the existing ambivalences about it. These forces may well lead to a diminishing demand long before any kind of official abolition of use could be effective. Those people moving into the tiny but growing middle class are more and more limiting their chewing to once a week (in addition to special occasions) and it is clear that their main motives for this are the reduction of expenses, so that cash may be used for radios, television sets, automobiles, and home improvements. Such trends will undoubtedly continue, bringing about a natural diminution of demand for qat. However, as we have seen the social rewards of qat sessions are complex; it will probably be a very long time before such natural forces could be expected to eliminate the culturally dynamic qat institution. Conducing to this is the fact that these modernizing trends will proceed slowly in this fairly stagnant agricultural economy.

The Yemenis have integrated the use of a stimulant drug into their social fabric in a most profound way, yet we need to remember that they are not alone in this. Perhaps most human groups have, to a greater or lesser degree, made similar integrations of psycho-active substances. We need only think of the ubiquitous uses of alcohol, tea, coffee, and tobacco to be assured of this, but there is a long list of other examples. In Euroamerican societies, and many others, frequent ingestion of synthetic tranquilizers and stimulants keeps millions of people in states other than ordinary reality. Cannabis (variously called marijuana, hashish, kif, ganja, etc.) has been used as a recreational social lubricant, but also a stimulant to work in Africa, the Middle East, Asia and the Caribbean throughout most of the known histories of these regions. The story of opium is well known. Other powerful psychoactive substances such as ayahuasca, certain snuffs, nutmeg, peyote, and the "magic mushrooms" of both Asia and the New World, not only contribute to the powerful imagery of indigenous religions, but help to intergrate these societies as well. (For an introduction to this literature see Dobkin de Rios 1979, Efron *et al.* 1968, Blum 1971, Rubin 1975, Rubin and Comitas 1975, Solomon 1966, Westermeyer 1982).

Of course, this brief listing is not at all a complete catalogue of the extensive uses of mind altering substances by social groups, societies and social classes. I only allude to it to remind the reader of the context of universal drug use within which the instutionalized use of qat in Yemeni society should be viewed. There are, however, two natural stimulant drugs which have even longer histories of use than does qat, which are ingested in a similarly natural manner (mastication of natural leaves), which have somewhat similar psychological effects, and have also served important social and economic functions within their societies. These are coca (*erythroxylon coca*) and betel nut (*areca catechu*).

The chewing of coca leaves among the Indians of Peru, Columbia and Bolivia, and of betel nut in India, Southeast Asia and the Pacific are practices which reach back more than 2000 years in each case (Martin 1970:422, Burton-Bradley 1979:481). Both of these plants contain complex combinations of alkaloids which, like those of qat act as central nervous system (CNS) stimulants. Like qat, they are highly regarded for promoting a sense of well being, driving away fatigue, assuaging feelings of hunger, sharpening concentration and memory, and relieving ailments of the body. Because of these features their uses have become ritualized, praised in poetry, and are incorporated into the religious systems of their areas. They are also symbols of social reciprocity and respect and are central to social gatherings. Their growth and trade are of great importance in the economic systems of their regions. Again, as with qat, both drugs are presently under pressure from Western medical authorities, and they have been subjected to attacks by orthodox religious forces at various times in their histories.

COCA

When the Spanish conquered the Inca and Chibcha civilizations of South America in the 16th century, the noble classes were found using the drug plant coca, which they regarded as divine. It was used in religious sacrifices, as the temple of the sun, employed for divination, and chewed at all religious ceremonies. It also was one of the finest gifts which could be bestowed on a person (Martin 1970). After the conquest the drug diffused to the masses, and it is now almost universally used by the populous Quechua and Aymara peoples which today make up the bulk of the peasantry of Peru and Bolivia. Coca is still of great ceremonial and social importance among these groups as well as among many smaller tribes such as the highland Kogi and the lowland Cubeo of Columbia (Martin 1970, Salser 1970). Among these groups it is still used in divination and sacrifice. It is still integral to all social gatherings, presented as a gift on many occasions, and remains a symbol of solidarity, friendship and general goodness.

Cocaine was isolated from coca leaves in 1860 and since that time most opinion has regarded it as the active ingredient which accounts for the psychoactive effects of coca chewing. However, Mortimer contested this oversimplified interpretation in 1901, and since then at least 14 alkaloids have been isolated from the plant. These fall under the ecognines, tropines, and hygrines (Martin 1970:422). Much of the bad press against coca has stemmed from the abuse of cocaine in Western societies and the assumption that coca and cocaine are identical. However, some research indicates that though some cocaine is present in the dried coca leaves, and that the lime chewed with coca leaves does facilitate the extraction of alkaloids, it also acts to *degrade* cocaine, i.e., the cocaine tends to undergo hydrolysis in the gastrointestinal tract before it gets into the bloodstream. Thus, ecognine, which is 80 times less toxic than cocaine, may be a more important active ingredient circulating in the coca chewer's blood (research by Nieschulz and Montesinos summarized in Burchard 1975). This matter is still unclear, however, since another study done on 6 subjects with powder made from coca leaves (doses containing 15 to 50 mg of cocaine) in the lower Amazon basin showed cocaine to be the principal extra ingredient in the blood after chewing (Holmstedt *et al.* 1979).

It may be that the chewing of whole leaves, as is the custom in the high mountains, releases less cocaine into the blood than does the more efficient ground coca powder of the Amazon (Fuchs 1978:281). However, the question remains as to why many of the behavioral effects of coca are different from those of cocaine, and why coca chewers not only do not resemble cocaine addicts, but have been able to build viable institutions around coca use which have lasted for thousands of years.

The Quechua and Aymara Indians, both of whom are credited with great feats of physical endurance, are reported to chew coca during work and after it from 3 to 6 times per day for periods of 15 to 30 minutes each. They may also chew during social gatherings for longer periods (Allen 1981, Martin 1970:425—430). However, despite some early laboratory studies showing that coca leaves in 20 to 90 gram doses produced increases in oral temperature, heart rate, blood pressure, and respiration rate (Hanna 1974:282), several field researchers reported that they observed no euphoric effects at all, in themselves or as reported by the Indians (Martin 1952 , Bolton 1976, Hanna 1974). Moreover, there are many reports of a lack of withdrawal symptoms on being deprived of the drug (Hanna 1974:283).

The Indians themselves usually claim that they chew to get energy for work, avoid fatigue, to keep warm in the high altitude climate, and to palliate their hunger (Bolton 1976:631). There is some preliminary experimental evidence which shows that coca use may increase working time, and some which shows that it tends to promote heat retention (Hanna 1974). The question of alleviation of hunger is important becuase, as in the case of qat, it has long been asserted that coca chewing replaces food and promotes a malnutrition cycle (Gutierrez-Noriega 1949:143, Wolff 1952:147).

One study comparing 47 coca chewers with 47 non-chewers cautiously interpreted its weak results as supporting this assumption (Buck *et al.* 1968). However, other studies do not support it (e.g., Chahud *et al.* 1969, Baker and Mazess 1964), and it has been pointed out that coca leaves contain relatively high levels of vitamins B and B2 and C, while the lime chewed with the leaves is a good source of calcium (Burchard 1975:480). Also, it is clear that coca does not prevent or inhibit eating, but only allays hunger if no food is available. The Indians usually eat immediately after chewing and often even chew with meals (Bolton 1976, Burchard 1975, Murphy *et al.* 1969:45).

A psychophysiological hypothesis proposed by Bolton which has potential for futhering the explanation of the universal persistence of coca chewing among Andean Indians, is that some active substances in the leaves, coupled with a high carbohydrate diet, raise blood sugar and so alleviate symptoms of borderline hypoglycemia promoted by high altitude stress (hypoxia) and other stresses. This was supported in a study by Bolton in which 17 hypoglycemic subjects consumed significantly more coca than did 17 normoglycemic ones (1976:632). Since both cocaine and the tropines in coca leaves are capable of raising and sustaining blood sugar levels (Bolton 1976, Burchard 1975), this is a very interesting hypothesis.

It has similarly been argued that coca chewing relieves the symptoms of polycythemia (the abnormal increases of red blood cells) which is a typical response to high altitude stress and other stresses. This is also plausible since not only are the polycythemia symptoms of headache and fatigue among those which the Indians report as being relieved by coca, but there is evidence that cocaine and ecognine both can act to reduce red blood cells (erythropoeiesis) (Fuchs 1978).

These psychophysiological hypotheses which attempt to account for the persistence of coca chewing are very suggestive. They have not been adequately tested, and with all the current interest in cocaine, one wonders why this research has not taken place. However, even if the links between these metabolical processes and the effects of coca were established beyond the shadow of a doubt, I do not think they could completely account for the widespread and persistent use of coca in the Andes. One cannot discount the fact that the chewing of coca enters into all aspects of ritual and is intensively involved in all social reciprocity patterns in many Andean communities. The use of coca also is an assertion of Indian cultural identity versus the Mestizo culture, and this in additional powerful motive for chewing, (see Allens' interesting paper 1981). It is too facile to attempt to account for the deep religious and social involvements of coca by citing only its physiological effects. As with qat, they are undoubtedly part of the picture, but powerful traditional cultural forces are also obviously important. After all, the Mestizos in the same high altitude stressful environment have not as a group adopted the use of coca while many Indians in low altitude environments have done so (e.g., see Salser 1970). The concatenation of forces sustaining coca chewing in the Andes must be complex. Just as the drug activity of coca and qat cannot be reduced to single alkaloids, so the persistence of the coca and qat "habits" cannot be reduced to single causes (see Bray and Dollery 1983 for further discussion of these issues).

BETEL

The mastication of a piece of areca palm nut with fresh piper betel leaves and a little lime is far more widespread in the world than the uses of both qat and coca combined. It is a common practice throughout India and all countries of Southeast Asia, the Philippine and Micronesian Islands. Betel nut chewing is also found in parts of China, Japan, and in Melanesia. A conservative estimate is that more than 200 million people chew betel nut (Burton-Bradley 1979:481, Lewin 1931:232). The areca (betel) nut is called *tambula* in most of India, but is known by local names, as are the betel leaves (mainly called *pan* in India (Gode 1961). This combination of ingredients for the chew is used by all social classes and religions, and is mentioned by Herodotus 340 B.C., in ancient Sanskrit works, and in Pali writings of Sri Lanka from more than 500 years BC (Raghavan 1958:316, Burton-Bradley 1979:481). In his travels between 1325 and 1354 A.D. Ibn Batuta described the chewing of betel in Dhofar, Mogadishu, the Maldive Islands, Burma, and Sumatra (Gode 1961:126—127).

Gode has documented the numerous ways in which betel nut has been used symbolically in India and Southeast Asia. There are many regional variations which we cannot reproduce here. It should only be indicated that, like qat and coca, it was regarded as an appropriate gift for royalty and was integral to weddings, birth ceremonies and special occasions. For example, in some areas the bride and groom each took one end of a rolled betel leaf with areca and lime in their mouths, biting it off at the appropriate time in the ceremony (Gode 1961:150). Lower caste individuals made gifts of betel chewing materials to Brahmins, and friends exchanged betel nut as a symbol of their relationship upon meeting. There are elaborate beliefs about how much should be given on certain occasions and how much should be used for certain purposes. Since it is a symbol of pleasure, those who are in mourning or religiously fasting should avoid it. I allude to these customs here only to illustrate the cultural and social significance which this stimulant drug has attained in the life of the people of Asia, a significance similar to those of coca and qat (see Gode 1961:111—190, Penzer 1952:187—300, for philological, cultural and historical data).

The betel nut also has a strong reputation as a medicine. Since ancient times it has been used against tapeworms, and in Ayurvedic medicine it has been used as a heart tonic, a laxative, a coolant for fever, to relieve urinary disorders, as an aphrodisiac, a treatment for open sores and bleeding gums etc. (*Ibid.*:338). In Papua New Guinea it is also prescribed for many physical ills and also used as therapy for severe mental illness (Burton-Bradley 1979:483—484).

In preparation for chewing, the betel leaf is generally smeared with lime, a piece of areca nut is placed on it, and then another leaf placed on top, before it is taken into the mouth. However, other "spices" such as tobacco, camphor, nutmeg are often added to the packet. In some areas the materials are crushed together in a mortar. The combination of basic ingredients produces a bright red saliva which stains the mouth and lips, and which is believed to make women more attractive. Chewing betel is also said to produce a pleasant smelling breath, and is associated with love-making. There are many variations on the basic theme of preparing the material for chewing and numerous special implements for its use (Charpentier 1977, Penzer 1952, Lewin 1931:235—236).

Though chewing of betel leaves and areca nuts is much older and more widespread than the mastication of qat and coca, even less modern research has been focused on it. However, at least six alkaloids have been isolated from the areca nut: arecoline, arcaidine, arecodine, guvacine, guvacoline, and isoguracine (Raghavan *et al.* 1958:335) It is thought that the primary CNS stimulant effects come from the arecoline and arecaidine. The combination of the alkaloids from the nut, which are released by the lime, and the aromatic oil from the betel leaves, seems to provide the euphoriant effects, and it also stimulates production of saliva, sweat and tears (Burton-Bradley 1979:482).

I was unable to locate any chemical or pharmacological studies on the betel leaves, or any controlled behavioral studies of the effects of betel nut chewing in general. However, there are many strong tannins in the areca nut, since they are each extracted for commercial tanning of leather in India. This use and utilization of the areca palm wood for construction, along with the mastication of the nuts for medical, recreational and ceremonial purposes, makes the areca palm a very significant factor in the economics of Asia.

There is also some food value in the areca nuts which have been shown to contain small amounts of carbohydrates, proteins, and vitamin A, as well as some calcium, phosphorous and iron (Raghaven *et al.* 1958:337). Thus, we may suppose that people chewing up to 12 or more nuts per day (Lewin 1931:236) are getting a significant fraction of their daily nutrient needs met by the custom. Of course, more studies of this are needed, as they are for qat and coca as well.

The subjective experience of betel nut chewers is said to be a mood of well being and even gaiety, as well as stimulation to mental or physical work (Orme 1914:326, Burton-Bradley 1979:484). On first chewing, nervousness, dizziness, red face, sweating and faintness may occur, but these pass with habituation. As with the other drugs described here, feelings of hunger are assuaged, but here the stimulation of saliva also relieves thirst. The sexual appetite is said to be stimulated and betel nut is much used as an aphrodisiac, though, as with qat, there is mixed opinion about this (Lewin 1931:239). The alkaloids and other ingredients, and thus in the strength of their effects vary from place to place as well as according to the maturity of the nuts when picked, the subspecies of areca, etc. For example, older nuts contain more arecoline and less tannins (Raghavan *et al.* 1959:1336—1337, Lewin 1931:241). Chewing areca nuts in excess is said to bring on intestinal cramps and diahrrea and dizzinesss. This may be the result of ingesting too much arecoline, which appears to be highly toxic in pure form (Raghaven *et al.* 1959:339). The question of withdrawal symptoms for betel chewers has not been much addressed, but Lewin, who made an early special study of betel made the following statement reminiscent of those of Western travellers cited earlier in this book concerning qat:

> The Siamese and Manilese would rather give up rice, the main support of their lives, than betel, which exercises a more imperative power on its habitues than does tobacco on smokers. To cease to chew betel is for the betel chewer the same thing as dying. The greatest privations of life, insufficient or bad nourishment, hard work, rough weather, and illness lose their disagreeable character before the comforting action of betel (1931:231).

However, I have found no evidence supporting the idea that betel chewing results in physiological dependence. It seems that, like qat, it assists attainment of a mood of well being which promotes sociability and is psychologically habituating. As with coca this uplift may fortify the user against the vicissitudes of life (Burton-Bradley 1979:484).

The long term institutionalization of these 3 natural stimulant substances in large populations for hundreds, even thousands of years, is suggestive of the hypothesis that these customs are adaptive for these groups on several levels. When the consideration is added to this that tobacco, coffee and tea, which are also clearly stimulants, have become nearly universal in the world, and the fact that marijuana is also used as a stimulant to work (Rubin and Lomitas 1975), and when we note the widespread and increasing use of amphetamines, it is plausible to propose that human beings crave (and perhaps latently "need") supporting stimulation. More than any desire to "escape", they may seek means of staving off boredom, the normal fatigue of daily labor, and the natural physiological letdowns which seem to universally occur in the human physiological cycle. The search for benign means to heighten faculties of attention and sociability, for assistance to engage life more actively and with all senses sharpened, could well be universal. In any case, it seems evident that this is a far more common goal than that of seeking radically altered states of consciousness where there is a loss of contact with ordinary reality, loss of motor abilities, etc., that is, the kinds of changes brought about by hallucinogenic substances.

Whether these speculations have merit, it is clear that a great deal of profitable and important research could be directed to natural stimulant substances with long histories of institutionalized use in their traditional settings. There can be no substitute for studies in natural settings because (1) the substances used in their crude forms (e.g., plant materials) contain many ingredients which appear to significantly interact with one another. Examinations of the complex constituents of qat, coca and betel show that it is a fallacy to assume that any one "active ingredient" is wholly responsible for all the effects with which such substances are credited, (2) the psychology and other conditions created in the natural social setting (natural limitations on use, temperature, physical relaxation, etc.) make their own contributions to physiological and other substance effects. Meaning and setting not only must be recognized as integral to the substance-assisted experience, they must be made part of research efforts.

Research on these substances in their natural settings is only beginning, and in fact it is surprising how little work has been done on the uses of *any* drugs in their everyday environments. Of course, it is much easier and more "clean" to do laboratory studies on a pure substance such as TCP, cocaine or cathinone using rats or a few subjects. I am not disparaging such research; it is important and necessary, but it does not substitute for studies of natural products under normal living conditions. It seems obvious that laboratory studies should go hand in hand with field studies.

Field studies, of course, are much more difficult. They take more time, requiring researchers to spend long periods away from their homes. It is difficult to control conditions, and great tolerance for the unexpected is necessary. People who are relied upon may not complete their agreed-upon research responsibilities, the subjects do not always cooperate, there are language barriers and work may be carried out under uncertain political conditions. Plans must be changed continually. These are all reasons why more of this research is not carried out. Such conditions also are not fully appreciated by funding agencies, and thus, if this kind of research is funded at all, the inherent problems are often exacerbated by lack of sufficient resources.

The relative research neglect of the natural psychoactive substances has brought about a condition where the few studies that have been done on them are all unique. Due to the lack of a coherent overall framework they have been dependent upon the whims, interests, and training of individual scholars. In most ways these studies are not comparable, and most of them are on botany, chemistry or are simply behavioral descriptions. For example, no study like the one reported here has been carried out for either coca or betel nut. I would very much like to see comparable systematic samples made of the chewers of these similarly institutionalized substances relating the opinions and experiences of users to frequency of use, economic levels, and health. At the same time, the as yet inconclusive studies which suggest relationships between environmental stress and coca use, and those measuring active coca ingredients in the bloodstream should be emulated in more refined form with qat and betel, as well as being continued with coca. It is curious that coca raises blood sugar levels, while qat appears to depress them, etc. For these stimulants it also would be extremely useful to adopt some of the physiological and psychological techniques used by Rubin and Lomitas in their study of marijuana (ganja) in Jamaica (1975) and the psychiatric case study methods developed by Westermeyer in his research on opium use in Laos (1982).

Having made a modest attempt to do field research on one of these natural substances, I am well aware of the pitfalls that lie in wait for future investigators. Yet I am even more convinced of the necessity and potential significance of research on natural institutionalized psychoactive substances than I was when I began. If much of mankind perceives the need for the regular assistance of stimulants to participate in life and work at intensified levels for at least brief periods, and if, as seems probable, people inevitably are going to continue to seek such stimulants, it behooves us to find the most healthful and socially beneficial ways of achieving this and to assess the costs. Perhaps one or more of these institutionalized natural stimulants is much superior to the caffeine, tobacco and amphetemines so widely used to achieve these purposes in Euroamerican societies. On the other hand, we may find that the physical, social and economic problems entailed are too great. Before making negative ethnocentric judgments, and before drastic socially and psychologically disruptive actions are precipitiously taken, much more extensive and careful research should focus on these great natural experiments of substance use. This book points the way to the tasks ahead.

BIBLIOGRAPHY

Abbasy, M.
1957 The habitual uses of 'Qat'. *International Journal of Prophylactic Medicine and Social Hygiene, 1*, May 31.

Abdullahi, M., Anania, M., and Nencini, P.
1983 Long-lasting analgesic effects of cathinone. *In* Shahandeh, *et al.*, *The health and socio-economic aspects of khat use* (pp. 144—147). Lausanne: Int. Council on Alcohol and Addictions.

Aden Colony
1958 *Report of the qat commission of inquiry*. Aden, Government Printer.

Adra, N.
1982 *Qabayla: The tribal concept in the central highlands of the Yemen Arab Republic*. Ph.D. Diss. Temple Univ., Ann Arbor Univ. Microfilm, Int.

Allen, C.
1981 To be Quechua: The symbolism of coca chewing in highland Peru. *American Ethnologist, 8*:157—171.

Alles, G., Fairchild, D., and Jensen, M.
1961 Chemical pharmacology of catha edulis. *Journal of Medicinal and Pharmaceutical Chemistry, 3*:323—352.

Andrews, G. and Solomon D. (eds.)
1975 *The coca leaf and cocaine papers*. N.Y.: Harcourt Brace Jovanovich.

Anonymous
1912 Chemistry of catha edulis. *The Pharmaceutical Journal and Pharmacist, 89*:675.

Anonymous
1911 Kat-Tee, *Tropenfflauzer* (Berlin), *12*:510—511.

Anonymous
1956 Khat. *Bulletin on Narcotics, 8*:6—13.

Anonymous
1883 Khat, cafta, or Arabian tea, originally published in Produce Markets Review, March 24, 1883. *Pharmaceutical Journal and Transactions, 42*:840.

Anonymous (ed.)
1945 Poisoning by khat or mirra. Catha Edulis, *East African Medical Journal, 22*:1—2.

Anonymous
1966 Twenty years of narcotics control under the United Nations — Review of the work of the Commission on Narcotics from its 1st to its 20th session. *Bulletin on Narcotics, 18*:1—67.

Arfaa, F.
1972 Studies on schistosomiasis in the Yemen Arab Republic. *American Journal of Tropical Medicine and Hygiene, 24*:421.

Ayoub, M.
Yemen between the qat and the corrupted rule before the revolution. Cairo: Dar al Ma'arif (Arabic).

Azais, R. and Chambard, R.
1931 Cinq années de recherches archéologiques en Éthiopie. Province du Harar et Éthiopia méridionale. Paris: Librairie Orientaliste Pane Geuthner.

Baird, D.
1951 Indian remedies for poor memory. *British Medical Journal*, p. 1522.
Baker, P. and Mazess, R.
1963 Calcium: Unusual sources in the highland Peruvian diet. *Science, 142*:1466—1477.
Bally, P.
1945 Catha edulis. *East African Medical Journal, 22*:2—3.
Barraduni, A.
1972 Al-Qat. *The new Yemen* (*Al Yaman al Jadid*). Third issue, in Arabic.
Becker, H.
1963 *Outsiders: Studies in the sociology of deviance.* N.Y.: MacMillan Ltd.
Beguinot, A.
1939 Notizie sula *catha edulis forsk.* Coltivata nel R. Orto Botanico di Genova. *Nuovo Giornale Botanico Italiano* (N.S.) *46*:332—334.
Beitter, A.
1900 *Pharmakognostisch-chemische Untersuchung der Catha Edulis.* Inaugural Dissertation der mathemat. und naturwissenschaftlichen Fakultät der Kaiser-Wilhelms-Universität. Strassburg: Schleisier & Schweikardt, 76 pp.
Beitter, A.
1901 Pharmakognostisch-chemische Untersuchung der Catha Edulis. *Archiv der Pharmazie, 239*:17—33.
Bidwell, R.
1983 *The two Yemens.* Boulder, Colorado: Westview Press.
Blum, R.
1969 *Society and drugs, social and cultural observations.* San Francisco: Jossey-Bass.
Bolton, R.
1976 Andean coca chewing: A metabolic perspective. *American Anthropologist, 78*:630—634.
Bolton, R.
1979 On coca chewing and high altitude stress. *Current Anthropology, 20*:418—420.
Bornstein, A.
1974 Food and society in the Yemen Arab Republic, F.A.O. Rome, Mimeo.
Bosworth, C.
1976 Kat. *Encyclopedia of Islam.* New Edition, Leiden, E. J. Brill.
Botta, P.
1880 *Relation d'un voyage dans l'Yémen, entrepris en 1837* pour le Musée d'Histoire Naturelle de Paris. Ancien Député. Paris: Duprat.
Braenden, O.
1980 Research on the chemical composition of khat. *In* L. Harris (ed.), *Problems of drug dependence*, Washington, D.C., NIDA Monograph 27.
Brauer, E.
1934 *Ethnologie der Jemenitschen Juden.* Heidelberg: Carl Winters Universitätsbuchhandlung.
Bray, W. and Dollery, C.
1983 Coca chewing and high altitude stress: A spurious correlation (plus commentaries). *Current Anthropology, 24*:269—282.
Brilla, R.
1962 *Über den zentral erregenden Wirkstoff der frischen Blätter von Catha Edulis Forskal.* Dissertation: Bonn.
Britton, E.
1939 The use of 'qat', appendix to Scott, H. article (1939). *Geographical Journal, 93*:121—122.
Brooke, C.
1960 Khat (*catha edulis*): Its production and trade in the Middle East. *Geographical Journal, 126*:52—59.

Brucke, F.
1941 Über die zentral erregende Wirkung des Alkaloides Cathin. *Archiv für experimentelle Pathologie und Pharmakologie, 198*:100—106.
Buck, A., Sasaki, T., Hewitt, J., and Macrae, A.
1968 Coca chewing and health. *American Journal of Epidemiology, 88*:159—177.
Bulletin on Narcotics
1957 The medical and social problems of khat in Djibouti. 9(4):34—36.
Bulletin on Narcotics
1966 Twenty years of narcotics control under the U.N. — Review of the work of the Commission on Narcotic Drugs from its 1st to 20th session. Vol. XVII, No. 1, January—March.
Bulletin on Narcotics
1969 Part III. The coca leaf and cocaine. Vol. XXI, No. 4, October—December.
Bulletin on Narcotics
1980 Special issue devoted to catha edulis (khat), Volume XXXII, No. 3.
Burchard, R.
1975 Coca chewing: A new perspective. *In* V. Rubin (ed.), *Cannabis and culture*. The Hague: Mouton.
Burrowes, R.
1978 State building in North Yemen: 1968—1976. Unpublished ms.
Burrowes, R.
1985 The Yemen Arab Republic and the Ali Abdallah Salih Regime: 1978—1984. *The Middle East Journal, 39*:287—316.
Burton, R.
1964 *Personal narrative of a pilgrimage to al-Madinah and Meccah*. Vol. 1 (first published in 1855). Dover.
Burton, R.
1966 *First footsteps in east Africa*. Edited by Gordon Waterfield. New York: Fredrich Praeger.
Burton-Bradley, B.
1979 Arecaidinism: Betel chewing in transcultural perspective. *Canadian Journal of Psychiatry, 24*:481—488.
Bury, W.
1915 *Arabia infelix: Or the Turks in Yemen*. London: MacMillan Co.
Cais, M., Ginsberg, D., and Mandelbaum, A.
1975 Constituents of catha edulis. Isolation and structure of cathedine D. *Tetrahedron, 31*:2727—2731.
Cambrony, H., Vincent, J., and Wierer, C.
1975 *Coffee culture in Yemen*. Technical Report to FAO/UNDP and Government of the Yemen Arab Republic. April 6—May 4.
Carothers, J.
1945 Miraa as a cause of insanity. *The East African Medical Journal, 22*:4—6.
Central Planning Organization.
1973 *Results of the first session for studying expenses of living of families in Sanaa*. Sanaa, Yemen: Central Planning Organization, Report #16, (Mimeo in Arabic).
Charpentier, C.
The use of betel in Ceylon. *Anthropos, 72*:107—118.
Chahud, A. *et al.*
1969 Seroproteinas en indigenas coqueros. *Revista Clinica Espanola, 115*:213—218.
Chelhod, J.
1970 L'organisation sociale au Yémen. *L'Ethnographie, 64*:61—86.
Chelhod, J.
1970 Recherches ethnologiques au Yémen: Problèmes et perspectives. *Objects et Mondes, 10*:119—134.

Chelhod, J.
1972 La société Yémenite et le kat. *Objets et Mondes*, Tome XII: 3—22.
Chelhod, J.
1973 La parente et le mariage au Yémen. *L'Ethnographie, 67*:47—90.
Chevalier, A.
1924 La culture de Cafeier et du cat en Arabic heureuse. *Revue de Botanique Appliquée et d'Agriculture Tropicale, 4*:693—694.
Chevalier, A.
1949 Les Cat's d'Arabie, d'Abyssinie et d'Afrique orientale. *Revue de Botanique Appliquée et d'Agriculture Tropicale, 29*:413—417.
Chevalier, J.
1911 Étude pharmacodynamique du catha edulis Forsk. *Bulletin des Sciences Pharmacologiques, 17*:264—275.
Chevalier, J.
1911 Le catha edulis: Pharmacologie et pharmacodynamie. *Bulletin Général de Thérapeutique Médicale, Chirurgicale, Obstétricale et Pharmaceutique, 161*:572—586.
Chinnery, E.
1922 Piper methysticum in betel chewing. *Man, 22*:24—27.
Christ, H.
1870 Über Catha Edulis. *Archiv der Pharmacie, 191*:67—71.
Cohen, J. and Lewis, D.
1979 *A review of the literature and analysis of rural development issues in the Yemen Arab Republic*. Working Notes #6, Rural Develop. Com. Res. Programs, Center for Int. Studies, Cornell University.
Collin, E.
1893 Le catha edulis. *Journal de Pharmacie et de Chimie*, Ser. 5, *28*:337—342.
Coon, C.
1936 *Measuring Ethiopia and flight into Arabia*. Boston: Little Brown.
Coon, C.
1943 Southern Arabia, a problem for the future. *Peabody Papers, 20.*
Costa, P. and Vicario, E.
1977 *Arabia felix, a land of builders*. New York: Rizzoli International Publications.
Cottevieille-Giraudet, R.
1935 Le catha edulis. Fut-il connu des Egyptiens? *Bulletin de l'Institut Français d'Archaéologie Orientale, 35*:99—113, Cairo.
Darby, W. *et al.*
1959 Khat. *Ethiopia nutrition survey*. A survey by the interdept. committee on nutrition for national defense. Washington, D.C., pp. 166—169.
Dequin, H.
1973 Land use map with monography of Yemen. In *World atlas of agriculture*.
Dequin, H.
1976 *Arabische Republik Jemen: Wirtschaftsgeographie eines Entwicklungslandes*, Riyadh: Saudi Arabien.
Dezani, S.
1918 Ricerche Farmacognostiche sulla 'Catha edulis'. *Archivio di Farmacognosis e Scienze Affini* (Rome). *7*:4—5.
Dobkin de Rios, M.
1984 *Visionary vine*. Illinois: Waveland Press.
Dorsky, S.
1986 *Women of Amran: A Middle Eastern ethnographic study*. Salt Lake City: Univ. of Utah Press.
Dostal, W.
1974 Socio-economic aspects of tribal democracy in northeast Yemen. *Sociologus, 24*:1—15 (German).

Dostal, W., Serjeant, R., and Wilson, R.
1983 Analysis of the San'a' market today. *In* Serjeant, R. and R. Lewcock (eds.), *San'a', an Arabian Islamic city* (pp. 241—275). London: World of Islam Festival Trust Press.
Dresch, P.
1981 The several peaces of Yemeni tribes. *Journal of the Anthropological Society of Oxford, 12*:73—86.
Eddy, N. and Halbach, H.
1965 Drug dependence: Its significance and characteristics. *Bulletin, W.H.O., 32*:721—733.
Efron, D., Holmstedt, B., and Kline, N.
1979 *Ethnopharmacologic search for psychoactive drugs.* New York: Raven Press.
El-Attar, S.
1964 *Le sous-développement économique et social du Yémen, perspectives de la révolution Yémenite.* Editions du Tiers-Monde Algier.
El-Baidani, A.
1962 *The Yemenite economy.* U.S. Joint Publications Research Service 12—36, January 18.
El-Guindy, M.
1971 Effects of catha edulis (khat) chewing on the human body. *Journal of the Egyptian Medical Association, 54*:230—234.
El-Mahi, T.
1961 A preliminary study on khat — together with the institutional history of coffee as a beverage in relation to khat. WHO Regional office for the Eastern Mediterranean, WHO document EM/RC 11/10 MS., Mimeo.
Elkiey, M., Karawya, M., and Ghourab, M.
1968 A pharmacognostical study of Catha Edulis Forsk grown in Egypt. *Journal of the Pharmaceutical Sciences of the United Arab Republic, 9*:127—145.
Elkiey, M., Karawya, M., and Ghourab, M.
1968 Estimation of the alkaloids of Catha Edulis Forsk grown in Egypt. *Journal of the Pharmaceutical Sciences of the United Arab Republic, 9*:159—169.
El-Sissa, H. and Abdulla, M.
1966 Polyphenolics of the leaves of catha edulis (Part I). *Planta Medica, 76*:83.
FAD/WHO/UNICEF
1971 Report on *Khat.*
Farrago, L.
1938 *Arabian antic.* New York: Sheridan House.
Fayein, C.
1957 *A French doctor in Yemen.* London: Hale.
Fluckiger, F. and Gerock, J.
1887 Contributions to the knowledge of catha leaves. *Pharmaceutical Journal and Transactions, 47*:221—224.
Forsskal, P.
1775 *Flora Aegyptico-Arabica,* (ed.) Niebuhr, C. Paris.
Friebel, H. and Brilla, A.
1963 Über den zentralerregenden Wirkstoff der frischen Blätter und Zweigspitzen von Catha Edulis Forsk. *Naturwissenschaften, 50*:354—355.
Fuchs, A.
1978 Coca chewing and high altitude stress: Possible effects of alkaloids in erythropoeiesis. *Current Anthropology, 19*:277—293.
Galante, E.
1948 L'azione Fisilogica del Ciat (Catha Edulis), *Rivista di Biologica Coloniale, 9*:111—121.
Gellert, M., Szendrei, K., and Reisch, J.
1981 Dihydromyricetin 3-0-rhom noside from leaves of catha edulis. *Phyto Chemistry, 20*:1759.

Gerholm, T.
1977 *Market, mosque and mafraj*. Stockholm: Department of Anthropology, Univ. of Stockholm.
Getahun, A. and Krikorian, A. D.
1973 Chat: Coffee's rival from Harrar: Ethiopia I. Botany, cultivation and use. *Economic Botany, 27*:353—377.
Ghaibah, H.
1976 Review and appraisal of progress in Yemen Arab Republic under the International Development Strategy. Prepared for CPO, Y.A.R., Mimeo.
Glaser, E.
1913 *Sammlung, Eduard Glaser I. Eduard Glaser's Reise nach Marib*. Hrsg. von D. H. Mutter und N. Rhodokanakis. Wien.
Gode, P.
1961 *Studies in Indian cultural history*. Hoshiarpur Visvestivaranond Vedei Research Institute.
Goitein, S.
1954 *Jemenica*, Leipzig.
Goitein, S.
1969 The Jews of Yemen. *In* Arberry, A. J. (ed.), *Religion in the Middle East* (pp. 226—235). Cambridge, Vol. 1, and Vol. 2, p. 663.
Goitein, S.
1951 The transplantation of the Yemenites: The old life they lead. *Commentary, 12*:24—29.
Greenway, P.
1947 Khat. *East African Agricultural Journal, 13*:98—102.
Guantai, A. and Maitai, C.
1982 Relative distributions of cathinone and norpseudoephederine in catha edulis growing in Kenya. *East African Medical Journal, 59*:394—398.
Guedel, L. and Marguet, J.
1957 The medical and social problems of khat in Djibouti. *Bulletin on Narcotics*, 9(4):34—36.
Gutierrez-Noriega, C.
1949 El habito de la coca en El Peru. *America Indigena, 9*:143—154.
Hakem, H.
1972 *Qat in Sudan*. The Criminology Laboratories in Sudan.
Halbach, H.
1971 FAO/WHO/UNICEF Group Meeting on khat.
Halbach, H.
1972 Medical aspects of chewing khat leaves. *Bulletin WHO, 47*:12—19.
Halbach, H.
1973 Defining drug dependence and abuse. In *Bayer Symposium IV*, Springer-Verlag.
Halliday, F.
1974 *Arabia without Sultans*. Middlesex, England: Penguin Books.
Hanna, J.
1974 Coca leaf use in southern Peru: Some biosocial aspects. *American Anthropologist, 76*:281—296.
Harris, L. (ed.)
1980 *Problems of drug dependence*. Washington, D.C., NIDA, Monograph #27.
Heacock, R. and Forrest, J.
1974 Khat. *Canadian Journal of Pharm. Sci., 9*:64—66. (From Biological Abstracts, 58:10).

Heisch, R.
1945 A case of poisoning by catha edulis. *East African Medical Journal, 22*:7—10.
Helfritz, H.
1936 *Land without shade*. New York: National Travel Club.
Helfritz, H.
1956 *The Yemen: A secret journey*. London: George Allen Unwin.
Hes, J.
1970 On the use of catha edulis among Yemenite Jews. *Journal of the Israel Medical Association, 78*(6):283—284.
Hess, J.
1927 and 1976 Kat. *Encyclopedia of Islam* II:808, London: Luzac & Co.
Heyworth-Dunne, G.
1952 *Al Yemen. A general social political and economic survey*. Cairo: Reconnaissance Book Shop.
al-Hibshi, A.
1972 Qat in the literature of Yemen. ("Al-qat ti l-adab al-Yemeni). *The New Yemen* (*Al Yaman al-Jedid*) 3rd Issue, (in Arabic).
Hill, B.
1965 Cat (Catha edulis Forsk). *Journal of Ethiopian Studies, 3*:13—23.
Hjort, A.
1974 Trading Miraa: From school-leaver to shop-owner in Kenya. *Ethnos, 39*:27—43.
Hobley, C.
1912 Catha edulis. *Journal of the East African and Uganda Natural History Society, 2*(4):126—127.
Hocking, G.
1963 Catha edulis (khat or kat). *Quarterly Journal of Crude Drug Research, 3*:338—344.
Hodgkinson, R.
1962 A study of the clinical effects of catha edulis (Khat, Miraa) in Kenya. *The Medical Journal of Australia*, June 9.
Holmstedt, B., Lindgarten, J., and Rivier, L.
1979 Cocaine in the blood of coca chewers. *Journal of Ethnopharmacology, 1*:69—78.
Horhammer, L.
1961 Über den qualitativen und quantitativen Flakongehalt von Arzneipflanzen im Hinblick auf ihre spasmolytische Wirkung. *Congr. Sci. Pharm. Conf. Comun. 21*:548—588.
Hughes, P.
1973 Khat chewing in Yemen. Paper presented at the 4th International Institute on the Prevention and Treatment of Drug Dependence, Lausanne, Switzerland: International Council on Alcoholism and Addictions, pp. 32—46.
Hughes, P. and Khan, I.
1979 Assessment of public health and social problems associated with khat chewing. *In* Louis S. Harris (ed.), *Problems of drug dependence*, NIDA Research Monograph, 27, 1979.
Ibn Batuta
1968 *The travels of Ibn Batuta*. N.Y.: Johnson Reprint Corp, (1929).
Ingrams, D.
1970 *A time in Arabia*. London: John Murray.
Ingrams, W.
1966 *Arabia and the Isles*. New York: Praeger, pp. 105—106.
Ingrams W.
1963 *The Yemen*. London: John Murray.

Ingrams, W.
1946 A journey in the Yemen. *Journal of the Royal Central Asian Society, 33*:58—69.
Isbell, H. and Chrusciel, T.
1970 Dependence liability of "non-narcotic" drugs. W.H.O. Supplement to Vol. 43 Bulletin of the W.H.O.
Kalant, O.
1966 *The amphetamines: Toxicity and addiction.* C. C. Thomas: Toronto.
Kalix, P.
1980 A constituent of khat leaves with amphetamine-like releasing properties. *European Journal of Pharmacology, 68*:213—215.
Kalix, P.
1981 The amphetamine-like releasing effect of the alkaloid (−) cathinone on rat nucleus accumbens and rabbit caudate nucleus. *Progress in Neuro-psychopharmacology and Biological Psychiatry, 6*:43—49.
Kalix, P.
1983 A comparison of the catecholemine releasing effect of the khat alkaloids (−) cathinone and (+) norpseudoephederine. *Drug and Alcohol Dependence, 11*:395—401.
Kalix, P.
1983 Mechanism of action of (−) cathinone, a new alkaloid from khat leaves. *Alcohol and Alcoholism, 18*:301—303.
Kalix, P.
1983 The pharmacology of the khat alkaloid cathinone. *In* Shahandeh, B., Geudah, Tongue, A., Tongue, E., Rolli, J. (eds.), *The health and socio-economic aspects of khat use* (pp. 140—143). Lausanne, International Council on Alcohol and Addictions.
Kalix, P.
1984 The pharmacology of khat, *General Pharmacology, 15*:179—189.
Kalix, P. and Braenden, O.
1985 Pharmacological aspects of the chewing of qat leaves. *Pharmacological Reviews, 37*:149—164.
Karawya, M., Elkiey, M. and Ghourab, M.
1968 A study of the alkaloids of Catha Edulis Forsk growing in Egypt. *Journal of Pharmaceutical Sciences of the U.A.R., 9*:147—157.
Kennedy, J.
1981 Erkenntnisse der medizinischen Qat-Forschung. *Rausch and Realität*, Drogen im Kulturvergleich, Teil 2, Koln: des-Rautenstrauch-Hoset-Museums für Völkerkunde der Stadt Köln.
Kennedy, J., Teague, J., and Fairbanks, L.
1980 Qat use in North Yemen and the problem of addiction: A study in medical anthropology. *Culture, Medicine and Psychiatry, 4*:311—344.
Kennedy, J., Teague, J., Rokaw, W., and Cooney, E.
1983 A medical evaluation of qat-use in North Yemen. *Social Science and Medicine, 11*:783—793.
Kervingant, D.
1959 The consumption of khat in French Somaliland. *Bulletin on Narcotics, 11*:42.
Khadduri, M.
1960 Khat. *Geographical Journal*, CXXVI.
Kielholz, P.
1973 Addictive behavior in man. In *Bayer Symposium IV* Springer-Verlag.
Knoll, J.
1980 Studies on the central effects of (−) cathinone. *In* Harris, L. D. (ed.), *Problems of drug dependence*. Washington, D.C., NIDA Monograph, #27.

Kopp, H.
1981 *Agrargeographie der Arabischen Republik Jemen.* Selbstverlag der Frankischen Geographischen Gesellschaft in Kommission bei Palm und Enke, Sonderband 11, Erlange. Geog. Arbeiten.

Krikorian, A.
1983 Khat and its use: An historical perspective. *In* Shanhandeh B. *et al.* (eds.), *The health and socio-economic aspects of khat use* (pp. 7—71). Lausanne, International Council on Alcohol, and Addictions.

Krikorian, A., and Getahun, A.
1973 Chat: Coffee's rival from Harrar: Ethiopia II. Chemical composition. *Economic Botany, 27*:378—389.

Kuntz, R., Malakatis, G., Lawless, D., and Strome, C.
1953 Medical mission to the Yemen, Southwest Arabia 1951: II. A cursory survey of the intestinal protozoa and helminth parasites in the people of the Yemen. *Journal of Tropical Medicine and Hygiene, 2*:13—19.

La Roque, J.
1726 A Voyage to Arabia the Happy by way of the Eastern Ocean and the Straits of the Red Sea, etc., London.

Laurent, J.
1962 Consequences médicales de la toxicomanie au cath. *Médicine Tropicale* (Marseille) *22*:477—483.

Laurent, J.
1962 Toxique et toxicomanie inconnus, 'Le Cath', *Annales Médico-Psychologiques Revue Psychiatrique, 120*:649–657.

Laurent, J.
1963 Toxique et toxicomanie inconnus: Le 'Cath'. *Lyon Médicale, 210*:91—100.

Le Bras, M. and Fretilliere, Y.
1965 Les aspects médicaux de la consommation habituelle du cath. A propos de 53 obvservations. *Médicine Tropicale 25*(6):720—732.

Leete, E.
1958 Biogenesis of d-norpseudoephedrine. *In* Catha edulis, *Chemistry and industry*, August 16, 1088—1089.

Leloup, C.
1890 Sur le catha edulis et ses effects thérapeutiques. *Bulletin Général de Thérapeutique Médicale, Chirurgique, Obstétricale et Pharmaceutique, 119*:216—227.

Lemordant, D.
1971 Contribution à l'ethnobotanique éthiopienne. *Journal d'Agriculture Tropicale et de Botanique Appliquée, 1—3*:1—55, *4—6*:142—179.

Lemordant, D.
1959 *Contribution à l'étude du khat C.E.F.* Thesis in Medicine and Pharmacology at U. of Marseille.

Lemordant, D.
1960 *Les plantes éthiopiennes.* Addis Ababa: Central Printing Press.

Lemordant, D.
1966 Toxicité et antagonistes du khat. *Médicine Tropicale, 26*:124—129.

Levey, M. and Al-Khaledy, N.
1967 *The medical formulary of al-Samarkandi*, Philadelphia: Univ. of Penn. Press.

Lewin, L.
1931 *Phantastica: Narcotic and stimulating drugs.* N.Y.: E.P. Dutton & Co.

Lobb, C.
1974 El uso de la coca como manifestacion de cultura indigena en las montañas occidentales de Sud america. *America Indigena, 34*:919—938.

Luftman, H. and Spitelle, G.
1974 Structure of cathidin from Catha edulis F. — Polyhydroxy basic compound. *Tetrahedron, 30*:2577—2578.
Luqman, F.
1970 *Yemen*. Aden.
Luqman, F.
1970 Qat. Aden Chronicle.
Luqman, W. and Danowski, T.
1976. The use of khat (Catha edulis) in Yemen: Social and medical observations. *Annals of Internal Medicine, 85*:246—249.
Macro, E.
1960 *Bibliography on Yemen and notes on Mocha*. U. of Miami, Press, Coral Gables.
Macro, E.
1968 *Yemen and the western world (since 1751)*. London: C. Hurst Co.
Maitai, C. and Mugera, G.
1975 Excretion of the active principle of Catha edulis (Miraa) in human urine. *Journal of Pharmaceutical Sciences, 64*(4).
Makhlouf, C.
1979 *Changing veils: Women and modernization in North Yemen*. Austin: University of Texas Press.
Makki, I.
1975 *Schleimhautkarzinome der Mundhöhle unter besonderer Berücksichtigung des Qat-und-Schama-Abusus*. Inaugural Dissertation. Erlangung der Doctorwürde in der Zahnheilkunde der Ruprecht-Karl-Universität zu Heilberg.
Mancioli, M. and Parrinello, A.
1967 Il qat (Catha edulis). *La Clinica Terapeutica*. V. 43, fasc. 2(269), 31 Ottobre.
Margetts, E.
1967 Miraa and myrrh in East Africa — Clinical notes about catha edulis. *Economic Botany*, p. 358—362.
Margetts, E.
1968 Corrigenda. *Economic Botany, 21*:123.
Martin, R.
1970 The role of coca in the history, religion, and medicine of South American Indians. *Economic Botany, 24*:422—438.
Messick, B.
1978 *Transactions in Ibb: Economy and society in a Yemeni highland town*. Ph.D. dissertation. Princeton Univ. Ann Arbor: Univ. Microfilms.
Millot, J.
1965 Inde et Bétel. *Objets et Mondes: La Révue du Musée de L'Homme, 5*:73—122.
Monge, M.
1982 The need for studying the problem of coca leaf chewing. *Bulletin on Narcotics, 4*:13—15.
Moser, C.
1917 The flower of paradise. The part which khat plays in the life of the Yemen Arab. *National Geographic, 32*:173—186.
Mosso, U.
1891 Azione fisiologica del prinicipo attivo del Celastrus edulis. *Rivista Clinica, 30*:65—79.
Mount, R. and Baranski, J.
1953 Medical mission to the Yemen, Southwest Arabia, 1951; III. A seriological and bacteriological survey. *J. Trop. Med. and Hyg., 2*:20—29.

Mount, R.
1953 Medical mission to the Yemen, Southwest Arabia, 1951; I. Geomedical observations. *American Journal of Tropical Medicine and Hygiene, 2*:1—2.

Mundy, M.
1979 Women's inheritance of land in highland Yemen. *Arabic Studies, V*:161—187.

Murphy, H., Rios, O., and Negrete, J.
1969 The effects of abstinence and of retraining the chewer of coca leaf. *Bulletin on Narcotics, 21*:41—47.

Mustard, M.
1952 Ascorbic acid content of some miscellaneous tropical and subtropical plants and plant products. *Food Research, 17*:31—35.

Myntti, C.
1979 *Women and development in the Yemen Arab Republic*. Eschborn, W. Germany: GTZ.

Nencini, P., Anania, M., Abdullahi, G., Amiconi, G., and Elmi, A.
1983 Physiological and neuroendocrine effects of khat in man. *In* Shahandeh, B. *et al.* (eds.), *The health and socio-economic aspects of khat use* (pp. 148—152). Lausanne, The Int. Council on Alcohol and Addictions.

Niebuhr, C.
1774 *Travels through Arabia and other countries in the east*. Trans. Robert Heron, 2 Vols. Beirut: Librarie du Libnan 1792.

Nordal, A.
1980 Khat: Pharmacognostical aspects. *Bulletin on Narcotics, 32*:51—64.

Nyrop, R. *et al.*
1977 *Area handbook for the Yemens*. Washington, D.C.: Gov. Printing Office.

O'Ballance, E.
1971 *The War in the Yemen*. Connecticut: Anchor Books.

Obermeyer, G.
1973 *Anthropological aspects of qat and the use of qat in the Y.A.R.* Report to the W.H.O., (Mimeo).

Orme, W.
1914 Makan Sirid (Betel Chewing). *Brit. Medical Journal, I*:325—324.

Owen, F.
1910 Catha edulis. *J. Society of Chemical Industry, 29*:1091.

Paris, M. and Moyse, H.
1958 Abyssinian tea (Catha edulis Forsk, Celastracae). A study of some samples of varying geographical origin. *Bulletin on Narcotics, 10*(2):29—34.

Paris, M. and Moyse, H.
1957 Essai de caractérisation du Kat ou thé des Abyssins (Catha edulis Forsk, Celastracae), drogue récémment inscrite au tableau B. *Annales Pharm. Ascétique Françaises, 15*:89—97.

Paul, B.
1887 Coffee husks and catha edulis. *Pharmaceutical Journal and Transactions, 46*:656.

Paul, B.
1887 Note on catha edulis. *Pharmaceutical Journal and Transactions, 46*:1009.

Peele, S.
1978 Addiction: The analgesic experience. *Human Nature*, pp. 61—67.

Penzer, N.
1952 *Poison damsels and other essays in folklore and anthropology*. London: Sawyer.

Peters, D.
1952 Khat: It's history, botany, chemistry and toxicology. *Pharmaceutical Journal, 5* July:16—18, *12* July:36—37, V. 169.

Peterson, J.
1982 *Yemen, the search for a modern state.* London: Croom Helm.
Petrie, P.
1942 San'a and the qat-eaters. *The Scottish Geographical Magazine, 58*(2):49—53.
Phillips, W.
1955 *Qataban and Sheba.* New York: Harcourt, Brace & Co.
Qedan, S.
1972 Catha Edulis, Eine wenig bekannte Rausch- und Genussdroge. *Planta Medica, 21*:113—126.
Qedan, S.
1972 Über das ätherische Öl Catha Edulis. *Planta Medica, 21*:410—415.
Radt, C.
1969 Contribution à l'histoire ethno-botanique d'une plante stimulante: le kat. Le Kat au Yémen. *Journal d'Agriculture Tropicale et de Botanique Appliquée, 16*:215—243.
Radt, C.
1971 Contribution à l'histoire ethno-botanique d'une plante stimulante: le kat. Le Kat en Éthiopie. *L'Ethnographie, 65*:38—65.
Radt, C.
1971 Le Kat en Yemen. *Journal d'Agriculture Tropicale et de Botanique Appliquée, 65*:38—65.
Raghavan, V. and Baruah, H.
1958 Areca nut: India's popular mascatory — History, chemistry and utilization. *Economic Botany, 12*:315—345.
Ramadan, M., Fathi, M., Tash, M. and Abu el-Kheir, F.
1979 Metabolic changes caused by khat consumption in Yemen. *Dirasat Yamaniyyah*, a Journal of the Yemen Centre for Studies and Research, No. 3.
Ramadan, M., Fathi, A., Abu el-Kheir, A., and Labib, S.
1978 Effects of catha edulis (khat) on glucose tolerance in diabetics. *Dirasat Yamaniyya*, No. 4.
Raymond-Hamet, M.
1965 Sur l'action sympathico-esthétique d'une Célastracée de l'Afrique orientale, le Catha edulis Forskal. *Comptes Rendus Hebdomadaires des Sciences de l'Académie des Sciences, 260*:1020—1022.
Revri, R.
1983 *Catha edulis Forsk. Geographical dispersal, botanical, ecological and agronomical aspects with special reference to Yemen Arab Republic.* Gottingen.
Rihani, A.
1930 *Arabian peak and desert: Travels in al-Yaman.* Boston: Houghton-Mifflin.
Ristic, S.
1962 Über die Inhaltsstoffe von Catha Edulis. *Archiv der Pharmazie, 295*/67:524—525.
Robertson, W.
1943 Yemen Journey. *Scottish Geographical Magazine, 59*:63—70.
Rodinson, M.
1977 Esquisse d'une monographie du qat. *Journal Asiatique, 265*:71—96.
Rosecrans, J., Campbell, O., Dewey, W. and Harris, L.
1979 Discriminative stimulus and neurochemical mechanisms of cathinone: A preliminary study. *In* Harris, L. S. (ed.), *Problems of drug dependence*, Washington, D.C., NIDA, Monograph #27.
Rosenthal, F.
1971 *The herb, hashish versus medieval muslim society.* Leiden, E. J. Brill.
Rubin, V. (ed.)
1975 *Cannabis and culture.* The Hague: Mouton.

Rubin, V. and Comitas, L.
1975 *Ganja in Jamaica*. The Hague: Mouton.
Rucker, G., Kroger, H., Schikarski, M., and Qedan, S.
1973 Über die Alkaloide im Catha Edulis. *Planta Medica, 24*:61—65.
Russo, J. (ed.)
1968 *Amphetamine abuse.*
Sage, C.
1944 Catha edulis. *Pharmaceutical Journal*, pp. 153—228.
Said, E.
1968 On some physiological aspects induced by khat administration (Catha edulis). *Proceedings of the Egyptian Academy of Sciences, 20*:65—68.
Salser, J.
1970 Cubeo acculturation to coca and its social implications. *Economic Botany, 24*:182—186.
Schmidt, D.
1968 *Yemen: The unknown war*. New York: Holt, Rinehart and Winston.
Schopen, A.
1978 *Das Qat: Geschichte und Gebrauch des Genussmittels Catha Edulis Forsk.*, in *Der Arabischen Republic Jemen*, Wiesbaden, Franz Steiner Verlag, GMBH.
Schorno, X. and Steinegger, E.
1979 The Phenalalkylamines of Catha edulis Forsk: The absolute configuration of cathinone. United Nations Document MNAR/3/1979.
Schorno, X., Brenneisen, R., and Steinegger, E.
1982 Qualitative und quantitative Untersuchung über die Verteilung in verschiedenen Organen von Catha edulis. *Pharm. Acta. Helv., 57*:168—176.
Schuster, C. and Johanson, C.
1980 Behavioral studies of cathinone in monkeys and rats. *In* Harris, L. S. (ed.), *Problems of drug dependence*. Washington, D.C., NIDA, Monograph #27.
Scott, H.
1942 *In the High Yemen*. London: John Murray.
Serjeant, R.
1983 The market, business life, occupations, the legality and sale of stimulants. *In* Sergeant, R. B. and Lewcock, R. (eds.), *San'a', An Arabian Islamic City* (pp. 161—178). London: World of Islam Festival Trust.
Serjeant, R.
1983 The post-medieval and modern history of San'a' and the Yemenis. *In* Serjeant, R. and Lewcock, R. (eds.), *San'a', An Arabian Islamic City* (pp. 68—107). London: World of Islam Festival Trust.
Serjeant, R. and al-Akwa, I.
1983 The statute of San'a' (Qanun San'a', with additional documents). In *San'a', an Arabian City*. R. Serjeant and R. Lewcock (eds.). London: World of Islam Festival Trust.
Serjeant, R. and Lewcock, R. (eds.)
1983 *San'a', An Arabian Islamic City*. London: World of Islam Festival Trust.
Shadan, P. and Shellard, E.
1962 An anatomical study of Ethiopian khat (leaf of Catha edulis Forsk). *J. of Pharmacy and Pharmacology, 14*:110—118.
Shaffer, R.
1952 *Tents and towers of Arabia*. New York: Dodd, Mead & Co.
Shahandeh, B., Geadah, R., Tongue, A., Tongue, E., and Rolli, J. (eds.)
1983 *The health of socio-economic aspects of khat use*. Lausanne: International Council on Alcohol and Addictions.

Sharafaddin, A.
1961 *Yemen: Arabia felix*. Rome: Daily American Press.
Siering, O.
1958 Über den Abessinischen Tee (kat). *Acta Psykotherapeutica, 5*:13—19.
Sissy, H. and Abdulla, M.
1972 Polyphenolics of catha edulis. *Planta Medica, 14*:76—83.
Solomon, D. (ed.)
1966 *The Marihuana Papers*. N.Y.: Bobbs Merrill.
Steele, R.
1963 Psychiatric observations in Aden. *Transcultural Psychiatric Research Review and Newsletter, 15*:69—70.
Steffen, H. *et al.*
1978 *Final report on the airphoto interpretation project of the Swiss technical cooperation service — Yemen Arab Republic*. Zurich.
Stevenson, T.
1985 *Social change in a Yemeni highlands town*. Salt Lake City: Univ. of Utah Press.
Stockman, R.
1912 The active principles of Catha edulis. *The Pharmaceutical J. and Pharmacist, 89*:676—678.
Stockman, R.
1912 Stimulant-narcotics, with a special account of Catha edulis. *The Pharmaceutical J. and Pharmacist, 89*:685—687.
Stockman, R.
1913 The pharmacological action of *Catha edulis* and its alkaloids. *J. of Pharmacology and Experimental Therapeutics, 35*:251—262.
Stookey, R.
1978 *Yemen: The politics of the Yemen Arab Republic*. Boulder, Colorado: Westview Press.
Stookey, R.
1974 Social structure and politics in the Yemen Arab Republic. *The Middle East Journal, 23*:*3*:248—60. (Part I), Summer 1974, (Part II), Fall *28*:409—418.
Swagman, C.
1985 *Social organization and local development in the western central highlands of the Yemen Arab Republic*, Doctoral Dissertation, U.C.L.A.
Swanson, J.
1979 *Emigration and economic development: The case of the Yemen Arab Republic*. Boulder, Colorado: Westview Press.
Sylvain, P.
1955 Le café du Yemen. *Agronomie Tropicale, 11*:62—73.
Szendrei, K.
1980 The chemistry of khat. *Bulletin on Narcotics. Special Issue devoted to Catha edulis* (*Khat*), *3*:5—36.
Szendrei, K.
1983 Recent progress in khat chemistry. *In* Shahandeh, Geadah, R., Tongue, A., Tongue, E., Roli, J., (eds.), *The health and socio-economic aspects of khat use* (pp. 91—109). Lausanne, Int. Council on Alcohol and Addictions.
Tanret, G.
1933 Le kat (Catha edulis). *La Presse Médicale, 22*:452.
Tarcici, A.
1972 *The queen of Sheba's land. Yemen*. (*Arabia felix*). Beirut: Nowfel, N.D.
Turner, V.
1974 *Dramas, fields, and metaphors*. London: Cornell Univ. Press.

Tutweiler, R. and Carapico, S.
1981 *Yemeni agriculture and economic change*. American Institute for Yemeni Studies, Sanaa, Yemen. Development Series, #1.

U.N.D.P. Report
1971 *Sociomedical study of some villages in Yemen Arab Republic*, by Hammarin Lars, M.D. Information Paper #9, AGS. SF/YEM 9.

U.N.D.P. Report
1970 *Nutrition health standards and home economics.*

U.N.D.P. Report
1971 *Report on agriculture in Yemen.*

United Nations Narcotics Laboratory.
1979 Report of an expert group, *The botany and chemistry of khat*, GE 79—10365.

U.S. Embassy in Taiz, YAR.
1964 *Economic report on the Yemen Arab Republic.*

Van der Meulen, D.
1961 *Faces in Shem*. London: John Murray.

Varisco, D.
1982 *The adaptive dynamics of water allocations in Al-Ahjar, Yemen Arab Republic.* Ph.D. dissertation, Univ. of Penn. Ann Arbor: Univ. Microfilms, Inst.

Varisco, D.
1986 On the meaning of chewing, the significance of qat (Catha edulis) in the Yemen Arab Republic. *Int. J. Middle East Stud. 18*:1—13.

Vaughan, J.
1852 Notes upon the drugs observed at Aden Arabia. *Pharmaceutical Journal, 12*:226—229, 268—271, 385—388.

Valterio, C. and Kalix, P.
1982 The effect of the alkaloid (−) cathinone on the motor activity of mice. *Archives Internationales de Pharmacodynamie et de Thérapie, 255*:196—203.

Von Brucke, T.
1941 Über die zentral erregende Wirkung des Alkaloides Cathin. *Naunyn Schmiedeberg's Archiv für Experimentelle Pathologie und Pharmakologie, 189*:100.

Von Euler, U. *et al.*
1945 Nicotine-like actions of arecoline. *Acta Pharmacologica, 1*:263—269.

Watt, J. Brandwijk-Greyer M.
1962 *The medicinal and poisonous plants of southern & eastern Africa*. Edinburgh: E.S. Livingstone.

Weil, A.
1972 *The natural mind*. New York: Houghton-Mifflen.

Weir, S.
1983 *Economic aspects of the qat industry in North West Yemen*. Paper presented at the Symposium on Contemporary Yemen, Exeter Center for Arab Gulf Studies.

Weir, S.
1985 *Qat in Yemen, consumption and social change*. London: British Museum Publications.

Weiss, B. and Laties, V.
1962 Enhancement of human performance by caffeine and amphetamines. *Pharmacology Reviews, 14*:1—36.

Wellman, F.
1961 *Coffee: Botany, cultivation and utilization*. New York: Interscience Publishers.

Wenner, M.
1965 *Yemen, a selected and annotated bibliography since 1960*. Washington, D.C., Library of Congress.

Wenner, M.
1967 *Modern Yemen: 1918—1966*. Baltimore: Johns Hopkins Press.
Westermeyer, J.
1982 *Poppies, pipes and people: Opium and its use in Laos*. Berkeley: U.C. Press.
Winterfeld, K. and Bernsmann, G.
1960 Zur Kenntnis der Inhaltsstoffe von Catha edulis Forskal. *Archiv der Pharmazie, 293*/65:991—1000.
Wolfes, O.
1930 Über das Vorkommen von d-nor-iso-Ephedrin in Catha edulis. *Archiv der Pharmazie, 268*:81—83.
Wolff, P. O.
1952 General considerations on the problem of coca leaf chewing. *Bulletin on Narcotics, 4*:2—5.
World Bank
1976 *Current economic positions and prospects of the Yemen Arab Republic*. Report #840a YAR.
Yacoub, S. and Akil, A.
1971 *A socio-economic study of Hujjuriyya district, Y.A.R.* Faculty of Agricultural Sciences, Publication #49, American University of Beirut.
Yanagita, T.
1979 Studies on cathinones: Cardiovascular and behavioral effects in rats and self-administration experimentation in rhesus monkeys. *In* Harris, L. S. (ed.), *Problems of Drug Dependence*, Washington, D.C., NIDA Monograph, #27.
Zabbal, S.
1971 Al Qat. *Al-Arabi, 147*:100—114.
Zwemmer, S.
1900 *Arabia: The cradle of Islam*. New York: Fleming. H. Revell Co.

NAME INDEX

SUBJECT INDEX

THE CULTURE, ILLNESS, AND HEALING BOOK SERIES

Leon Eisenberg and Arthur Kleinman (eds.), *The Relevance of Social Science for Medicine,* 1981, x + 422.
ISBN 90–277–1176–3 (HB) / 90–277–1185–2 (PB).

Arthur Kleinman and Tsung-yi Lin (eds.), *Normal and Abnormal Behavior in Chinese Culture,* 1981, xxiv + 436.
ISBN 90–277–1104–6.

Carolyn Fishel Sargent, *The Cultural Context of Therapeutic Choice,* 1982, xii + 192.
ISBN 90–277–1344–8.

Anthony J. Marsella and Geoffrey M. White (eds.), *Cultural Conceptions of Mental Health and Therapy,* 1982, xii + 414.
ISBN 90–277–1362–6 (HB) / 90–277–1757–5 (PB).

Noel J. Chrisman and Thomas W. Maretzki (eds.), *Clinically Applied Anthropology,* 1982, viii + 437.
ISBN 90–277–1418–5 (HB) / 90–277–1419–3 (PB).

Robert A. Hahn and Atwood D. Gaines (eds.), *Physicians of Western Medicine,* 1985, ix + 345.
ISBN 90–277–1790–7 (HB) / 90–277–1881–4 (PB).

Ronald C. Simons and Charles C. Hughes (eds.), *The Culture-Bound Syndromes,* 1985, xv + 516.
ISBN 90–277–1858–X (HB) / 90–277–1859–8 (PB).

L. L. Langness and Harold G. Levine (eds.), *Culture and Retardation,* 1986, xv + 212.
ISBN 90–277–2177–7 (HB) / 90–277–2178–5 (PB).

Craig R. Janes, Ron Stall, and Sandra M. Gifford (eds.), *Anthropology and Epidemiology*, 1986, ix + 349.
ISBN 90–277–2248–X (HB) / 90–277–2249–8 (PB).

John G. Kennedy, *The Flower of Paradise,* 1987, xii + 268.
ISBN 1–55608–011–5 (HB) / 1–55608–012–3 (PB).